RELIGION AND CULTURE IN

Medieval Virg

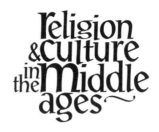

RELIGION AND CULTURE IN THE MIDDLE AGES

Medieval Virginities

Edited by

ANKE BERNAU, RUTH EVANS and SARAH SALIH

UNIVERSITY OF WALES PRESS
CARDIFF
2003

British Library Cataloguing-in-Publication Data
A catalogue record for this book is available from the British Library.

ISBN 0–7083–1763–4 hardback
     0–7083–1762–6 paperback

Typeset by Bryan Turnbull
Printed in Great Britain by MPG Books Limited, Bodmin

CONTENTS

List of Illustrations   vii

Series Editors' Preface   viii

Acknowledgements   ix

Notes on Contributors   xi

Abbreviations   xiv

1   Introduction: Virginities and Virginity Studies
     SARAH SALIH, ANKE BERNAU and RUTH EVANS   1

2   When is a Bosom Not a Bosom?
     Problems with 'Erotic Mysticism'
     SARAH SALIH   14

3   The Sheela-na-Gig: An Incongruous Sign of Sexual
     Purity?
     JULIETTE DOR   33

4   Virginity and Chastity Tests in Medieval Welsh Prose
     JANE CARTWRIGHT   56

5   Four Virgins' Tales: Sex and Power in Medieval Law
     KIM M. PHILLIPS   80

6   The Labour of Continence:
     Masculinity and Clerical Virginity
     JOHN H. ARNOLD   102

7   Edward the Celibate, Edward the Saint:
     Virginity in the Construction of Edward the Confessor
     JOANNA HUNTINGTON   119

8   Alchemy and the Exploration of Late Medieval Sexuality
     JONATHAN HUGHES   140

9   The Jew, the Host and the Virgin Martyr:
     Fantasies of the Sentient Body
     RUTH EVANS   167

10   Can the Virgin Martyr Speak?
     ROBERT MILLS   187

11   'Saint, Witch, Man, Maid or Whore?':
     Joan of Arc and Writing History
     ANKE BERNAU   214

12   Virginity Now and Then: A Response to
     Medieval Virginities
     JOCELYN WOGAN-BROWNE   234

Bibliography   254
Index   289

List of Illustrations

1   Sheela-na-Gig   34

2   'Melusine' from the *Ripley Scroll*   158

3   'The burning of St Agnes', scene from the lid of the Royal Gold Cup   198

4   'The miracles of St Agnes', scene from the lid of the Royal Gold Cup   198

5   'St Agnes Cycle', Pamplona Bible   199

6   'St Agnes Cycle', Pamplona Bible   200

7   'Barbara's trial', panel from Meister Francke, *Martyrdom of Saint Barbara*   205

8a   *Gray's Anatomy*: ventral aspect of the penis   246

8b   *Gray's Anatomy*: female external genitalia   246

SERIES EDITORS' PREFACE

Religion and Culture in the Middle Ages aims to explore the interface between medieval religion and culture, with as broad as possible an understanding of those terms. It puts to the forefront studies which engage with works that significantly contributed to the shaping of medieval culture. However, it also gives attention to studies dealing with works that reflect and highlight aspects of medieval culture that have been neglected in the past by scholars of the medieval disciplines. For example, devotional works and the practice they imply illuminate in remarkable ways our understanding of the medieval subject and its culture, while studies of the material space designed and inhabited by medieval subjects yield new evidence on the period and the people who shaped it and lived in it. In the larger field of religion and culture, we also want to explore further the roles played by women as authors, readers and owners of books, thereby defining them more precisely as actors in the cultural field.

The series as a whole investigates the European Middle Ages, from *c.*500 to *c.*1500. Our aim is to explore medieval religion and culture with the tools belonging to such disciplines as, among others, art history, philosophy, theology, history, musicology, the history of medicine, and literature. In particular, we would like to promote interdisciplinary studies, as we believe strongly that our modern understanding of the term applies fascinatingly well to a cultural period marked by a less tight confinement and categorization of its disciplines than the modern period. However, our only criterion is academic excellence, with the belief that the use of a large diversity of critical tools and theoretical approaches serves for a deeper understanding of medieval culture. We want the series to reflect this diversity, as we believe that, as a collection of outstanding contributions, it offers a more subtle representation of a period that is marked by paradoxes and contradictions and which necessarily reflects diversity and difference, however difficult it may sometimes have proved for medieval culture to accept these notions.

ACKNOWLEDGEMENTS

We would like to thank all at University of Wales Press, especially our editor Susan Jenkins, and also the anonymous reader who reported on the proposal with discerning enthusiasm. But thanks are due mainly to the contributors for their unwavering commitment to the project. Thanks too to everyone who has joined in conversations about virginity over the years.

NOTES ON CONTRIBUTORS

JOHN H. ARNOLD is a Lecturer in Medieval History at Birkbeck College, London. He is the author of *History: A Very Short Introduction* (Oxford University Press, 2000) and *Inquisition and Power: Catharism and the Confessing Subject in Medieval Languedoc* (Pennsylvania University Press, 2001).

ANKE BERNAU is a Lecturer in Medieval and Renaissance English Literature, Cardiff University. She has worked extensively on medieval virginity and her current research focuses mainly on female foundation myths as well as issues of historiography, translation and gender in medieval and early modern literature.

JANE CARTWRIGHT is Lecturer in Welsh at the University of Wales, Lampeter. She is the author of *Y Forwyn Fair, Santesau a Lleianod: Agweddau ar Wyryfdod a Diweirdeb yng Nghymru'r Oesoedd Canol* (University of Wales Press, 1999) and editor of *Celtic Hagiography and Saints' Cults* (University of Wales Press, 2003). She has published various articles on Middle Welsh hagiography and feminine sanctity.

JULIETTE DOR is Professor of Medieval English Language and Literature at the University of Liège, Belgium. She has published widely on French in medieval England, Chaucer, myths and mythology, Arthurian literature, the texts of the *Katherine Group* and gender studies. She has edited two volumes of essays on feminist approaches to medieval literature and/or medieval literary women: *A Wyf Ther Was* (L3, 1992) and *New Trends in Feminine Spirituality: The Holy Women of Liège and their Impact* (Brepols, 1999). She also extensively translates Middle English into Modern French.

RUTH EVANS is Senior Lecturer in English Studies at the University of Stirling, Scotland. She has published articles on medieval English drama, courtly literature, virginity literature, Margery Kempe, Chaucer and translation. She has contributed to *The Cambridge Guide to Women's Writing in English* (Cambridge University Press, 1999) and *The Cambridge Companion to Medieval Women's Writing* (Cambridge University Press, 2003). She is co-editor (with Jocelyn Wogan-Browne, Nicholas Watson and Andrew Taylor) of *The Idea of the Vernacular: An Anthology of Middle English Literary Theory, 1280–1530* (Penn State, 1999). She is currently writing a book on Chaucer for Palgrave.

JOANNA HUNTINGTON is a Ph.D. candidate at the Centre for Medieval Studies, University of York. Her current research interests include the construction of lay male sanctity in twelfth-century England.

JONATHAN HUGHES is a Wellcome Research Fellow in the School of History in the University of East Anglia. He is the author of *The Religious Life of Richard III* (Sutton, 1996) and *Arthurian Myths and Alchemy: The Kingship of Edward IV* (Sutton, 2002). He is currently working on a history of alchemy and medicine in late medieval England.

ROBERT MILLS is a Lecturer in English at King's College London. His research is interdisciplinary, spanning literary studies, art history, religious history and cultural studies. To date, he has mainly been concerned with representations of the punished body in the late Middle Ages and, within that broad theme, constructions of pain, pleasure, gender and sexual identity. He is currently working on a study of erotic responses to the art and literature of medieval Christian devotion.

KIM M. PHILLIPS is a Lecturer in History at the University of Auckland. She is the author of articles on rape in English common law, gesture and gender in normative literature and aspects of women's youth in late medieval England. She is a co-editor of *Young Medieval Women* (Sutton, 1999) and of *Sexualities in History: A Reader* (Routledge, 2001). Forthcoming publications include *Medieval Maidens: Young Women and Gender in England, c. 1270–1530* (Manchester University Press).

SARAH SALIH is a Lecturer in English Literature, University of East Anglia, Norwich. She is the author of *Versions of Virginity in Late Medieval England* (D. S. Brewer, 2001) and co-editor of *Gender and*

Holiness: Men, Women and Saints in Late Medieval Europe (Routledge, 2002). She is currently working on a study of medieval paganities.

JOCELYN WOGAN-BROWNE is an Associate Professor at Fordham University, New York, and is one of the leading experts on virginity in the middle ages. She has published numerous articles on virginity and hagiography: she is also the co-editor of *Virgin Lives and Holy Deaths: Two Exemplary Biographies for Anglo-Norman Women* (Everyman, 1996) and author of *Saints' Lives and Women's Literary Culture, c.1150–1300: Virginity and its Authorizations* (Oxford University Press, 2001).

LIST OF ABBREVIATIONS

Bible   *The Holy Bible: Translated from the Latin Vulgate and Diligently Compared with Other Editions in Divers Languages (Douay, AD 1609; Rheims AD 1582).* London: Burns Oates and Washbourne, 1914.

BL   British Library

EETS   Early English Text Society.
ES   extra series.
OS   original series.
SS   supplementary series.

PL   *Patrilogiae Cursus Completus: Series Latina*, 217 vols, ed. J. P. Migne, Paris, 1844–64.

Introduction: Virginities and Virginity Studies

SARAH SALIH, ANKE BERNAU and RUTH EVANS

Medieval virginity is currently the subject of considerable scholarly and popular interest. In the six years since we began to plan this collection, monographs, articles and collections on virgins and virginity have appeared regularly enough to constitute a mini-discipline of medieval virginity studies, and we are already in the enviable position of being able to review and take stock of a growing body of material. Meanwhile, popular interest in virginity has grown, reflected in the media presence of (usually North American) virginity movements and high-profile individual virgins from Ann Widdecombe to Britney Spears.[1] In the horror-film genre the virginal young woman is a ubiquitous presence, a central narrative device – a fact ironically acknowledged in the self-reflexive movie *Scream*.[2] Even medieval virgins have a presence in current popular culture: Christine Carpenter, the runaway anchoress of Shere, is the subject of a recent film and novel.[3] Virginity's association with the medieval speaks to deep-rooted myths about both: the Middle Ages are imagined as the location of chastity belts and *droit de seigneur*, while a popular conception of the whole period sees it as virginal in an uncontaminated innocence which is then frequently opposed to a present constructed as jaded, knowing – and more sophisticated. As Sarah Salih puts it in this collection: 'Sweeping statements about the alterity of medieval people . . . have a tendency to turn out on closer inspection to be based on a desire for a Middle Ages which is other in every way to the modern.'

Medieval virginity, however, is no more self-evident than the medieval itself. It is precisely because medieval virginity so often fantasizes itself (and is fantasized by others) as self-identical and ahistorical that we need to theorize and historicize its various manifestations. The chapters in this collection both make major theoretical claims for virginity and examine its complications and compromises in individual lives and texts. The variety of subjects and disciplines represented here testifies to the elusiveness of virginity. Virginity is a paradoxical condition, both perfect and monstrous, defined by both absence and presence. It is often visible only insofar as it is under threat: as Margaret W. Ferguson writes, 'the virgin item's cultural value lies partly in the fact that it has *not yet* been used'.[4] Analyses of virginity necessarily engage with a wide range of matters and disciplines. The study of virginity requires discussions of gender identity, subjectivity, conceptions of the body, of truth and of representation. Virginity is a key to the analysis of sex–gender systems. Depending on how it is deployed, it may confirm or disrupt sexual difference, sexual hierarchy and the sexual economy. This collection addresses a number of questions about virginity: what does virginity do? How is virginity attained? How is virginity recognized? How is virginity used? The critical languages used include feminist, queer, psychoanalytic, poststructuralist and postcolonial: the plurality of voices mimics the plurality of virginities. The frameworks employed as well as the questions raised equally reflect back onto those writing about virginity, both past and present. In engaging with virginities we are always also confronted with our own desires, our own investments. This collection not only shows how a range of scholarly and theoretical approaches lend themselves productively to an engagement with historically distant texts, but also reveals that this is an unpredictable process which frequently results in a rethinking of the critical paradigms employed. Virginity refuses to be a passive object of study, faithfully mirroring the critic's cherished preconceptions.

Our title insists that virginities are multiple. Secular virginity is not identical to religious virginity, nor male virginity to female virginity. Virginity as a permanent identity is not the same as virginity as a normally temporary stage in a life cycle. Virginity performs various functions in a number of genres and discourses. This collection includes numerous different virginities: virginity is a permanent masculine sexual identity in the chapters by John Arnold and Joanna Huntington; a stage in the female life cycle in those by Jane Cartwright and Kim Phillips; a troublesome discursive effect in those by Anke Bernau and Robert Mills.

Although not all the virginities discussed in this collection are primarily religious concepts, virginity is one of the great inventions of medieval Christian culture, theorized and practised from early Christianity.[5] Virginity in this discourse is the image and practice of perfection, the highest form of life, an imitation of the angels. It is in religious texts that the idea that virginity may constitute a gender in itself is most clearly articulated – though it is also here that it is most clearly contained – and it is religious texts which have been most thoroughly discussed in recent scholarship. Virginity, removing individuals from the sexual economy, may function as a challenge to binary gender and heterosexuality: as St Jerome famously wrote, 'while a woman serves for birth and children, she is different from man as body is from soul. But when she wants to serve Christ more than the world, then she shall cease to be called a woman and shall be called man.'[6] Chaste clerics could be categorized as a third gender; the virgin body differed from the female body in its wholeness and perfection.[7] Virginity may even produce relative female autonomy in historical practice: Dyan Elliott has shown that unconsummated marriages were associated with the moderation of the husband's authority.[8]

Hagiography, and especially the cults and vernacular legends of virgin martyrs, has so far been one of the prime sites for the discussion of virginity.[9] Critics have considered the question of what kinds of role-models these legends of rebellious and articulate saints offered to medieval women and whether they were primarily regarded as models for imitation or intercessionary figures.[10] Katherine J. Lewis expanded the scope of such questions with a contextual study of the cult of Katherine of Alexandria in its multiple manifestations, exploring the saint's appeal to men as well as women and her patronage of entities as diverse as scholars, marriageable girls and the city of Bath.[11] Karen Winstead and Gail Ashton have produced large-scale analyses of the whole genre, Winstead focusing on changes to the genre during the later Middle Ages and Ashton on the question of the relations of virgin's and hagiographer's voices.[12] The violent torture which is so prominent a feature of the legends has been much debated: condemned as pornographic by some critics, it is read as a discursive system by others.[13] The possibility that it could be both is beginning to be investigated: Evelyn Birge Vitz argues that medieval women readers may have taken pleasure in rape narratives, and the analysis could be transferred to hagiography.[14] Mills's comparisons of hagiographic and pornographic torments advance the argument by using hagiography to investigate the category of pornography and to posit various pleasurable responses to these scenes.[15] In this collection Mills and Ruth Evans revisit the torture of virgins to make analyses which go beyond the question of whether or not virgin martyrs are good role-models for women readers. Awareness of virginity's theoretical potential to undermine binary gender and enjoyment of the assertive and articulate virgins of hagiography may produce the impression that virginity is inherently enabling for women. This collection nuances and corrects this view: Cartwright and Phillips find that, once the virgin becomes available for exchange in the secular world, the concept of virginity is most likely to be used to constrain the behaviour of women and maintain the gender status quo.

Virginity studies developed from women's studies, and has often had a strong feminist commitment.[16] This has been an area of study in which women are, unusually, the privileged term. The extent to which this privilege is produced by the disciplinary categories of modern scholarship is one of our areas of enquiry. Some virginity texts idealistically imply that gender ceases to matter as virginity removes men and women alike from the sexual economy. At other times, gender oppositions are not undermined but replicated and reconfirmed through virginity, with clear differences in the conception and enactment of male and female virginal identities. Sometimes, for instance, virginity really is a condition relevant only to women: Phillips could not have written on virginal men in legal discourse, because virginity is a legal category for women only.

Male virginity has received less attention, though work in this area is increasing. In two well-received recent collections, for example, *Menacing Virgins*, edited by Kathleen Coyne Kelly and Marina Leslie, and *Constructions of Virginity and Widowhood*, edited by Cindy Carlson and Angela Jane Weisl, only one essay deals with medieval masculine virginity.[17] Another collection explores in detail historical and theological aspects of one particular form of masculine virginity, clerical celibacy.[18] Other discussions of male virginity occur within the context of larger ones of female virginity: Elliott discusses virgin men within her study of marital abstinence and Jocelyn Wogan-Browne discusses the lives of clerics alongside those of chaste widows.[19] A major development of the field occurs in Kelly's *Performing Virginity*, the most wide-ranging study to date of medieval virginity, which asks the wonderfully resonant question, 'Do men have a hymen?' of the 'oxymoronic bodies' of male virgins.[20] In this volume Arnold investigates and qualifies Kelly's analysis. Kelly is not the only critic to find male virginity especially problematic. Maud Burnett McInerney, studying male virginity in the writings of Hildegard of Bingen, argues that the male virgin is, strictly speaking, non-existent, for virginity feminizes the male body.[21] Katherine Lewis suggests Richard II attempted to claim the mystique of masculine virginity: if so, the strategy evidently failed.[22] Nevertheless, this collection aims to take part in the shift from women's studies to gender studies by paying attention to various forms of masculine virginity: embattled clerical virginity appears in the chapters of Arnold and Salih and the problems of kingly virginity in those of Hughes and Huntington.

Virginity and virgins may also be treated as tokens or signs which signify something other than themselves. Karen Winstead has argued that virgin saints may represent clerics in their privileged access to religious truth and heretics in their subjection to religious persecution.[23] Kelly has analysed the inviolability of virgin saints as a figure for the inviolable mystic body of the Church, a claim extended by Evans in this volume.[24] In a comparable argument, Cindy Carlson aligned the virgin body of Mary with the social body.[25] That virginity is itself already a fantasy of wholeness and perfection makes it a suitable figure for other imaginary bodies. A particularly exciting argument is Wogan-Browne's for the dotality of virgins, which is likely to inform the next wave of virginity studies.[26] Such analyses allow a movement from asking what the virgin *is* to asking what s/he *is for*. Though the virgin is, at least rhetorically, removed from the sphere of sexual exchange, the idea of the virgin is too valuable a cultural property to keep out of circulation; virgins are good to think with. Such analyses enable more far-reaching accounts of virginity than those which treat virgins only as images of women. Here virginity is bound up with discourses of nation and historiography in the chapters by Bernau, Hughes and Huntington; Evans and Mills further examine the identification of the virgin with the imaginary whole of Christianity.

Virginity is difficult to define or pin down: in the discourse of the church fathers, as Kelly writes, 'chastity is best maintained by a deliberate non-play of signifiers: by absence and silence'.[27] A virgin described and seen is thereby no virgin. Virginity has no ontological security. Physical tests for women's virginity are widely distrusted as destroying what they seek to confirm, and there is no consensus about

the nature of the masculine virgin body.[28] The hymen, we learn from
Giulia Sissa, is an invention, and one which may turn up in unexpected
places – as part of the body of Christ, for example, in *Hali Meiðhad*.[29]
Several contributors to this volume address the difficulties and paradoxes of virginity. Bernau focuses not on Joan's virginity but on its contestation; Juliette Dor on virginity as signified by its apparent other, the
exhibitionist sheela-na-gig; Hughes on the identification of virginity with
fertility; Salih on the doubts about virginity which hagiographic texts
occasionally betray. Phillips's chapter shows that virginity is most likely
to appear in legal records in relation to its loss and Cartwright details
tests for virginity which refuse to look directly at the woman's body.

   The difficulty of virginity enables virginity studies to meet another
currently popular topic, monstrosity.[30] The virgin is constructed with
reference to the monster: according to Tertullian, the virgin woman
who evades masculine control is 'a third generic class, some monstrosity with a head of its own'.[31] This aspect of virginity is highlighted in
the deliberate ambiguity of titles such as *Ravishing Maidens* and
Menacing Virgins: in so far as virginity is monstrous, it challenges
order and hierarchy. It also functions like a monster in the sense of
portent, a heterogeneous (sometimes repellent, sometimes baffling)
sign that demands to be interpreted. Fear of the virgin and desire for
her are often intimately connected. Dor's Sovereign Lady and the
virgins with serpent-bearing vaginas mentioned by Wogan-Browne and
Salih demonstrate how the virgin can be a frightening figure who
nonetheless must be approached. Undoubtedly, some medieval depic-
tions of virginity – the self-castrating beaver, the sexually aggressive,
alluring and terrifying virgin-dragon of *Mandeville's Travels* – are
extremely strange: virginity is stalked by mutilation, hermaphroditism,
unnaturalness.[32] This collection both confirms and questions the
monstrosity of virginity. Dor and Hughes examine further examples of
monstrous virginity, the sheela-na-gig and the mercurial Melusine.
Other contributors provide different perspectives: Phillips and Cartwright show the mundanity of virginity in much historical practice, and
the use of virginity to control women's behaviour, a use which
continues in much of the modern virginity movement. The identification of the monstrousness of virginity can obscure its more authoritarian and hegemonic deployments. Mills and Evans examine the use
of virginity to promote exclusionary fantasies of Christian unity and to
naturalize hierarchies of class, race and religion. The virgin can do
violence as well as suffer it.

This collection aims to trace some of the specific manifestations of virginity in late medieval culture. We aim both to build on current work on medieval virginities and to start to delineate some of the other virginities which have received less attention: masculine, legal and medical virginities are investigated as well as the more common literary and art-historical treatments of virgin women. Of course, gaps in the coverage remain: secular masculine virginity is treated only briefly; the virginity of Christ and Mary appears only in reflection; the virginity of holy children, as in *Pearl* or *The Prioress's Tale*, is worthy of further attention. We hope others will fill these gaps.

This collection is both interdisciplinary and multidisciplinary, employing literary, historical and art-historical approaches to a range of material. The topic of virginity seems to have encouraged contributors to test their own disciplinary limits. Two historians, Arnold and Huntington, have produced textual analyses; Bernau, a literary critic, has written on historiography; Cartwright mixes literary, legal and medical documents; Hughes, scientific, political and romance texts; Salih questions conceptual as well as interpretative categories. All show that virginity is a subject which resists containment within boundaries, be they disciplinary, generic or both. The variety of the collection asks, finally, whether virginity is an object at all, or whether the varieties of virginity delineated here might be discrete phenomena. The 'integrated whole' of discourses of virginity may be as elusive as that of virginity itself.

Sarah Salih examines critically the associations between the terms 'eroticism' and 'mysticism' in mystical and hagiographic narratives in order to think through the indeterminate relationship of the erotic to virginity, for, as she argues, the erotic 'can be read either as inimical to virginity or as constituent of it'. By problematizing the erotic, Salih shows how interpretative paradigms – here specifically psychoanalytic and theological – can run the risk of reducing or even eliding the multiple and complex intersections between categories. The oversimplification of concepts such as the erotic – and its relationship to other figures, such as virginity – is shown to have profound implications for those who engage with the past.

Juliette Dor focuses on carvings of exhibitionist sheela-na-gigs, pointing to the need to consider material evidence alongside textual. She argues that non-mimetic theories of representation enable sheelas to be read as paradoxical representations of virginity as well as sexuality, open to both Christian and non-Christian readings. More fundamentally, reading the sheelas raises questions about the nature, the limits – even the possibility – of representation, particularly the representation of virginity.

Jane Cartwright offers a Welsh perspective on tests of female virginity in mythology, romance, law and medicine. She links the common European motif of the embarrassing mantle, which magically raises itself to display the bodies of unchaste women, with the treatment prescribed in Welsh law for the non-virginal bride, whose shift is cut to expose her genitals. She concludes that virginity in medieval Wales was a valuable commodity which belonged as much – if not more so – to family or community as to the virgin herself.

Kim Phillips shows that legal documents provide a perspective in virginity quite distinct from that found in literary treatments. Virginity is elusive in legal texts, most likely to appear as it is lost, but it is not conceptually difficult: it can function unproblematically as a female identity, and its value when lost can be assessed with some precision – Isabella Alan's was worth 20 marks. Phillips argues that 'the ideal of premarital virginity formed a key part of the control and appropriation of female sexuality', offering a valuable corrective to the tendency of some literary studies to celebrate virginity as enabling female autonomy. She also produces an important new interpretation of leyrwite, a manorial fine for premarital loss of virginity, as being in some cases exacted in order to suppress peasant resistance.

John Arnold identifies masculine, and especially clerical, virginity as a performative production. He finds that various ways of conceptualizing masculinity and virginity coexist within twelfth- and thirteenth-century ecclesiastical discourse. Arnold tests Kelly's hypothesis that male virginity is not investigated but 'assayed', modifying it to argue that in some instances such virginity is investigated through being tested. He distinguishes male chastity, the control of desire which is always vulnerable to failure of the will, from the much rarer state of male virginity in which desire is eliminated entirely.

Joanna Huntington traces the development of the (probably fictive) virginity of Edward the Confessor through three early *vitae*, as it becomes more central to the texts and to the construction of his sanctity. She locates virginity firmly in the material world, remarking on the economic and spiritual value of a virginal saintly corpse to Westminster Abbey. Her findings confirm Arnold's: while Osbert of Clare represents Edward as an achieved and transcendent virgin, Aelred of Rievaulx returns him to the far more fragile state of chastity.

Jonathan Hughes draws virginity away from its traditional religious confines, and away even from medicine, exploring the ways in which it underlies symbolic alchemical and political bodies. He shows that alchemical thought desires and produces both an untrammelled female virginal potential and an imperative to control and appropriate it: virginity is needed so that it can be eliminated. Virginity is an ambiguous quality in the body politic, signifying virile prowess in the young Edward IV, or Sir Galahad, but impotence in the prematurely aged Henry VI. The range of discourses and materials cited in this chapter mimics the resistance of virginity to easy categorization.

Ruth Evans connects two forms of *imitatio Christi*, the passions of the virgin martyrs and the anti-Semitic fantasy of host-desecration, to examine the connections and oppositions between the virgin and the Jew, both figures fundamental to the process of imagining Christendom. She sees the virgin as 'metonymically both Church and eucharist': violent assault is necessary to test the integrity of all three, and thus violent assailants, Jews and pagans, must be supplied.

Robert Mills also revisits the virgin martyr legend, a favourite genre of many recent students of virginity, to resist the polarization of 'empowering' and 'oppressive' readings of the figure of the martyr. He makes an ambitious connection between martyrdom and sati to argue that the virgin's identity 'is predominantly an effect of discourse, rather than a clearly identifiable, self-evident reality'. Mills reminds us that to read with the virgin may implicate the reader in the marginalization of non-elite and non-Christian persons: the virgin may speak as the oppressor. His argument complements Phillips's warning against uncritical celebration of the virgin.

Anke Bernau moves beyond the ontology of virginity to its deployment, looking beyond the usual period boundary to examine the troubled reception of medieval virginity in Renaissance England. Newly Protestant England's need to mark its break with the Catholic past while retaining a narrative of continuous nationhood is a struggle which became located in contestation of the virginity of Joan of Arc. Virginity is revealed as the trope concealed beneath idealizations of nation and history: national history is fantasized as whole and self-evident in terms which show it to be in fact a fragile construct. Virginity itself is revealed as an aporia, meaning that 'writing about virginity . . . is never just that'.

Finally, Jocelyn Wogan-Browne, whose publications and personal encouragement of other scholars have done so much to constitute the field of virginity studies, gives her response to the collection and reminds us why medieval virginity is very much a current issue.

Notes

[1] Elizabeth Abbott, *A History of Celibacy: From Athena to Elizabeth I, Leonardo da Vinci, Florence Nightingale, Gandhi, and Cher* (New York: Scribner, 2000) speaks to the non-academic interest in virginity. The new virginity movement, which revives the most authoritarian and exclusionary aspects of medieval virginity, has produced numerous texts and websites. Kathleen Coyne Kelly, *Performing Virginity and Testing Chastity in the Middle Ages* (London: Routledge, 2000), pp. 119–41, offers an entertaining survey of virginity in North American popular culture.

[2] Carol J. Clover's characterization of this figure as the 'Final Girl' has often been cited in discussions of medieval virgins; Clover, *Men, Women and Chainsaws: Gender in the Modern Horror Film* (Princeton: Princeton University Press, 1992), p. 40; *Scream,* dir. Wes Craven (1996).

[3] *Anchoress*, dir. Chris Newby (1993); Paul L. Moorcraft, *Anchoress of Shere* (Shere: Millstream Press, 2000).

[4] Margaret W. Ferguson, 'Foreword', in Kathleen Coyne Kelly and Marina Leslie (eds), *Menacing Virgins: Representing Virginity in the Middle Ages and Renaissance* (London: Associated University Presses, 1999), pp. 7–14 (p. 7).

[5] See Peter Brown, *The Body and Society: Men, Women and Sexual Renunciation in Early Christianity* (New York: Columbia University Press, 1988) for the early history of the theology of virginity.

[6] Jerome, *Commentarium in Epistolam ad Ephesios, PL,* 26, cols 459–554 (col. 533); translation quoted in Jocelyn Wogan-Browne, 'The virgin's tale', in Ruth Evans and Lesley Johnson (eds), *Feminist Readings in Middle English Literature: The Wife of Bath and All her Sect* (London: Routledge, 1994), pp. 165–94 (p. 166).

[7] P. H. Cullum, 'Clergy, masculinity and transgression in later medieval England', in D. M. Hadley (ed.), *Masculinity in Medieval Europe* (London: Longman, 1999), pp. 178–96; Karma Lochrie, *Margery Kempe and Translations of the Flesh* (Philadelphia: University of Pennsylvania Press, 1991), p. 4.

[8] Dyan Elliott, *Spiritual Marriage: Sexual Abstinence in Medieval Wedlock* (Princeton: Princeton University Press, 1993), pp. 55–8.

[9] Jocelyn Wogan-Browne's steady flow of articles has been particularly influential in calling attention to this body of material: see in particular 'Saints' lives and the female reader', *Forum for Modern Language Studies*, 27 (1991), 314–32; 'The apple's message: some post-conquest accounts of hagiographic transmission', in Alistair Minnis (ed.), *Late Medieval*

Religious Texts and their Transmissions (Cambridge: Brewer, 1993), pp. 39–53; '"Clerc u lai, muine u dame": women and Anglo-Norman hagiography in the twelfth and thirteenth centuries', in Carol M. Meale (ed.), *Women and Literature in Britain 1150–1500* (Cambridge: Cambridge University Press, 1993), pp. 61–85; 'Chaste bodies: frames and experiences', in Sarah Kay and Miri Rubin (eds), *Framing Medieval Bodies* (Manchester: Manchester University Press, 1994), pp. 24–42; 'The virgin's tale'.

[10] See Eamon Duffy, 'Holy maydens, holy wyfes: the cult of women saints in fifteenth- and sixteenth-century England', in W. J. Shiels and Diana Wood (eds), *Women in the Church*, Studies in Church History, 27 (Oxford: Blackwell, 1990), pp. 175–96, and Wogan-Browne, 'Saints' lives and the female reader', for two different answers to the question.

[11] Katherine J. Lewis, *The Cult of St Katherine of Alexandria in Late Medieval England* (Woodbridge: Boydell, 2000).

[12] Karen Winstead, *Virgin Martyrs: Legends of Sainthood in Late Medieval England* (Ithaca, NY: Cornell University Press, 1997); Gail Ashton, *The Generation of Identity in Late Medieval Hagiography: Speaking the Saint* (London: Routledge, 2000).

[13] Simon Gaunt, *Gender and Genre in Medieval French Literature* (Cambridge: Cambridge University Press, 1995), p. 197; Kathryn Gravdal, *Ravishing Maidens: Writing Rape in Medieval French Literature and Law* (Philadelphia: University of Pennsylvania Press, 1991), p. 24; Katherine J. Lewis, '"Lete me suffre": reading the torture of St Margaret of Antioch in late medieval England', in Jocelyn Wogan-Browne et al. (eds), *Medieval Women: Texts and Contexts in Late Medieval Britain: Essays for Felicity Riddy* (Turnhout: Brepols, 2000), pp. 69–82; Sarah Salih, *Versions of Virginity in Late Medieval England* (Cambridge: Brewer, 2001), pp. 74–97.

[14] Evelyn Birge Vitz, 'Rereading rape in medieval literature: literary, historical and theoretical reflections', *Romanic Review*, 88 (1997), 1–26.

[15] See also Robert Mills, 'Visions of excess: pain, pleasure and the penal imaginary in late medieval art and culture' (unpublished Ph.D. thesis, University of Cambridge, 2000) and Mills, 'A man is being beaten', in Rita Copeland, David Lawton and Wendy Scase (eds), *New Medieval Literatures*, vol. 5 (Oxford: Oxford University Press, 2002), pp. 115–54. See Mills, '"Whatever you do is a delight to me!": masculinity, masochism and queer play in representations of male martyrdom', *Exemplaria*, 13 (2001), 1–37, on how the male, like the female, martyr is sexualized.

[16] The major exception is the pre-feminist analysis of John Bugge, *Virginitas: An Essay in the History of a Medieval Ideal* (The Hague: Martinus Nijhoff, 1975).

[17] Kathleen Coyne Kelly, 'Menaced masculinity and imperiled desire in Malory's *Morte Darthur*', in Kelly and Leslie (eds), *Menacing Virgins*, pp. 97–114.

[18] Michael Frasetto (ed.), *Medieval Purity and Piety: Essays on Medieval Clerical Celibacy and Religious Reform* (New York: Garland, 1998).

19 Elliott, *Spiritual Marriage*, esp. pp. 113–28; Jocelyn Wogan-Browne, *Saints' Lives and Women's Literary Culture c.1150–1300: Virginity and its Authorizations* (Oxford: Oxford University Press, 2001), ch. 5.

20 Kelly, *Performing Virginity*, pp. 91–118.

21 Maud Burnett McInerney, 'Like a virgin: the problem of male virginity in the *Symphonia*', in McInerney (ed.), *Hildegard of Bingen: A Book of Essays* (New York: Garland, 1998), pp. 133–54 (pp. 147–50).

22 Katherine J. Lewis, 'Becoming a virgin king: Richard II and Edward the Confessor', in Samantha J. E. Riches and Sarah Salih (eds), *Gender and Holiness: Men, Women and Saints in Late Medieval Europe* (London: Routledge, 2002), pp. 86–100.

23 Winstead, *Virgin Martyrs*, pp. 69, 137.

24 Kathleen Coyne Kelly, 'Useful virgins in medieval hagiography', in Cindy L. Carlson and Angela Jane Weisl (eds), *Constructions of Widowhood and Virginity in the Middle Ages* (Basingstoke: Macmillan, 1999), pp. 135–64, and Kelly, *Performing Virginity*, pp. 40–62.

25 Cindy L. Carlson, 'Like a virgin: Mary and her detractors in the N-Town cycle', in Carlson and Weisl (eds), *Constructions of Widowhood and Virginity*, pp. 199–217.

26 Wogan-Browne, *Saints' Lives and Women's Literary Culture*, ch. 2.

27 Kelly, 'Useful virgins', p. 156.

28 Joyce E. Salisbury, *Church Fathers, Independent Virgins* (London: Verso, 1991), p. 30; Kelly, *Performing Virginity*, pp. 91–4.

29 Giulia Sissa, *Greek Virginity*, trans. Arthur Goldhammer (Cambridge, MA: Harvard University Press, 1990); *Hali Meiðhad*, in Bella Millett and Jocelyn Wogan-Browne (eds and trans.), *Medieval English Prose for Women from the Katherine Group and Ancrene Wisse* (Oxford: Clarendon Press, 1990), pp. 2–44, pp. 8–9; Kelly, *Performing Virginity*, pp. 22–33. On hymens, see Jocelyn Wogan-Browne in this volume.

30 Recent scholarship on medieval monstrosity includes: Bettina Bildhauer and Robert Mills (eds), *The Monstrous Middle Ages* (Cardiff: University of Wales Press, forthcoming); Michael Camille, *Mirror in Parchment: The Luttrell Psalter and the Making of Medieval England* (London: Reaktion, 1998), pp. 232–75; Jeffrey Jerome Cohen (ed.), *Monster Theory: Reading Culture* (Minneapolis and London: University of Minnesota Press, 1996); Cohen, *Of Giants: Sex, Monsters, and the Middle Ages* (Minneapolis: University of Minnesota Press, 1999); Timothy S. Jones and David A. Sprunger (eds), *Marvels, Miracles and Monsters: Studies in the Medieval and Early Modern Imaginations* (Kalamazoo: Medieval Institute Publications, 2002); Liz Herbert McAvoy and Teresa Walters (eds), *Consuming Narratives: Gender and Monstrous Appetites in the Middle Ages and Renaissance* (Cardiff: University of Wales Press, 2002); David Williams, *Deformed Discourse: The Function of the Monster in Mediaeval Thought and Literature* (Exeter: University of Exeter Press, 1999).

31 Tertullian, *Liber de virginibus velandis*, PL, 2, cols 887–914 (col. 898); 'On

the veiling of virgins', *The Writings of Tertullian*, vol. 3, ed. Alexander Roberts and James Donaldson, trans. S. Thelwell (Edinburgh: Clark, 1895), pp. 154–80, ch. 7.

[32] *Bestiary: Being an English Version of the Bodleian Library, Oxford MS Bodley 764*, trans. Richard Barber (Woodbridge: Boydell, 1999), pp. 43–4; *Mandeville's Travels, Translated from the French of Jean d'Outremeuse, Edited from MS. Cotton Titus C. XVI in the British Museum*, ed. P. Hamelius, EETS, os, 153 (London: Oxford University Press, 1919), pp. 14–16.

2

When is a Bosom Not a Bosom?
Problems with 'Erotic Mysticism'

SARAH SALIH

'It's a great theme in women's poetry, the waiting. That marvellous Rossetti poem about lying there and waiting for the knock on the door. It's meant to be Christ, but it's not, of course.'[1] But what if it *were* Christ? Germaine Greer's 'of course' exemplifies what David Lawton characterizes as 'the rather glib modern attitude that we find to the Song of Songs': a belief that we can read its language confident that its referent is not religious but erotic.[2] This assumption highlights a more widespread problem modern commentators have with what we call 'erotic mysticism': what, exactly, is the relation of the two terms? Should we privilege the erotic or the mystic? Are texts which speak of longings, ecstasies, penetrations 'really' sexual or 'really' religious? To what extent can the two modes coexist? Recent scholarship has explored the slipperiness and difficulty of the term 'mysticism' and interrogated the investments in deciding which texts, persons, experiences are permitted to qualify as mystical.[3] However, the equally crucial and, I would suggest, equally difficult category of the erotic remains largely unquestioned and is regularly treated as if it were self-evident. It needs to be interrogated in the same way as the category of the mystical: what are our grounds for deciding that a text claims or signifies erotic experience, and what are our investments in such a decision? Whether given passages in mystical texts should be read as sexual is not self-evident: commentators lack generally agreed principles of decoding. Michael Camille identifies some common medieval visual codes for sexual activity, but if there is an equivalent, culture-specific verbal code, I am not aware that it has been defined.[4] Julie B. Miller comments that in much current scholarship the erotic language of, in particular, medieval women mystics 'is not thought to be merely allegorical. Rather, the religious experience of medieval and early modern women mystics is often regarded as intrinsically erotic; moreover, the erotic is often considered to be an inherently positive, stable and self-explanatory category.'[5] The article makes an important intervention in current work on mystical writing. Miller's interest is in problematizing the violent strands of women's erotic mysticism: mine here is in the apparently naive question of how we can identify the erotic at all. My argument at first addresses mystical texts, as these tend to be the privileged examples in the critical debate, before moving on to two hagiographic texts which offer usefully different articulations of the problem.

Why this question should appear in a collection on virginities requires some explanation. Sexuality and virginity are intimately but unpredictably related topics, of which the medieval versions sometimes appear alien to modern readers. As argued in the introduction to this volume and by several of its contributors, virginity can be an object difficult to locate, and so one of the methods used by both medieval and modern writers is to outline it by delineating what it is not. In the case of erotic mysticism, the erotic can be read either as inimical to virginity or as constitutive of it. Enjoying erotic experience with God can be one of the defining marks of virginity, as I have previously argued in relation to the early Middle English anchoritic texts.[6] Eroticism which can be labelled as carnal and not mystical, however, can destroy virginity, as in the tale of the assaulted or masturbating monk discussed elsewhere in this volume by John Arnold: in this case, the question is, precisely, does this experience constitute sex and is this man a virgin?[7] Theologians of mysticism were divided as to whether mystical rapture resembled or was entirely other than carnal rapture, making discernment harder still.[8] Jean Gerson reports that

> I heard a Carthusian tell that he had heard from an important figure, who thereby showed his foolishness, that mortal sin does not always destroy charity, nor does it block out the love of God above all things. Instead, it sometimes inflames with a divine sweetness and thanksgiving in admiration, praise and delight. He gave as an example delight in fornication. This person was indeed out of his mind in his error.[9]

The error may indeed seem a surprising one, but Gerson must have thought it common or plausible enough to merit warning his readers against it.

If erotic desires and experiences can present a pressing interpretative problem for the medieval would-be virgin, it becomes imperative for both medieval and modern commentators to be able to identify them with some certainty. Modern critics frequently attempt to do so by deploying interpretative paradigms derived from sources outside the text: in this chapter, therefore, I aim to examine modern criticism as well as medieval texts. This chapter is in part a response to one such paradigm proposed by Nancy Partner's provocative question, 'Did mystics have sex?' Partner argues that mysticism is fundamentally a description of sexual experience, even in cases where erotic language is not foregrounded:

> Medieval mysticism wants to tell us about the heavy weight of sexual restriction, sexual guilt, and conformity to difficult rules of self-constraint carried by monks and nuns, and by all women, but especially those whose religious compunctions were sensitive and genuine . . . Frankly using a psychoanalytic language of libidinal drives, sublimations and displacements, acknowledging in medieval people the full mental structure of the unconscious as well as conscious personality, will restore to the life stories we write of and for them the depth, complexity, and fellowship with ourselves they deserve.[10]

Thus, Partner argues, if mystics appear to use sexual language to talk of God, that is because they are actually talking about sex, whether they know it or not. Sex with God is not a metaphor for the ineffability of contact with the divine: mystics are expressing sexual feelings in sexual language, though God must be named to enable the real erotic plot. This argument relies on a theoretical acceptance of Freudian and post-Freudian psychology, aligned with an ethical demand for the acknowledgement of our common humanity with medieval people. It also requires a rejection of alterity, claiming that 'the deep structure of human experience' is largely unchanged.[11]

My doubts about this argument are also a self-critique, as I have previously described Margery Kempe's relation with Jesus as erotic without, I now think, enough interrogation of the underlying assumptions of that categorization.[12] Despite the commonsensical appeal of Partner's case, it has its problems as an interpretative key. Some readers may feel that the claim that 'It might be seriously considered that the mystical "ineffable" is the orgasm, volatilized beyond sensation and projected into an objectified reality' fails to demonstrate the continuity of human sexuality.[13] Nor does the approach always convince at the level of textual analysis. For example, Partner comments on Margery's habit of falling to the ground and crying out when overwhelmed by thoughts of Jesus: 'Unself-consciously describing passionate love-making, Margery's seizures mimic the orgasm in dramatic exaggeration.'[14] This is Margery's description of one such moment:

> whan þei cam vp on-to þe Mownt of Caluarye, sche fel down þat sche mygth not stondyn ne knelyn but walwyd & wrestyd wyth hir body, spredyng hir armys a-brode, & cryed wyth a lowde voys as þow hir herte xulde a brostyn a-sundyr, for in þe cite of hir sowle sche saw veryly & freschly how owyr Lord was crucifyed.[15]

Admittedly, there is room for differing interpretation here: as Partner argues, the language of sexual experience is inherently metaphorical, because 'there is no literal language which directly describes the union of associational thought and emotion with bodily sensation which is the complex experience of sexual love'.[16] The range of critical reactions to Margery's text proves her point. Rosalynn Voaden remarks of Margery's embrace of God: 'The bodily contact was specifically non-genital – a kind of cosmic cuddle', citing a passage which other commentators have identified as unambiguously erotic: Jesus tells Margery 'þu mayst boldly take me in þe armys of þi sowle & kyssen my mowth, myn hed, & my fete as swetly as thow wylt'.[17]

There is insufficient space here for a detailed survey of verbal codings of sexual pleasure in various medieval genres, but those that come to mind – the stylized crudity of fabliau, the soft-focus generalities of romance, even the comically obscene allegory of the climax of the *Romance of the Rose* – do not sound much like Margery's text. Whether medieval women did writhe or scream in orgasm is not easily ascertainable, though this brief overview suggests that there was no normative expectation that they should do so. Other evidence is fragmentary and non-consensual: Albert the Great thought that humans alone amongst animals had sex silently, but a witness at a church court in York testified that 'she saw John and Alice lying together in the same bed and heard a noise from them like they were

making love together'.[18] Nevertheless, I would accept that falling,
writhing, screaming might refer to sexual pleasure. Then again, they
might not. To me at least Margery's behaviour at Calvary does not
appear to be unambiguously or even primarily a description of sexual
pleasure, however dramatic the exaggeration. As David Aers argues,
the detail of Margery's spreading her arms suggests that she is
performing *imitatio Christi* and re-enacting the Crucifixion.[19] Admittedly, *imitatio* may be productive of eroticism, as it is in Þe *Wohunge of
ure Lauerd*: 'My body hangs with your body nailed to the cross . . . Oh
Jesus, it is so sweet to hang with you.'[20] Nevertheless, Margery's text is
less clear. The witnesses to her behaviour offer various interpretations:
'summe seyd it was a wikkyd spiryt vexid hir; sum seyd it was a
sekenes; sum seyd sche had dronkyn to mech wyn . . . and so ich man as
hym thowte. Oþer gostly men louyd hir & fauowrd hir þe mor.'[21] It
does not appear, therefore, that the writhing and the sobbing registered
as sexual to any of the hostile observers of Margery's performance,
who suggest that she is ill, demoniac or drunk.[22] The 'gostly men',
meanwhile, would presumably not have favoured her if they had
interpreted her behaviour as orgasmic, and if her priestly scribe had
made the connection he would surely have edited the incident out of
the text. The significance of Margery's behaviour was evidently
contestable, and contested, so to read it as necessarily sexual, on the
grounds that mysticism is always sexual, is to obscure the text. Despite
Partner's demand for respect for the full humanity of medieval people,
this interpretative method requires overwriting what our subjects said
they experienced in favour of what we know it was that they really
experienced. This is not to make the claim that psychoanalytic critique
is an inherently invalid tool for the study of medieval culture but to
make a more local argument that the particular version of it which
claims access to the psyches of medieval individuals does not solve the
problem of religious eroticism.[23]

Partner explicitly rejects the idea that medieval sex is significantly
different from modern sex. In the recent discovery and development of
the history of the body, sexual behaviour has often been identified as
the sign of such historical otherness.[24] The invocation of *imitatio
Christi* to explain Margery's writhings introduces an alternative
hermeneutic key to mysticism, that of theology, which has been one of
the most commonly used codes for articulating sexual alterity. Perhaps
the most influential current expression of this view is Caroline Walker
Bynum's:

Twentieth-century viewers tend to eroticize the body and to define themselves by the nature of their sexuality. But did medieval viewers? For several reasons, I think we should be cautious about assuming that they did. Medieval people do not, for example, seem to have defined themselves by sexual orientation . . . Nor did medieval people understand as erotic or sexual a number of bodily sensations which we interpret that way.[25]

If, however, we persist in reading some medieval religious language as having erotic reference, this may be due to 'a modern tendency to find sex more interesting than feeding, suffering or salvation'.[26] Medieval sexuality in this view is markedly different from the modern version: not constitutive of personal or categorical identities, more diffuse, less genital. Bynum's essay is subtitled 'A reply to Leo Steinberg', emphasizing her contestation of Steinberg's views, but, as Richard Rambuss and Robert Mills argue, Bynum and Steinberg are in agreement that theology is the appropriate interpretative paradigm for apparently erotic language and imagery when it occurs in religious contexts.[27] Sexual language can never be sexual language, but must always signify something else.

Bynum's argument is a sophisticated reinterpretation of an older claim that medieval people were simply less interested in sex than we are – a claim which asserts a far more radical alterity of sex and human personality than that found by self-avowed social constructionists. In this older view, the Middle Ages are constructed as prelapsarian: medieval people were innocent, while we moderns, sadly, have fallen into a post-Freudian obsession with matters sexual. The classic and often-quoted locus for this view is Jean Leclercq's remark: 'In such matters we must be careful not to project on to a less erotically preoccupied society the artificially stimulated and commercially exploited eroticism of our own sex-ridden age.'[28] The thesis certainly ventriloquizes a medieval orthodoxy that erotic and mystic experience are mutually exclusive precisely because of their superficial similarity, found in, for example, Bernard of Clairvaux's instruction: 'Your affection for your Lord Jesus should be both tender and intimate, to oppose the sweet enticements of sensual life. Sweetness conquers sweetness as one nail drives out another.'[29] However, its application to particular instances may be questioned. To cite a representative example of criticism informed by such views: Douglass Roby, introducing Aelred of Rievaulx's *Spiritual Friendship*, suggests that 'Aelred was not, of course, troubled by the twentieth century's pervasive consciousness of sexual drives.'[30] '*Of course*'? Leaving aside the vexed question of Aelred's personal sexual experience, I would suggest that *Spiritual Friendship* is well aware of sexual drives: it addresses itself to a reader posited as one who 'might be too eager for friendship and be deceived by its mere semblance, mistake the counterfeit for the true, the imaginary for the real, the carnal for the spiritual'.[31] The treatise needs to exist because this is a difficult judgement to make. If this is not pervasive enough, it can be supplemented with a rather later text, *Ancrene Wisse*: ' "But do you think" [the anchoress asks], "that I will leap on [a man] just because I look at him?" God knows, dear sister [the author replies], stranger things have happened.'[32] The author of *Ancrene Wisse* emphatically has and desires his readers to have a pervasive consciousness of sexual drives: it is hard to imagine how this text could be any more erotically preoccupied. As Anke Bernau argues, 'virginity in *Ancrene Wisse* demonstrates the proliferation of multiple sexual possibilities as it warns the anchoresses against desiring not only men, but also their sisters and even themselves'.[33] It is surely unsurprising that people whose lives required the regulation of sexuality should have had – or have been constructed as having – a pervasive awareness of it. Women were excluded from public religious roles precisely because of the perceived pervasiveness of sexual drives (amongst other reasons): it was argued that women's visibility would inevitably produce erotic arousal in men.[34] It was not Freud, but St Augustine, who defined sexuality – specifically, the male capacity for erection – as the marker of humanity's fallen state.[35] If we sometimes find medieval sexuality familiar, we are not necessarily projecting our post-Freudian obsessions back onto the innocent past: we may be recognizing a common post-Augustinian heritage.[36]

Thus, both theologically and psychoanalytically based interpretative strategies potentially produce totalizing explanations. They divide, systematically, on the question of whether sex is the vehicle, or the tenor of mystical writings. In a theological reading, mystical experience may express itself in erotic language as a gesture to the unrepresentability of the divine. Certain versions of psychoanalytic criticism may counter that erotic language refers to erotic content, which, however, is consciously or unconsciously coded as religious. Thus each interpretation obliterates one aspect of the texts as illusory, and risks a reductive overwriting of textual specificity. If mysticism is taken to be a genre, a historically sited cultural product, then interpretative master-keys are inappropriate, and an awareness of the variability of local effects more useful. This is not to suggest that every critical identification of religious texts as erotic or not-erotic is driven by a commitment to either of these ideologies: such choices are as likely to be made for the sake of local interpretative coherence. Nevertheless, such decisions bring with them the shadow of one or the other of these theorizations. That medieval subjects were aware of the theological but not the Freudian code may initially suggest that the theological readings should be accorded greater privilege. However, some of them also knew that erotic desire might manifest itself in devotional guises. Gerson warned that 'divine love' had to be carefully scrutinized 'because of the deceptive or fake golden colour of empty or carnal love. Thus it has happened that certain women, although out of ignorance, have been affected by a harmful love toward God.'[37] Gerson did not, of course, name the process 'repression' or 'sublimation', but would nevertheless have understood the concepts without difficulty.

The current self-conscious opposition between theological and pathological readings of mysticism dates from the late nineteenth century, 'as exemplified by the Salpêtrière doctor and hysteria expert Henri Legrand du Saulle: "Many *women Saints* and *Blesseds* were none other than simple hysterics!"'[38] Although the two interpretative strategies are thus produced as competing and radically incompatible with one another, they nevertheless also have their moments of complicity, such as Lacan's appropriation of the mystic ineffable as the unrepresentability of woman.[39] Both thus may silence the mystic/hysteric by obliterating what she actually says in favour of a master-narrative of her inability to signify without interpretative help.

In the current critical climate, the question, 'Is this about sex?', when asked in a sceptical tone, thus tends to come from a position which assumes the radical innocence and alterity of the Middle Ages. Meanwhile, many of the most interesting and thought-provoking recent analyses of medieval erotic mysticism come from a position which does not ask the question at all, accepting that texts may be both erotic and religious without feeling it necessary to investigate the relation between the terms. I think that asking the question is a valuable exercise: our subjects asked it and we can learn from their difficulties. I want to ask how to define the erotic without implying that it is an inherently illegitimate category in this context: indeed, such a question seems to me to be entirely necessary to establish the legitimacy of 'erotic mysticism' or 'erotic language' as objects of enquiry. If everything is

erotic, then nothing is. In this chapter I accept that sex and religion
overlap, and accept also that discerning them is difficult: my interest is
in examining the slippage between them rather than attempting to
reinforce any secure distinction. If, as Simon Gaunt argues, medieval
culture does not know a 'purely secular' sphere, neither does it know a
purely sacred one.[40] I will be examining here some moments when
medieval texts stage the same anxiety as the modern critical debate: is
this a carnal or spiritual experience? Is virginity at risk here? Many
medieval texts think that the carnal and the mystical erotic are self-
evidently distinct, but there are also a few which betray an uncertainty
as to whether a given emotion, image, experience is or is not carnal.
Hagiographic texts, to which I now turn, include some particularly
interesting articulations of this problem.

   One such moment of uncertainty appears in the *vita* of St Gilbert of
Sempringham, the twelfth-century founder of the monastic double
order of Sempringham. The *vita* is committed to establishing the perfect virginity of its hero. It recounts that, after Gilbert's death, a canon
of his order had a vision which confirmed that Gilbert, 'chaste [*uirgo*]
in body and mind', had been placed in the choir of virgins in honour
both of his own virginity and of his protection of virgin women.[41] His
virginity evidently requires such confirmation, for there were moments
in his lifetime when it might have been seen to be compromised. In
particular, an incident which occurred when Gilbert was a young clerk
in minor orders is most informative about both Gilbert's personal
virginity and his investment in virgin women.

> He occupied a dwelling in the churchyard of St Andrew's at
> Sempringham, and with a chaplain of proven virtue called Geoffrey he too
> led a solitary and commendable existence. Earlier they had both lodged
> with a family in the town. But a hidden infection stole upon them both
> from the beauty of the daughter of the household, who looked after them
> attentively; for Gilbert dreamt that he put his hand into the girl's bosom
> and was unable to draw it out. The most chaste of men was terrified that,
> human frailty being what it is, his dream foretold a sin of fornication, and
> so he immediately described his temptation and dream to the priest. In his
> turn this man confessed to him that he was being afflicted by the same
> trouble. Accordingly, following the apostle's advice, they speedily left
> those lodgings and built a house for themselves in the churchyard . . . But
> what he saw in his dream heralded not future sin, but glorious merit, for
> this girl was one of the seven original persons with whom the father
> founded the communities of his whole Order. Her bosom into which our

pastor and assiduous friend put his hand was like the mysterious peace of the church, of which he was a foundation.[42]

Gilbert and his hagiographer face essentially the same interpretative problem as do modern commentators on the mystical erotic: is his dream about sex, or about God? Their readings of the dream rehearse both strategies outlined above. Gilbert's initial reaction indicates that his first interpretation of the dream was that it was erotic and, therefore, dangerous to his virginity. The hagiographer's language of 'hidden infection' (*occulta . . . contagio*) supports his analysis. Gilbert's behaviour belongs to what Arnold identifies elsewhere in this volume as the second type of male chastity narrative, tending towards the undramatic end of that category.[43] Temptation occurs, but Gilbert promptly takes the proper steps to master it without too much difficulty. It is not clear whether Gilbert thought the dream itself, as an erotic experience, damaging to his virginity, as some of his contemporaries certainly would have, or whether it actually rescued his virginity by prompting him to flee to safety before anything worse occurred.[44] The second interpretation would suggest a conception of degrees of virginity comparable to that of *Hali Meiðhad*: 'Virginity is the blossom which, if it is once completely cut off, will never grow again (but though it may wither sometimes through indecent thoughts, it can grow green again nevertheless).'[45] The dream would function as both a withering and a salutary warning, which enabled Gilbert's flight and the regeneration of his virginity: nevertheless, in itself it is a clearly erotic experience.

The hagiographic and retrospective interpretation of the dream, however, is that it was not erotic but prophetic. The allegorization of the dream takes us into the familiar world of biblical exegesis, in particular the disembodying of the Bride of the Song of Songs into a figure for the soul or the Church.[46] Quite properly, Gilbert placed his hand into the bosom of Mother Church, an action erotic only on the surface level. When this surface level is properly read – that is, when it is obliterated – the girl is revealed to be actually constitutive of, not threatening to, Gilbert's virginity, for she is to become one of the women whom Gilbert recruits to his order, thus earning his eventual place in the choir of virgins. The text thus draws attention away from the still unanswered questions about Gilbert's dream (did it, for example, provoke nocturnal emission? Was Geoffrey's 'trouble' equally prophetic?) and its implications for his virginity by substituting

allegorical for literal readings and apparently unproblematic female
virgin bodies for a problematic male one. The virginity of the Church,
the girl and her six companions is brought to the foreground, occluding
and substituting for Gilbert's own.[47] His reaction to the dream
anticipates that of the women: they, like he, will preserve their virginity
by withdrawal from society into a same-sex community attached to the
church of St Andrew.[48] There is a series of substitutions, driving one
another out like Bernard's nails. First Gilbert is replaced by the girl,
who is then herself subsumed into abstract entities. She becomes
identified with her enclosure, in the overlaying of closed body and
enclosed space made by Gilbert himself when he referred to the key to
the virgins' lodging as 'the seal of their purity' (*pudoris earum
signaculum*).[49] Virginity has been moved away from Gilbert himself,
evidently a troublesome site, into an idealized abstraction, secured by
assimilating body to architecture.

If the *vita* sees this abstraction as the proper location of virginity, its
apparent insouciance about the possible compromising of its hero's
virtue becomes more explicable. Whether Gilbert experienced the
physical symptoms of desire or not is unimportant if his virginity is
primarily a vicarious condition, held safely by the virgin women of his
order. This reading also elucidates the *vita*'s omission of two tales
about Gilbert, current in contemporary sources, which on the face of it
might seem good material to illustrate his energetic defence of women's
virginity and his masculine sexual purity by contrast with errant nuns.
One is the case of the Nun of Watton, known from a letter of Aelred of
Rievaulx, in which Gilbert oversees the punishment and redemption of
an unchaste nun.[50] The second is the anecdote told by Gerald of Wales
that Gilbert responded to a nun's confession of desire for him by
stripping naked to preach to the nuns about the snares of lechery.[51] The
pragmatic rationale for the exclusion of these tales may well be that
they reveal an inherent structural problem of Gilbert's double order,
but this shades into their deeper misfit with the *vita*'s logic. They
problematize the security of the location of virginity in the bodies of
monastic women. The second is especially difficult, returning the focus
to Gilbert's body in circumstances which would certainly compromise
his virginity were he a woman, for it is a commonplace of virginity texts
that to be seen and desired is to be unchaste.

Gilbert's response to the dream, however, indicates that he had no
privileged access to its meaning at the time, having, at this stage in his
life, no virgin women under his protection. In addition, he continued to

be mistaken about its significance for some years. The two interpretations are mutually incompatible: the prophetic tenor of the dream
obliterates its erotic vehicle. A bosom is no longer a bosom, but the
mysterious peace of the Church. If the second interpretation alone
were recorded, scholars following Leclercq's line would no doubt
reproach the anachronistic assumptions of any critic who read erotic
matter into the sanctified metaphor of Gilbert's dream. And yet as
both interpretations are presented in the text, a stable understanding of
the dream is difficult. Surely the hagiographer did not intend to
reassure his clerical readers that their erotic dreams would probably
turn out to be prophecies in disguise. In many cases, such doubtful
incidents were probably tidied away somewhere in the process of
producing hagiography, with either the first interpretation or the whole
incident being omitted altogether. This, indeed, is what happens in
John Capgrave's 1451 abridgement of Gilbert's life, which passes over
the incident in silence, though it does reproduce the *vita*'s earlier statement that Gilbert 'touched he neuer woman'.[52] Capgrave's omission
points to a fear that the potential carnality of the dream is not
thoroughly contained by the hagiographer's allegorization.

A near-contemporary text, *The Life of Christina of Markyate*, offers
a comparable moment of uncertainty as to sexual status. The situation
here is slightly different: Christina and her biographer did not have to
distinguish between erotic and prophetic experience, but to determine
whether experiencing sexual temptation compromised her virginity.
Christina's struggle with sexual temptation was ended when she was
granted a vision of the infant Christ:

> And with immeasurable delight she held Him at one moment to her
> virginal breast, at another she felt His presence within her even through
> the barrier of the flesh . . . From that moment the fire of lust was so
> completely extinguished [*libidinis ardor ita extinctus defecit*] that never
> afterwards could it be revived.[53]

The paradox of describing the elimination of desire in the language of
desire lends itself to the theological reading outlined above and accords
with Bernard's metaphor of the nails which drive each other out: this
text intends a statement about the incompatibility of the erotic and the
mystical. Its difficulties lie elsewhere. Christ's visit is recognizable as a
'mystic castration' as discussed by Jacqueline Murray.[54] Most such
stories concern male subjects: Christina's is also unusual in that it does

not completely suffice to confirm her virginity. She remained uncertain as to whether she was truly a virgin: 'For she was mindful of the thoughts and stings of the flesh with which she had been troubled, and even though she was not conscious of having fallen in deed or desire, she was chary of asserting that she had escaped unscathed.'[55] This is hagiography, of course, so the doubts are resolved by heavenly affirmation, just as Gilbert's virginity was confirmed by a vision: in both cases, however, it is acknowledged that normal human interpretative strategies may have considerable difficulty discerning the limits of the erotic. Even in cases when the principal actors are certain of the difference between carnal and spiritual friendship, such relationships are open to misreading. Christina's chaste spiritual affection for the hermit Roger must be kept secret 'for they feared scandal to their inferiors' and ill-wishers suspect that her friendship with her 'beloved' (*dilecti*) Abbot Geoffrey is one of 'earthly love'.[56] Christina, lacking Gilbert's resource to substitute locations of her virginity, continues to be a focus of sexual anxieties.

I cannot offer here a universally reliable interpretative key to erotic language in religious contexts, but I can suggest that it is informative to trace incidents of sexual trouble to consider how individual texts and persons defined the difference between sex and religion. The persistence of confusion – and indeed of the desire to distinguish – suggests that the two are not now and were not then discrete realms of discourse or of experience. Sweeping statements about the alterity of medieval people – that they had no conception of childhood; that they were innocent of both inter- and intra-personal conflict; that they had no sense of individuality – have a tendency to turn out on closer inspection to be based on a desire for a Middle Ages which is other in every way to the modern. As Ruth Mazo Karras argues in relation to the classical past, 'A healthy respect for the alterity of the past need not make us deny all similarity or continuity': alterity should not become an imperative.[57] I acknowledge that this is a difficult topic to quantify, but to judge from the evidence of medieval writing, including medical treatises, romance, lyric, fabliau, sermons and penitentials, medieval people seem to have found sex quite as interesting a topic as we do, and to have discussed it, in various discourses, humorously, tenderly, pornographically and moralistically. Medieval people were not so other that they were not also fascinated by the alterity of sex in other times, as we see in, for example, Thomas Malory's famous meditation (in contradiction with his narrative) on 'love in kynge Arthurs dayes', or of sex in other cultures, as in the account of 'Sir John Mandeville' of the bridegrooms who employ professional deflowerers because they believe that 'of olde tyme men hadden ben dede for deflourynge of maydenes þat hadden serpentes in hire bodyes þat stongen men vpon hire both ȝerdes'.[58] I would suggest that examples such as those of Gilbert and Christina indicate also that medieval people were not so different that they did not sometimes have the same interpretative problems as ourselves in deciding whether sex was indeed sex and whether virgins were indeed virgins.

Notes

This chapter is part of an ongoing conversation with Robert Mills. I am grateful to him, Anke Bernau and Ruth Evans for their comments on drafts. I would also like to thank everyone who listened and responded to earlier versions of this material both at 'Seeing Gender', the January 2002 Gender and Medieval Studies Conference organized by Emma Campbell and Robert Mills, and at the University of East Anglia Literature Seminar.

[1] Germaine Greer, interviewed by Joseph Kestner in Jan Todd (ed.), *Women Writers Talking* (New York: Holmes & Meier, 1983), p. 154.

[2] David Lawton, *Faith, Text and History: The Bible in English* (Charlottesville: University Press of Virginia, 1990), p. 154.

[3] For investigations of the category of 'mysticism', see Sarah Beckwith, 'A very material mysticism: the medieval mysticism of Margery Kempe', in David Aers (ed.), *Medieval Literature: Criticism, Ideology and History* (Brighton: Harvester, 1986), pp. 34–57; Beckwith, 'Problems of authority in late medieval English mysticism: language, agency and authority in *The Book of Margery Kempe*', *Exemplaria*, 4 (1992), 171–99; Amy Hollywood, *Sensible Ecstasy: Mysticism, Sexual Difference, and the Demands of History* (Chicago: University of Chicago Press, 2002); Nancy F. Partner, 'Reading *The Book of Margery Kempe*', *Exemplaria*, 3 (1991), 29–66; Partner, 'Did mystics have sex?', in Jacqueline Murray and Konrad Eisenbichler (eds), *Desire and Discipline: Sex and Sexuality in the Premodern West* (Toronto: University of Toronto Press, 1996), pp. 296–311; Nicholas Watson, 'Censorship and cultural change in late medieval England: vernacular theology, the Oxford translation debate, and Arundel's Constitutions of 1409', *Speculum*, 70 (1995), 822–64.

[4] Michael Camille, 'Manuscript illumination and the art of copulation', in Karma Lochrie, Peggy McCracken and James A. Schultz (eds), *Constructing Medieval Sexuality* (Minneapolis: University of Minnesota Press, 1997), pp. 58–90. See, however, John W. Baldwin, 'Five discourses on desire: sexuality and gender in northern France around 1200', *Speculum*, 66

(1991), 797–819, for a more general discussion of medieval erotic
discourses; Simon Gaunt, 'A martyr to love: sacrificial desire in the poetry
of Bernart de Ventadorn', *Journal of Medieval and Early Modern Studies*, 31
(2001), 477–506, for an investigation of the relation of erotic and religious
language; Jeffrey J. Kripal, *Roads of Excess, Palaces of Wisdom: Eroticism
and Reflexivity in the Study of Mysticism* (Chicago: University of Chicago
Press, 2001) for a comparative erotics of mysticisms; and Richard Rambuss,
Closet Devotions (Durham, NC: Duke University Press, 1998) for readings
of seventeenth-century writing as simultaneously religious and erotic.

5 Julie B. Miller, 'Eroticized violence in medieval women's mystical literature:
a call for a feminist critique', *Journal of Feminist Studies in Religion*, 15
(1999), 25–49 (25).

6 Sarah Salih, 'Queering *sponsalia Christi*: virginity, gender and desire in the
early Middle English anchoritic texts', in Rita Copeland, David Lawton
and Wendy Scase (eds), *New Medieval Literatures*, vol. 5 (Oxford: Oxford
University Press, 2002), pp. 155–76.

7 This volume, pp. 104–14. The incident is also discussed by Jacqueline
Murray, 'The law of sin that is in my members: the problem of male
embodiment', in Samantha J. E. Riches and Sarah Salih (eds), *Gender and
Holiness: Men, Women and Saints in Late Medieval Europe* (London:
Routledge, 2002), pp. 9–22 (p. 13).

8 Dyan Elliott, 'The physiology of rapture and female spirituality', in Peter
Biller and A. J. Minnis (eds), *Medieval Theology and the Natural Body*
(Woodbridge: York Medieval Press, 1997), pp. 141–73 (pp. 147–8).

9 Jean Gerson, 'On distinguishing true from false revelations', in Gerson,
Early Works, trans. Brian Patrick McGuire (New York: Paulist Press,
1998), pp. 334–64 (p. 357).

10 Partner, 'Did mystics have sex?', pp. 307–8.

11 Partner, 'Reading *The Book of Margery Kempe*', 61. Although not all
psychoanalytic critics use the code in this way, Partner's approach is not
unique, and is explicitly supported by, for example, Madeline H. Caviness,
*Visualizing Women in the Middle Ages: Sight, Spectacle and Scopic
Economy* (Philadelphia: University of Pennsylvania Press, 2001), p. 24.

12 In *Versions of Virginity in Late Medieval England* (Cambridge: Brewer,
2001), pp. 224–40.

13 Partner, 'Reading *The Book of Margery Kempe*', 38.

14 Ibid., 56. This is not an idiosyncratic reading: see also Wendy Harding,
'Body into text: *The Book of Margery Kempe*', in Linda Lomperis and
Sarah Stanbury (eds), *Feminist Approaches to the Body in Medieval
Literature* (Philadelphia: University of Pennsylvania Press, 1993), pp.
168–87 (p. 173), and Hope Phyllis Weissman, 'Margery Kempe in
Jerusalem: *Hysterica Compassio* in the late Middle Ages', in Mary J.
Carruthers and Elizabeth D. Kirk (eds), *Acts of Interpretation: The Text in
its Contexts* (Norman, OK: Pilgrim Books, 1982), pp. 201–18 (p. 212), for
further identifications of such behaviours as reminiscent of orgasm.

[15] *The Book of Margery Kempe*, ed. Sanford Brown Meech and Hope Emily Allen, EETS, os, 212 (London: Oxford University Press, 1949), p. 68.

[16] Partner, 'Reading *The Book of Margery Kempe*', 37.

[17] Rosalynn Voaden, 'Beholding men's members: the sexualizing of transgression in *The Book of Margery Kempe*', in Biller and Minnis (eds), *Medieval Theology and the Natural Body*, pp. 175–90 (p. 181), citing *Margery Kempe*, p. 90. The same passage is considered 'specifically sexual' in Garrett P. J. Epp, 'Ecce homo', in Glenn Burger and Steven F. Kruger (eds), *Queering the Middle Ages* (Minneapolis: University of Minnesota Press, 2001), pp. 236–52 (p. 239), and 'strongly erotic' in A. C. Spearing, '*The Book of Margery Kempe*; or, the diary of a nobody', *Southern Review*, 38 (2002), 625–35 (629).

[18] Albert, cited in Michael Camille, *Images on the Edge: The Margins of Medieval Art* (London: Reaktion, 1992, repr. 1995), p. 48; *Women in England c.1275–1525: Documentary Sources*, ed. and trans. P. J. P. Goldberg (Manchester: Manchester University Press, 1995), p. 62.

[19] David Aers and Lynn Staley, *The Powers of the Holy: Religion, Politics and Gender in Late Medieval English Culture* (University Park: Pennsylvania State University Press, 1996), p. 55.

[20] *Þe Wohunge of ure Lauerd*, ed. W. Meredith Thompson, EETS, os, 241 (London: Oxford University Press, 1958), ll. 590–602. My translation.

[21] *Margery Kempe*, p. 69.

[22] See Nancy Caciola, 'Mystics, demoniacs, and the physiology of spirit possession in medieval Europe', *Comparative Studies in Society and History*, 42/2 (2000), 268–306, on the external similarity of divine and demonic possession.

[23] See Louise O. Fradenburg, 'Analytical survey 2: We are not alone: psychoanalytic medievalism', in Rita Copeland, David Lawton and Wendy Scase (eds), *New Medieval Literatures*, vol. 2 (Oxford: Clarendon Press, 1998), pp. 249–76; Fradenburg, '"Be not far from me": psychoanalysis, medieval studies and the subject of religion', *Exemplaria*, 7 (1995), 41–54; Lee Patterson, 'Chaucer's Pardoner on the couch: Psyche and Clio in medieval literary studies', *Speculum*, 76 (2001), 638–80; and Paul Strohm, *Theory and the Premodern Text* (Minneapolis: University of Minnesota Press, 2000), pp. 165–214, for some recent contributions to the much larger question of the place of psychoanalytic language in medieval studies.

[24] Alain Boureau, *The Lord's First Night: The Myth of the droit de cuissage*, trans. Lydia G. Cochrane (Chicago: University of Chicago Press, 1998), p. 16.

[25] Caroline Walker Bynum, *Fragmentation and Redemption: Essays on Gender and the Human Body in Medieval Religion* (New York: Zone Books, 1992), pp. 85–6. For further discussion of the still open question of whether and, if so, how, sexual orientation can be conceptualized in medieval culture, see Ross Balzaretti, 'Michel Foucault, homosexuality and the Middle Ages', *Renaissance and Modern Studies*, 37 (1994), 1–12; Carolyn Dinshaw, *Getting Medieval: Sexualities and Communities, Pre- and Postmodern*

(Durham, NC: Duke University Press, 1999); Allen J. Frantzen, *Before the Closet: Same-Sex Love from* Beowulf *to* Angels in America (Chicago: University of Chicago Press, 1998); David M. Halperin, 'Forgetting Foucault: acts, identities, and the histories of sexuality', *Representations*, 63 (1998), 93–120; Mark D. Jordan, *The Invention of Sodomy in Christian Theology* (Chicago: University of Chicago Press, 1997); Karma Lochrie, *Covert Operations: The Medieval Uses of Secrecy* (Philadelphia: University of Pennsylvania Press, 1999).

[26] Bynum, *Fragmentation and Redemption*, p. 92. This is not necessarily Bynum's only position on the question: see also her argument that in mystical pleasure 'sexual feelings were . . . not so much translated into another medium as simply set free', which seems close to Partner's argument: *Holy Feast and Holy Fast: The Religious Significance of Food to Medieval Women* (Berkeley: University of California Press, 1987), p. 248.

[27] Rambuss, *Closet Devotions*, p. 44; Robert Mills, 'Ecce homo', in Riches and Salih (eds), *Gender and Holiness*, pp. 152–73 (p. 155). They refer to Leo Steinberg's *The Sexuality of Christ in Renaissance Art and Modern Oblivion*, 2nd edn (Chicago: University of Chicago Press, 1995).

[28] Jean Leclercq, *Monks and Love in Twelfth-Century France: Psycho-Historical Essays* (Oxford: Clarendon Press, 1979), p. 100.

[29] Bernard of Clairvaux, *On the Song of Songs I: Sermons 1–20*, trans. Killian Walsh (Kalamazoo: Cistercian Publications, 1981), sermon 20, p. 150.

[30] Aelred of Rievaulx, *Spiritual Friendship*, trans. Mary Eugenia Laker, intro. Douglass Roby (Kalamazoo: Cistercian Publications, 1977), p. 21. The spectre of homosexuality is particularly likely to produce such claims: see M. J. Ailes, 'The medieval male couple and the language of homosociality', in D. M. Hadley (ed.), *Masculinity in Medieval Europe* (London: Longman, 1999), pp. 214–37, for another example, and Kripal, *Roads of Excess*, esp. pp. 64–81, 185–93; Karma Lochrie, 'Mystical acts, queer tendencies', in Lochrie, McCracken and Schultz (eds), *Constructing Medieval Sexuality*, pp. 180–200; and Mills, 'Ecce homo', for critiques of the heterosexist presumptions of much scholarship in this area.

[31] Aelred, *Spiritual Friendship*, p. 73. I accept Katherine M. Yohe's point that Aelred's sense of 'carnal' is not coterminous with 'sexual', but would argue that the sexual is not thereby excluded from the carnal; Yohe, 'Sexual attraction and the motivations for love and friendship in Aelred of Rievaulx', *American Benedictine Review*, 46 (1995), 283–307 (287–9).

[32] *Anchoritic Spirituality:* Ancrene Wisse *and Associated Works*, trans. Nicholas Watson and Anne Savage, preface by Benedicta Ward (New York: Paulist Press, 1991), p. 68.

[33] Anke Bernau, 'Virginal effects: text and identity in *Ancrene Wisse*', in Riches and Salih (eds), *Gender and Holiness*, pp. 36–48 (p. 41).

[34] A. J. Minnis, '*De impedimento sexus*: women's bodies and medieval impediments to female ordination', in Biller and Minnis (eds), *Medieval Theology and the Natural Body*, pp. 109–39 (pp. 122–3).

35 Augustine of Hippo, *The City of God Against the Pagans*, trans. George E. McCracken, Philip Levine and William M. Green, 7 vols, Loeb Classical Library (London: Heinemann; Cambridge, MA: Harvard University Press, 1966), bk 13, ch. 13.

36 Kripal comments that medieval cabbalistic writers 'were applying "Freudian" principles within their distinctively mystical worldview centuries before Freud'; *Roads of Excess*, p. 273.

37 Gerson, 'On distinguishing true from false revelations', p. 356.

38 Quoted in Cristina Mazzoni, *Saint Hysteria: Neurosis, Mysticism and Gender in European Culture* (Ithaca, NY: Cornell University Press, 1996), p. 3. See also Hollywood, *Sensible Ecstasy*, pp. 236–73, for an important investigation of the desire to read medieval holy women as hysterical.

39 Mazzoni, *Saint Hysteria*, pp. 29, 49.

40 Gaunt, 'A martyr to love', 479.

41 *The Book of St Gilbert*, ed. Raymonde Foreville and Gillian Keir (Oxford: Clarendon Press, 1987), pp. 128–9.

42 Ibid., pp. 16–19.

43 This volume, pp. 105–6.

44 For discussion of the problem of nocturnal emissions, see Dyan Elliott, *Fallen Bodies: Pollution, Sexuality and Demonology in the Middle Ages* (Philadelphia: University of Pennsylvania Press, 1999), pp. 14–34; Jacqueline Murray, 'Mystical castration: some reflections on Peter Abelard, Hugh of Lincoln and sexual control', in Murray (ed.), *Conflicted Identities and Multiple Masculinities: Men in the Medieval West* (New York: Garland, 1999), pp. 73–91; Murray, 'Law of sin'; C. Leyser, 'Masculinity in flux: nocturnal emission and the limits of celibacy in the early Middle Ages', in Hadley (ed.), *Masculinity in Medieval Europe*, pp. 103–20.

45 *Hali Meiðhad*, in Bella Millett and Jocelyn Wogan-Browne (eds and trans.), *Medieval English Prose for Women from the Katherine Group and* Ancrene Wisse (Oxford: Clarendon Press, 1990), pp. 2–44 (pp. 8–11).

46 For analyses of Song exegesis, see Ann W. Astell, *The Song of Songs in the Middle Ages* (Ithaca, NY: Cornell University Press, 1990); E. Ann Matter, *The Voice of my Beloved: The Song of Songs in Western Medieval Christianity* (Philadelphia: University of Pennsylvania Press, 1990); Denys Turner, *Eros and Allegory: Medieval Exegesis of the Song of Songs* (Kalamazoo: Cistercian Publications, 1995).

47 Samantha J. E. Riches, 'St George as virgin martyr', in Riches and Salih (eds), *Gender and Holiness*, pp. 65–85 (pp. 75–7), makes a comparable argument that the presence of female virgin bodies in hagiography may indicate male virginity.

48 *Book of St Gilbert*, pp. 31–5.

49 Ibid., pp. 34–5.

50 Aelred of Rievaulx, *De sanctimoniali de Wattun*, *PL*, 195, cols 789–96; trans. in John Boswell, *The Kindness of Strangers: The Abandonment of Children in Western Europe from Late Antiquity to the Renaissance*

(Harmondsworth: Penguin, 1989), pp. 452–8. For further discussion of this, see Giles Constable, 'Aelred of Rievaulx and the nun of Watton: an episode in the early history of the Gilbertine Order', in Derek Baker (ed.), *Medieval Women*, Studies in Church History, Subsidia, 1 (Oxford: Blackwell, 1978), pp. 205–26; Elizabeth Freeman, 'Nuns in the public sphere: Aelred of Rievaulx's *De Sanctimoniali de Wattun* and the gendering of authority', *Comitatus*, 27 (1996), 55–80; Sarah Salih, 'Monstrous virginity: St Aelred writes the nuns of Watton', in Kate Boardman, Catherine Emerson and Adrian Tudor (eds), *Framing the Text: Reading Tradition and Image in Medieval Europe*, *Mediaevalia*, 20 (2001), 49–72.

[51] Gerald of Wales, *The Jewel of the Church: A Translation of* Gemma Ecclesiastica *by Giraldus Cambrensis*, ed. and trans. John J. Hagen (Leiden: Brill, 1979), p. 188.

[52] *Book of St Gilbert*, pp. 14–15; *John Capgrave's Lives of St Augustine and St Gilbert of Sempringham and a Sermon*, ed. J. J. Munro, EETS, OS, 140 (London: Kegan Paul, Trench, Trübner, 1910), p. 64.

[53] *The Life of Christina of Markyate: A Twelfth-Century Recluse*, ed. and trans. C. H. Talbot, Medieval Academy Reprints for Teaching, 39 (Toronto: University of Toronto Press, 1998), pp. 118–19.

[54] Murray, 'Mystical castration'.

[55] *Christina of Markyate*, p. 127.

[56] Ibid., pp. 103, 156–7, 173.

[57] Ruth Mazo Karras, 'Review essay: Active/passive, acts/passions: Greek and Roman sexualities', *American Historical Review*, 105 (2000), 1250–65 (1254).

[58] Thomas Malory, *Works*, ed. Eugène Vinaver (Oxford: Oxford University Press, 1971), p. 649; *Mandeville's Travels, Translated from the French of Jean d'Outremeuse, Edited from MS. Cotton Titus C. XVI in the British Museum*, ed. P. Hamelius, EETS, OS, 153 (London: Oxford University Press, 1919), p. 190.

3

The Sheela-na-Gig: An Incongruous
Sign of Sexual Purity?

JULIETTE DOR

Sheela-na-gig is the name given by anthropologists, folklorists and art historians to a type of ancient grotesque carved stone (in a few cases, wooden) sculpture of a naked woman displaying her oversized genitals (Fig. 1). These carvings date from the twelfth to the seventeenth centuries. Though related to the exhibitionist female figures found along the pilgrim routes in France and Spain, sheela-na-gigs are peculiar to England, Wales and Ireland (the country where they are most prevalent). Originally set high up in churches, or on the walls of castles or tower-houses, many of them were placed above the entrance, often as keystones. They could also be positioned on quoins, pillar-stones, windows or corbels. Their obscenity has caused offence: over time a number of the figures were displaced, buried, damaged (either deliberately, or by weathering) or completely destroyed.[1]

What have these explicitly sexualized figures, with their obscenely gaping vulvas, to do with virginity? If the virgin in the Middle Ages and early modern period represents a sacred ideal of the pure, enclosed and unbreachable body, then the sheela-na-gig appears to point to its opposite: a sacrilegious caricature of the impure, open and permeable body. Her image advertises the dangerous power of female sexuality: it seems the very reverse of the ideal of virginity. But is the grotesque body really the polar opposite of the virginal body? Some examples suggest otherwise: Giulia Sissa argues that the virgin prophetess Pythia of ancient Greek tradition was obscene because she invokes 'what

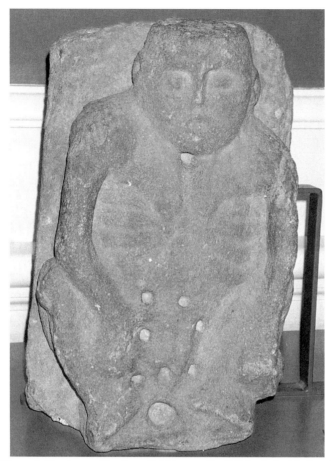

Figure 1 Sheela-na-Gig, from Seirkieran, Co. Offaly. © the National Museum of Ireland, Dublin. Photograph by Juliette Dor.

ought not to be seen: an inspired pregnant woman in a temple – a woman who simultaneously opens her mouth and her vagina'; like the sheela, she embodies the grotesque in holy space.[2] Freud theorizes that virginity itself is a fearful category. In his essay 'The taboo of virginity', Freud explores a puzzling practice of so-called 'primitive' societies: the husband's shunning of the performance of defloration.[3] He finds it puzzling, because the prevailing early twentieth-century middle-class ideology holds that the only possible bride must be a virgin. So 'naturalized' is this belief, Freud claims, that it is hard to understand why defloration in other cultures is taboo. Various explanations present themselves (the taboos against blood and menstruation; the fear of being 'infected with . . . femininity'),[4] but for Freud the most persuasive is not primarily anthropological but psychical: the husband is protecting himself against a peculiar female hostility, one rooted in penis envy and the castration complex: 'a woman's *immature sexuality*', he airily declares, 'is discharged on to the man who first makes her acquainted with the sexual act'. 'This being so', he continues, 'the taboo of virginity is reasonable enough [!] and we can understand the rule which decrees that precisely the man who is to enter upon a life shared with this woman shall avoid these dangers.'[5]

Of course it is difficult not to be more than a little irritated by Freud's blatant sexism and racism. His essay reveals more about early twentieth-century male fears of female sexuality than it does about women's 'true' sexual responses. But that is partly the point: in trying to unravel the complex weave of cultural meanings within which the sheela-na-gigs signify as paradoxical representations of virginity, I will argue that their representations tell us more about their (male) creators than they do about 'femininity'. Freud's essay is nevertheless instructive because it points to how the threat of the grotesque, of the dangerously erotic – perhaps, indeed, of some kind of female *jouissance* – haunts the idealized virgin body as an integral part of its cultural meaning, and not as a thing apart. This chapter seeks to extend the potential meanings of the sheela-na-gigs, especially their capacity to signify various attributes of virginity, within the minutely detailed context of Celtic iconography and mythology, Christian symbolism, Romanesque art and late medieval misogyny. In particular, it will argue for the need for new intellectual frameworks, derived from literary and textual approaches, to enrich our understanding of their significance.

Scholars still cannot agree about the meanings of these curious and enigmatic carvings. Jørgen Andersen repeatedly emphasizes the lack of information about the exact etymology of their name.[6] Although there is a growing body of scholarship on the sheela-na-gigs, the mystery of their origins remains almost intact.[7] Despite the fairly large number of sheela-na-gigs that survive from the Middle Ages, the term is apparently not recorded before the early seventeenth century, when it often referred to women of loose morals, or simply old hags.[8] Current interpretations of its meaning fluctuate between two possible Irish etymologies: 'the old hag of the breasts' (*Sighle na gCíoch*) or 'sheela [an old woman] on her hunkers' (*Síle-ina-Giob*).[9] Sheela-na-gigs were brought to scientific attention around the middle of the nineteenth century by certain Irish antiquarians, who were puzzled by these grotesque carvings abounding in holy places.[10] It is clear that the sheelas' functions and meanings have changed through the ages, which partly explains why they were destroyed or defaced by the Victorians while they once may have had a central, positive role for others, such as their Celtic ancestors. As Emma Rees rightly claims:

> Sheela does not change. Readings of her do. Hence the possibility that she was revered as a pagan goddess of fertility by the Celts, was a moral and didactic Christian emblem for Kilpeck's builders [there is a sheela on one of the corbels of the Romanesque parish church of Kilpeck, near Hereford], warning against sexual promiscuity, became imbued with apotropaic qualities in the later Middle Ages, and was erased generations later by Lewis [G. R. Lewis published, in 1842, a series of drawings representing sculptures of the church, significantly removing any suggestion of immodesty].[11]

Their gratuitously obscene (to patriarchy, at any rate) poses and gestures may have hindered serious scholarly analysis. With very few exceptions, they have been discussed almost exclusively by antiquarians, art historians, historians and anthropologists. But they have also caught the attention of a few specialists of Celtic mythology, and more recently of feminist critics.[12] And they are also part of 'popular' culture: not only are they the subject of various books aimed at the general reader, but several web-pages are devoted to them, and more are under construction.[13] They have also become a subject for Irish artists (painters, jewellers, sculptors). Until a few years ago, 'sheela-na-gig' was the name of a Galway feminist bookshop.

Rigorous discussion of the sheelas' historical functions and meanings is also hampered by the lack of certainty about their cultural origin. Two major and opposing hypotheses have been put forward. According to what I would call the Celtic one, their earliest forms are survivals of paganism; in Anne Ross's words, they 'portray the territorial or war-goddess in her hag-like aspect'.[14] Their grossly exaggerated sexual characteristics suggest less an erotic/pornographic aesthetic (although as Sarah Salih points out in this volume, the category of the erotic – and our investment in it – is highly problematic) than a connection with fertility or and/or apotropaic rites. While many ancient societies shared the belief in a divine Mother, that in mother-goddesses associated with plenty and fecundity was a pan-Celtic phenomenon, and its ubiquity implies that it was already present during Celtic prehistory. Furthermore, as Ross explains, 'the land, the locality, were of first importance to the Celts . . . it is thus not surprising that the Celtic goddesses tended to be particularly concerned with, or connected with the place or places in which they were venerated'.[15] The close association of those goddesses with the land is indeed frequently exemplified (for instance, the Rhineland Mothers[16] and the Irish myth in which the Sovereignty goddess also personifies the land itself).[17] The prototype of these female deities may have been the so-called Venus figurines of Upper Palaeolithic art, found on a wide arc extending from southern Russia to the Pyrenees.[18] According to Paul Mellars, they were 'small statuettes of rather well-developed (in some cases obese) female figures, with heavily accentuated sexual features and, usually, very attenuated or schematic representations of the heads, arms, and feet'.[19] Fertility was of course a major preoccupation of most early societies, and one of its most basic images was the mother.[20] In Catherine Johns's words, 'deities who symbolize and represent motherhood and who protect women in the dangers which this function involves are virtually universal'.[21]

The alternative view is that the sheela-na-gigs are a medieval Christian phenomenon that originated in France and northern Spain and was subsequently introduced into the British Isles by the Normans. Continuations of the male and female sexual exhibitionist figures that are a common motif of the corbels in French Romanesque churches, they are repeatedly encountered in the company of other grotesque and ugly acrobats such as mouth-pullers, tongue-protruders, mermaids or musicians. Most of these acrobats adopt undignified poses, indecently displaying their sexual anatomy. A high proportion of these voraciously leering female figures are situated along the pilgrim routes, especially to Santiago de Compostela and Rome. Their function was evidently apotropaic: to warn male pilgrims against the sins of the flesh. Mermaids, especially the two-tailed version, or melusine, were often carved in the company of other sexual(ized) symbols.[22] In line with the anti-feminism of the twelfth-century Church, with its patristically sanctioned misogyny and its emphasis upon biblical texts that fulminated against women, they embody the temptations, dangers and deceits of sensuality. They are versions, perhaps, of Freud's fear-inducing virgins.

But these two traditions – the Celtic and the Christian – do not exhaust the potential meanings of the sheela-na-gigs. As several contributors to this volume argue, virginity is also a problem of representation: it exemplifies the difficult relation between signifier and signified. Its 'truth' cannot be spoken by the body. One way in which the grotesquely sexualized sheelas stand for virginity is by enacting its opposite. For what can we know of the body's abstract spiritual attributes? What are virginity, sexual purity, femininity, motherhood? Any of their signifiers is notorious for its inadequacy. Since debates over how to represent such concepts had been raging for centuries, it is unsurprising that at some stage the Church resorted to using their grotesque negation. In particular, Celtic sacred depiction shows a marked tendency overtly to reject the Graeco-Roman ideal of mimesis with its tradition of 'matching' art, to use E. H. Gombrich's term.[23] Deliberately avoiding verisimilitude, this Celtic aesthetic tradition makes extensive use of non-mimetic forms, and often plays on multiplication, addition, exaggeration and synecdoche. So the sheela-na-gigs, with their distorted bodies, their lack of modesty, their uncompromising stare, their lack of frailty (many have Herculean shoulders), and above all their splayed vaginas, could figure as paradoxical signs for the powerful concept of virginity. Both the medieval Celtic religion and the Christian Church could articulate meaning not only through classical traditions of mimetic resemblance but also through a vast syntax of indirection, incongruity, inversion and negation; contradictory signifiers that acknowledge and play with the limits of representation.

This is seen clearly in the patriarchal myth of the Medusa's head. For Freud the decapitated head of Medusa figures what is both horrifying and seductive about the sight of the female genitalia.[24] An uncanny symbol of the ambivalence of women's nature, Medusa's head is the fetish par excellence since it represents both castration and its denial. As Camille Dumoulié says, 'woman occupies two antagonistic poles: evil (castration, the witch) and remedy (the phallus, the Virgin); abyss and the Ideal Thing'.[25] In her analysis of the function of witches, Claude Kappler quotes from the fifteenth-century *Malleus maleficarum* to demonstrate how the Middle Ages were haunted by the fear of the malevolent power of the sexual organs of these castrating women.[26] Kappler's argument provides an instructive historical parallel to Freud's observations about the taboo against virginity. When witches were tortured their pubic hair was shaved in order to make sure they could not hide anything in their sexual parts. According to Kappler, this bespeaks the desire to unveil the female genital organs in order to exorcize their secrets. A sense of anguish could arise from the clash between the fear of female sexuality, and an irresistible desire for it. Such a perverse desire endeavours to find some form of expression, sometimes assuming the shapes of monsters.[27]

Gilbert Lascault has argued that psychoanalysts and specialists of aesthetics need to collaborate on the construction of an 'atlas' of the phantasms associated with monsters.[28] One of the major chapters would deal with the *continent noir de la sexualité féminine*, and of femininity in general. Lascault argues that western culture despises and fears the female sex and the body in general, as the embodiment of the threat of castration, the abyss in which men could be swallowed up, Freud's *vagina dentata*. Literature abounds in this motif: for example, Michel Leiris reports his hero's sense of a frightful fall after having been trapped in the Ingénue's womb: 'Then I saw the ingénue who indicated to me the porch to her thighs with an obscene gesture of her hand . . . The only thing I could remember was a leap, a quick ascension, and that vertiginous fall through the coils of a womb whose indefinitely multiplied meanders had taken me here.'[29]

This uncanny and monstrous female body finds its forms within traditions of Celtic depiction (and I am aware here of the dangers of homogenizing a long and varied history, and disparate geographical areas), for which mimesis is viewed as inappropriate for the divine. As Miranda Green observes, the Celts strove to 'come to terms with the vagaries and capricious elements of the supernatural'.[30] They would honour deities, Joanne McMahon and Jack Roberts observe, by playing on 'plurality, exaggeration or schematism'.[31] In other words, the deliberate departure from the realistic often indicated an incursion into the world of the supernatural, an area in which the actual world of nature could be contradicted. By juxtaposing symbols that did not represent anything extant in reality it was possible to signal ambivalence. As a rule, duality was one of the most fundamental aspects of the pagan Celts' thought; in Ross's words, 'everything had, for them, a double meaning; many of their artistic forms are meant to be seen in two different ways; and also to possess a duality of significance – naturalistic and symbolic'.[32] The portraying of antagonistic features within the iconography of the Celts also recurs throughout their literature, where a similar conjunction of incompatible shapes and functions can be observed.

The same fundamental polysemy applies to their female gods. According to Ross, '[t]he basic Celtic goddess type was at once mother, warrior, hag, virgin, conveyor of fertility, of strong sexual appetite which led her to seek mates amongst mankind equally with gods, giver of prosperity to the land, protectress of the flocks and herds'.[33] The Great Celtic Goddess was indeed both a virgin and a mother; she figures a number of seemingly contradictory attributes, such as virginity, sexuality, war, death and sovereignty. Her various epiphanies reveal several of those traits, and also shift between them.[34] Maidenhood and motherhood were fused in the mythical figure of Aranrhod in the *Fourth Branch of the Mabinogi*'s Tale of Math.[35] Like the Virgin Mary, she was able to conceive a divine son while still sexually intact.[36] Most ancient patriarchal societies set a high value on virginity, and assumed that purity and fertility were concentrated in that exceptional state.[37] For instance, the goddess Diana originally embodied similar contradictions, since she stood for both fecundity and chaste maidenhood. Rome eventually rationalized her symbolism and differentiated her myth into two distinct goddesses, Juno (motherhood) and Minerva-Pallas (the virgin).[38]

Likewise, the legendary practice of female virgin foot-holders reflected the magic power of maidenhood; the king's strength was preserved by a close contact with a virgin's lap.[39] In Miranda Green's words, '[a] maiden was perhaps perceived as a powerful source of fertility, precisely because her sexuality was particularly intense, being undiluted, undissipated and thus entire'.[40] The myth of the cauldron of regeneration in the thirteenth-century Welsh poem *Preiddeu Annwn* is underwritten by a similar assumption. It can be heated only by the breath of nine virgins, which confirms the intensity of virginal sexual potential. According to Proinsias Mac Cana, '[p]agan traditions and cults . . . were accommodated under the capacious mantle of the Church . . . Pagan deities were canonized out of number.'[41] Amongst several famous examples of those smooth transitions from pagan female deities associated with abundance and motherhood to Christian virgin saints is Ana/Anu (wealth, abundance). She used to be the mother, the nourisher, of the principal family of pre-Christian deities who occupied Ireland before the Gaels, the dé Danaan.[42] Like many Celtic symbols, she possessed a dual nature and could be alternately beneficent or maleficent. St Brigid is an uncontroversial illustration of the shift from Celtic deity (*mater omnium deorum hibernensium*, according to the Irish late ninth-century *Cormac's Glossary*) to

Christian saint.[43] Her pagan avatar is closely associated with fertility and performs numerous functions, including the protection of women in childbirth. The transition from the goddess to the Christian Brigid is evidenced by the fact that both were celebrated on 1 February, a date that used to be that of the Celtic fertility ritual known as Imbolc.[44] Since the Irish saint was also able to cure female frigidity, she became a patron of pregnant women; but, at the same time, like so many Celtic goddesses, she remained sexually intact. Brigid's monastery at Kildare retained an ever-burning fire: a vestige, so to speak, of the Roman vestals. A substantial number of such female deities were sanctified or adapted to the Christian religion. As Ross observes, this capacity to signify in both pre-Christian and Christian terms is signalled by the polysemy of the Scottish Gaelic word *cailleach*, which designates both a hag and a nun.[45]

The contradictory nature of Celtic goddesses also led, paradoxically enough, to the inclusion of war as another important aspect of female fertility symbolism in Ireland. As Green explains, 'Most of the goddesses chronicled in the Irish vernacular tradition combine attributes of fertility and sexuality with that of war.'[46] The triple goddess Macha was a prophet, a warrior and a matriarch, and she stood for Ireland's sovereignty and fertility. Similarly, the Morrigan combined sex and war roles. Medieval Irish literature is rich in references to the mythological motif of the old and evil-looking hag who is transformed by a kiss into a lovely young maiden and reveals that she is Lady Sovereignty.[47] The twelfth-century *Adventure of the Sons of Echu Muigmedóin* provides a detailed description of the repulsive hag:

> Fergus found a well, but there was an old woman guarding it. She was as black as coal. Her hair was like a wild horse's tail. Her foul teeth were visible from ear to ear and were such as would sever a branch of green oak. Her eyes were black, her nose crooked and spread. Her body was scrawny, spotted and diseased. Her shins were bent. Her knees and ankles were thick, her shoulders broad, her nails were green. The hag's appearance was ugly.[48]

She agrees to give Fergus water, provided he kisses her. He refuses, preferring to perish. His other brothers experience the same repulsion; only Niall, his half-brother, accepts her conditions, kisses the loathsome lady and lies down with her. Suddenly the hag is transformed into a beauty and declares that she is Sovereignty. The Irish sovereignty figure is also known as *Cailleach Bhéirre* ('the old hag of Bear'): she appears to a knight or hero as an ugly old woman asking to be loved, and if he accepts her advances, she turns into a most beautiful young maiden. In Welsh literature crones – of covert divine rank – are intimately related to the cauldron of regeneration, and hence to regeneration itself. In *The Tale of Branwen*, Cymidei Cymeinfoll, the giant woman of a monstrous pair of cauldron-bearers, conceives and gives birth to a fully armed warrior every six weeks.[49] A similar myth is contained in *The Book of Taliesin*, in which goddess and magical cauldron are, again, closely associated. Ceridwen, a shape-shifting hag, was the keeper of the Cauldron of Inspiration and Knowledge.[50]

Elsewhere, the beautiful young maiden/ugly hag is a harbinger of death (another version of the Medusa's head). The *banshee* of Gaelic tradition is alternately the former, in which case she weeps for the coming death of a loved one; or the latter, and then she gruesomely foretells it. The occult power of females, and especially of their nakedness, also recurs. Cúchulainn, for example, endeavours not to see Richie's nakedness in order not to become an easy prey to her. In the early Irish saga known as the *Destruction of Da Derga's Hostel*,[51] a hideous female seer makes the legendary King Conaire violate the *geis* under which he must not allow a lone man or woman to visit his residence after sunset.[52] Her form is monstrous and there is an overt allusion to her sexual parts: Her 'beard – not the beard of her chin – reached her knees, and her mouth was on one side of her head', and she cast a baleful eye upon the king.[53] She also has other destructive behaviours, such as standing on one foot, a magical position to be taken in order to cast spells.[54]

The sheela-na-gigs are closely associated with those polysemous Celtic goddesses that combine opposite traits such as virginity and motherhood, peace and war. Reminders of the powers and dangers of female sexuality, they bear witness to the ambivalent cultural understanding of virginity that Freud tapped into. However, these curious stone figures have hardly been studied at all from a literary point of view. This may be due to the fact that they have not been conspicuous in literary sources, which has militated against interdisciplinary investigation. But things are changing. Lorraine K. Stock's recent identification of them as analogues for the construction of Morgan le Fay's character in *Sir Gawain and the Green Knight* bridges the gap between visual and textual evidences, opening up new lines of research.[55] A more complete inventory of the sheela-na-gigs is still badly needed, but to consider them as only of antiquarian, art-historical or anthropological interest is to neglect those literary frame-works in which the figure of the simultaneously fearful and seductive virginal female functions in a more ambivalent and multivalent way. The existence and typology of these 'witches on the wall' remain virtually unknown to literary specialists.

But what of their geographical specificity? Rather than identifying sheela-na-gigs with the continental exhibitionist figures, we need to sort out why they have developed into a specific phenomenon in the British Isles. In my view they result from the merging of the continental and insular traditions. When the Normans imported them, the exhibitionist representations were highly successful in places where they were reminiscent of a pagan tradition onto which they could be grafted. Little wonder then that male exhibitionist figures did not flourish in Ireland, while their female equivalents were conveniently adapted to the local artefacts. The continental imports came over with their original signification and were then redefined within the Celtic background. I fully subscribe to Eamonn P. Kelly's statement that 'in a European feudal context, the function of sheela-na-gigs was one which portrayed a negative view of women's sexuality, but the evidence suggests that this view was not fully endorsed by the native Irish, or, later, by the gaelicized Anglo-Irish'.[56]

Pope Gregory famously recommended that British pagans be converted to Christianity with diplomacy. There was no question of openly eradicating pre-Christian practices; they had to be preserved and incorporated into the Church's rituals under other labels. He advocated, for instance, transforming pagan temples into churches, or celebrating Christian feasts on the days of ancient festivals.[57] There was an uncontroversial 'willingness to reconcile pagan teachings with the new faith', explains H. R. Ellis Davidson.[58] There are numerous illustrations of the process of reconciliation of Christianity with the pagan heritage; the carved crosses of the Viking age or the Franks Casket (juxtaposing scenes of the cult of Woden with Christian ones) are outstanding examples. The introduction of Christianity into Ireland was even more seamless and peaceful. McMahon and Roberts explain that the similarities between the tenets of the old religion and the new meant that many of the pre-Christian idols and practices were easily Christianized; they conclude that 'it is not possible simply to categorise the Sheelas as either Christian demon or pagan idol but perhaps . . . [they are] representative of the merging of Christian and pagan ways'.[59] They have never been wholly exempt from superstition (some of them are still rubbed by those who believe in their efficacious magic), and a number of them have eventually been regarded as saints. Green, whose final chapter of *Celtic Goddesses* is entitled 'From goddess to saint', claims that the phenomenon was particularly clear 'in Ireland and Wales, for it is here that there is substantive evidence for early female saints, whose powers and character show marked resemblances to those which are identifiable in the goddesses of pagan tradition'.[60] The outcome of such a 'conversion' of the signified most often yielded an object of the utmost complexity, open to clashing interpretations. For example, in the specific case of the sheelas in the churches, they were, of course, survivals of an ancient pagan cult and symbolism, but they had also become part and parcel of the surrounding sermon in stone designed for the uneducated.

The construction of the monstrous sheelas as an incongruous sign of virginity may also be indebted to the negative theology of the Middle Ages. In *Deformed Discourse: The Function of the Monster in Medieval Thought and Literature*, David Williams has explored how medieval monsters developed a signification widely differing from those of omen and magical sign of the earlier period. 'The Middle Ages', he argues, 'made deformity into a symbolic tool with which it probed the secrets of substance, existence, and form incompletely revealed by the orthodox rational approach through dialectics.'[61] He relates the concept of the medieval monster to Pseudo-Dionysius' negative theology, and to the theologian's warnings against an overconfidence in rational constructs and the dangers of anthropomorphism in the processes of understanding and representation:

> Just as the senses can neither grasp nor perceive the things of the mind, just as a representation and shape cannot take in the simple and the shapeless, just as the corporeal form cannot lay hold of the intangible and incorporeal, by the same standard of truth beings are surpassed by the infinity beyond being, intelligences by that oneness which is beyond intelligence.[62]

The form cannot contain the being, and especially not in the case of the shapeless. Positive assertions are unfitting to express the divine because the latter is secret, invisible and ineffable.[63] According to that theory of cognition and symbolism, the mysteries of God and of heaven ought to be revealed by symbols that do not bear resemblance to their signified, which is the best way to make sure that nobody mistakes allegories for celestial essence. The more incongruous a sign was, the less it could be equated with what it represented. Because of its deformity, the monstrous sign did not stand for itself, and making use of it was guaranteed to avoid the medieval confusion between sign and referent: 'The sheer crassness of the signs is a goad so that even the materially inclined cannot accept that it could be permitted or true that the celestial and divine sights could be conveyed by such shameful things.'[64] The point was that those signs contributed to the elevation of the mind in the latter's apprehension of the divine. This primarily theological approach was extended to a wide range of contexts. The parallel between the mystification of God and that of Woman was easily drawn, a point highlighted by Lacan's 'Encore' seminar.[65] The mysteries of female sexuality and hence virginity could quite logically be expressed in the terms of negative theology.

The subsequent shift was from theology to aesthetics. Monstrosity and deformity became a symbolic language used in reaction to rational and logical affirmations; their role was to upset and hence call into question the adequacy of the signs traditionally used to signify, as well as the relationship between signifier and signified. The deformed became, in Williams's words, 'the sign of this superior form of unknowing'.[66] No system of representation is wholly unambiguous. The limits of the verbal are obvious, and medieval writers were highly sensitive to this issue.[67] They believed that words were often less adequate and rich than images, and presumably even more so if the signified was complex. In addition, in Romanesque art

> the natural world, and especially the animals and birds, yielded a dual symbolism in which lions may stand for good or evil, eagles may stand for St John or nobility of character or cruelty and rapaciousness, snakes may symbolize poison or healing, and peacocks may be a device against the Evil Eye or tell of immortality and incorruptibility. The phantasmagoria summoned up by the imagination gave an even more complicated symbolism, often dualistic also, so that griffins might equally indicate Christ or Satan.[68]

Or to put this in another way, because the lion was, on the one hand, the terrifying animal of the Old Testament and, on the other hand, the image of God (it could bring stillborn children back to life), both its name and its iconographic representation could express opposed concepts.[69] Because symbols are not static, their meaning has to be deciphered. But the point is that the key to interpretation is not always overt and, also, that symbols can embody different values and be highly ambivalent.

The grotesque has developed within the horizon of this historically specific understanding of representation. The construction of highly deformed and transgressive signs prevents the mind from taking them at face value. The presence of strange distortions evidences the use of a symbolic language. 'The bizarre and grotesque, the misshapen and ugly' also permeate Romanesque art.[70] They were the mirror of a world in which people lived in terror, frightened by the Christian doctrine of sin and redemption: 'The function of church art was to secure awe and apprehension, to define the narrow path, to bring awareness of divine retribution.'[71] Medieval hagiography, Williams also argues, could provide useful illustrations of how appropriate the monstrous was in order to reveal the divine. As he explains,

> The dynamic of the cult of the saint, in this and other cases, involves the iconographic representation of the opposite of the prayer . . . The interplay of cult and icon – prayer and picture – is based on the devotee's ability to recognize in the grotesque sign its contrary and the contrary of its signified.[72]

Michael Camille's seminal work on marginal representations is also highly pertinent here. By examining the counter-language inserted in a number of medieval spaces, he shows how these subversive marginalia juxtapose the sacred and the profane within some form of carnival-esque polyphony,[73] echoing Mikhail Bakhtin's discussion of the coexistence, among medieval people, of serious and comic approaches to life.[74] He argues that what is drawn, written or sculpted in the margins (that is, in the margins either of the page or of some more concrete location) brings an additional dimension to the 'centre', that is, the official spaces. What is marginal can question, parody or gloss the official discourse. In an essay published a year later, Camille explores a more specific case of interaction between signs.[75] He deals with the *sorplus* (the excess, additional meaning) of the kiss to highlight what he calls 'intervisuality – a process in which images are not stable referents in some ideal iconographic dictionary, but are perceived by their audiences to work across and within different and even competing value-systems'.[76] The medieval iconography of the kiss reveals a plural semantics; kisses can, for instance, be lecherous, spiritual, legal, courtly, treacherous or mystical. Such a polysemy can generate confusion and it can become impossible to ensure that images initially aimed at stimulating a prohibition do not also have the effect of stimulating transgression.

Critics have suggested a number of theories about the origins and functions of the sheelas. These range from their being signs of the castigation of lust or warnings against the temptations of the flesh, to their being magical fertility figures used as a cure for barrenness, or attempts to ward off evil. It is also clear that, insofar as they represent the Christianization of apotropaic or fertility magic, some of them are the by-products of religious syncretism. It is undeniable that the sheelas were not a static genre, and that their meanings gradually changed. Furthermore, depending on specific periods, some gestures, attributes or facial expressions were added which conferred a second-ary meaning on the carvings, and invited additional interpretations. Andersen has convincingly argued, for example, that the gesture of the hand beside the ear might signify that the sheela-na-gig was the guardian of the place.[77] But the crucial point is that all of them are nude, and that the gesture of their hands (sometimes from behind their flexed legs) clearly concentrates the viewer's whole attention upon their vulvas. Their genitals are presented in such a way that they are bound to fascinate the gaze. The marked disproportion between their pudenda and their abbreviated bodies (often with very short legs) is another indication that the central reference is to their sex. Since 'the fertility-bias of Celtic religion does not generally manifest itself in the exaggeration of the sexual/generative parts of the human body',[78] the emphasis on their genitals is of crucial importance. They lack other exaggerated female sexual characteristics. Almost all of them are conspicuously bald, and their breasts, if not omitted, are never larger than normal, or are rudimentary. All might be considered grotesque, ugly and repulsive. While a few are obese and can be regarded as akin to the Baubo type of Ptolemaic Egypt (small, fat, female figurines seated and displayed), most of them are bony and display emaciated ribs; most have large heads, bulging or crossed eyes; some leer, some grimace.[79] By pulling open their vaginas they show the object of the mythic fear that women might devour their partner's penis during sex, the dreadful *vagina dentata*. This may also be what Tertullian meant when he accused women of being the devil's gateway.[80] In other words, those carved figures were probably not intended as objects of pornography, but rather as a remedy to encourage chastity or virginity. But what is true of Camille's kissing couple is also true of the sheelas' possible distorted expression of virginity; their incongruous body can be understood in terms of a Bakhtinian dialogue between the virgin's traditional classical vs the grotesque body. This interpretation accounts for the paradoxical presence of obscene and, at first sight, sacrilegious, sculptures on the walls of churches.

Finally, whose gaze do they fascinate? Sarah Salih highlights the complexity of the spectacle of the violent torture of the female virgin martyrs' bodies in the Katherine group.[81] All three virgins are indifferent to being naked in public; their behaviour, Salih reminds us, is identical to that of their early Christian prototypes. Traditionally unashamed of their nakedness, they use it, in Margaret Miles's words, 'as a symbolic rejection, not only of sexuality, but also of secular society's identification of the female body with male desire, its relegation of the female naked body to spectacle and object'.[82] Salih argues that they deny that they are sexually desirable females: '[t]hey make their nakedness mean not sexuality, but virginity.'[83]

I am, of course, not arguing that the sheelas took some active part in the construction of their symbolism. But, *mutatis mutandis*, we might strive to find out the various viewpoints that they embody. The Normans thought that they were importing the castigation of lust and, in a way, they were.[84] Some of their sculptors might have enjoyed carving the details of their grotesque nudity and indecent gestures, but that cannot have been the message they were meant to convey. In fact the message was not single. First it depended on the viewer's sex. Their official purpose was to warn male viewers about the traps of female sexuality and to remind their female audience that they must abjure their own sexuality in order to embrace chastity, and, if possible, virginity. But this did not prevent viewers from remaining free to construct their own meanings. By cunningly fusing sexual aggressiveness and the absence of sexually arousing traits in their female characters, in a way their creators certainly wanted their signification to remain open. Salih argues that in the Katherine group the lack of mention of the virgins' breasts serves to distinguish them from other women.[85] While the sheelas were definitely not asexual beings, they too lacked conspicuous breasts, and could simultaneously reflect old age and virginity. This construction is not surprising in the Celtic world of shapeshifting women who can be simultaneously beautiful virgins and ugly old crones. However, the function of the sheelas is all the more difficult to define since they are also the by-products of a vast textual interweave that includes Celtic symbolism, the conjoining of opposites, grotesque art and negative theology. But even if the ancient fertility goddess had been partly deconstructed, she was only to be reconstructed with additional significance. The polysemous gaze of the sheela-na-gigs did not only perform a dangerous female sexuality in order to frighten women and to fascinate the eyes of the misogynistic clerks of a male-dominated society. It also reactivated a hoard of Celtic myths that portrayed a different view of womanhood and knew that 'femininity' covered and fused all its facets of womanhood; the ugly hag and the beautiful maiden, the mother and the virgin. Their demonstrative bodies proclaim a rejection of the passive role that patriarchy had assigned to them, but this did not mean that they aimed to seduce or that they reveal an authentic femininity. As Irigaray scornfully observes about Lacan's discussion of the secrets of female *jouissance* in his notorious 'Encore' seminar:

> And to make sure [that a non-masterful, non-masculinist logic] does not come up, the right to experience pleasure is awarded to a statue. 'Just go look at Bernini's statue in Rome, you'll see right away that St Theresa is coming, there's no doubt about it.'
>   In Rome? So far away? To look? At a statue? Of a saint? Sculpted by a man? What pleasure are we talking about? Whose pleasure?[86]

Just as Irigaray questions Lacan's capacity to make Bernini's statue signify as a model for female sexuality, so we should resist making the sheela-na-gigs signify as models for an unspoken female *jouissance* beyond the symbolic. Their gaze and gesture brook silence. Rejecting the social stereotype of 'femininity' and the proprieties of the virginal ideal, they bear witness to the impossibility of the representation of either 'woman' or 'virginity'.

Notes

Now that this chapter is eventually completed, it is difficult to be fully aware of my indebtedness to a number of friends and colleagues, not to mention the information digested during my repeated stays in Ireland. Let me, however, thank Dr Anke Bernau for inviting me to contribute to this collection of essays on virginity, a topic to which I became particularly sensitive when I examined her Ph.D. dissertation. I also want to express my thanks to Dr Sarah Salih, whose scrupulous checking of my manuscript made me check and rewrite a few points. Last, but not least, Dr Ruth Evans's highly relevant and friendly suggestions concerning further reading made me discover different directions, and also helped me avoid a number of ambiguities.

[1] According to Eamonn P. Kelly, *Sheela-na-Gigs: Origins and Functions* (Dublin: Country House, in association with The National Museum of Ireland, 1996), destruction of the figures appears to have begun in the seventeenth century (1631 provincial statutes for Tuam ordered parish priests to hide them away; 1676 diocesan regulations issued at Ossory and Waterford ordered wooden ones to be burnt; there are also accounts of more recent violence against them) (ibid., p. 14). For examples of cases of destruction or disfigurement of the figures, see Jørgen Andersen, *The Witch on the Wall: Medieval Erotic Sculpture in the British Isles* (Copenhagen: Rosenkilde & Bagger; London: George Allen & Unwin, 1977), pp. 27–31.

[2] Giulia Sissa, *Greek Virginity*, trans. Arthur Goldhammer (Cambridge, MA: Harvard University Press, 1990), p. 51.

[3] Sigmund Freud, 'The taboo of virginity' (1918 [1917]), in *On Sexuality: Three Essays on the Theory of Sexuality and Other Works*, trans. James Strachey, ed. Angela Richards (Harmondsworth: Penguin, 1977), pp. 261–83. For medieval awareness of this practice, see this volume, pp. 27, 247.

[4] Freud, 'Taboo of virginity', p. 271.

[5] Ibid., p. 280. Emphasis in original.

[6] Andersen, *Witch on the Wall*, esp. pp. 22–3.

[7] See, for instance, Lorraine K. Stock: 'The etymological provenance and meaning of the term . . . are uncertain': 'The hag of Castle Hautdesert: the Celtic Sheela-na-gig and the *Auncian* in *Sir Gawain and the Green Knight*', in Bonnie Wheeler and Fiona Tolhurst (eds), *On Arthurian Women: Essays in Memory of Maureen Fries* (Dallas: Scriptorium Press, 2001), pp. 121–48 (pp. 121–2); Emma L. E. Rees: 'Use of the term "Sheela-na-Gig" entered antiquarian circles in Ireland in the 1840s. Its origins are unclear': 'Sheela's voracity and Victorian veracity', in Liz Herbert McAvoy and Teresa Walters (eds), *Consuming Narratives: Gender and Monstrous Appetite in the Middle Ages and the Renaissance* (Cardiff: University of Wales Press, 2002), pp. 116–27 (p. 120).

[8] In *Images of Lust: Sexual Carvings on Medieval Churches* (London: Routledge, 1999), pp. 14–15, Anthony Weir and James Jerman provide a number of references to Irish sheelas from diocesan and provincial statutes.

[9] For example, see Kelly, *Sheela-na-Gigs*, p. 5.

[10] John O'Donovan called the figure of Kiltinane church a *Sheela Ny Gigg* in his *Ordnance Survey Letters, Co. Tipperary* (Dublin: typed copy, 1840); the name was also used in the *Proceedings of the Royal Irish Academy* (1840–4) to describe the exhibitionist carving in a church at Rochestown. The Royal

Irish Academy catalogue of Irish antiquities printed in 1857 describes three of them and makes a number of comments upon other carvings in Ireland; see Andersen, *Witch on the Wall*, esp. pp. 10–14.

[11] Rees, 'Sheela's voracity', p. 124.

[12] In his *Dictionary of Celtic Mythology* (Oxford: Oxford University Press, 1998), James MacKillop states that 'Recent feminist commentators have suggested that they may be reminders of the primal earth mother whose rule over life and death predated Christianity' (under 'Sheela-na-gig'). This view informs the work of Anne Ross, 'The divine hag of the pagan Celts', in Venetia Newall (ed.), *The Witch Figure* (London: Routledge & Kegan Paul, 1973), pp. 139–64. It is also drawn on by Eamonn P. Kelly and Miranda Green, especially in Green's *Celtic Goddesses: Warriors, Virgins and Mothers* (London: British Museum, 1995). However, MacKillop's dictionary article fails to mention the current, more general trend of feminist interest in the topic (for example, Stock, 'Hag of Castle Hautdesert'; Rees, 'Sheela's voracity'; Kathryn Price Theatana, 'Síla na Géige: Sheela na Gig and sacred space' (http://www.bandia.net/sheela/ Language Note); Ann Pearson, 'Reclaiming the *sheela-na-gigs*: goddess imagery in medieval sculptures of Ireland', *Canadian Woman Studies/Les Cahiers de la femme*, 17/3 (1997), 20–4, to name only a few).

[13] The following random examples are representative of their typology. These websites were all checked on 28 July 2002:

http://www.geocities.com/Wellesley/1752/sheela.html   [Larissa Brown's Website]

http://www.jharding.demon.co.uk/index.htm [Megalithica]

http://www.members.tripod.com/~taramc/sheelas.html [Tara McLoughlin's Sheela-na-gig Website]

http://www.sheelanagig.org/ [The Sheela Na Gig project]

http:///www.upnaway.com/~pixiecat/cat/Sheela.html [The Sheela page]

[14] Ross, 'Divine hag of the pagan Celts', p. 148.

[15] Ibid., p. 139.

[16] The cult of the matrons/*matres*/*matronae* (the Gaulish mother-goddess Matrona, who has given her name to the French river Marne, is one of them) is widely attested in many regions of the Roman Empire settled by both the Celts and the Germanic tribes, especially the Lower Rhine. See, for example, MacKillop, *Dictionary of Celtic Mythology*, and Rudolf Simek, *Dictionary of Northern Mythology* (Cambridge: Brewer, 1993). It is generally assumed that their cult must have had its origin during Celtic prehistory; see Miranda Green, *The Gods of the Celts* (Stroud: Sutton, 1986), p. 76.

[17] The goddess of Sovereignty was the personification of the power and authority of a kingdom as a woman to be won sexually, a belief predating Celtic written literature. There is a rich documentation of the forms of the myth in Ireland; see, for example, MacKillop, *Dictionary of Celtic Mythology*, under 'Sovereignty, Lady'.

[18] Paul Mellars, 'The Upper Palaeolithic revolution', in Barry Cunliffe (ed.), *The Oxford Illustrated Prehistory of Europe* (Oxford: Oxford University Press, 1994), pp. 42–79 (pp. 68, 69, 72).

[19] Ibid., p. 69.

[20] See, for instance, the chapter 'Arts et symboles, ou quand terre et femme ne faisaient qu'un' of Jean Guilaine, *La Mer partagée: La Méditerranée avant l'écriture, 7000–2000 avant Jésus-Christ* (Paris: Hachette, 1994), pp. 361–423.

[21] Catherine Johns, *Sex or Symbol? Erotic Images of Greece and Rome* (London: British Museum, 1982), p. 39.

[22] See Weir and Jerman: 'two-tailed mermaids whose tails curl up on either side, with the fins held at shoulder level, often touching the abacus and giving support to it. Like that of the acrobat, it is an attitude which gives the sculptor scope for sexual detail'; *Images of Lust*, p. 44. They add that '[the two-tailed version] strikes an attitude that strongly suggests exhibitionism. She is, moreover, always in the company of other sexual figures and allied symbols, so that there cannot be any doubt that the carvers were interested in her for reasons more cogent than mere decorative ornament' (p. 48).

[23] E. H. Gombrich, *Art and Illusion: A Study in the Psychology of Pictorial Representation*, 4th edn (London: Phaidon, 1972), p. 99.

[24] Sigmund Freud, 'The Medusa's head', *The Complete Psychological Works*, standard edition, 23 vols, trans. James Strachey (London: Hogarth, 1953–64), vol. 18, pp. 273–4.

[25] 'Méduse', in *Dictionnaire des mythes littéraires*, ed. Pierre Brunel (Paris: Éditions du Rocher, 1988), pp. 1018–27, p. 1023.

[26] Claude Kappler, *Monstres, démons et merveilles à la fin du Moyen Âge* (Paris: Payot, 1980), p. 271.

[27] Jean Chevalier and Alain Gheerbrant (eds), *Dictionnaire des symboles* (Paris: Laffont, Bouquins, 1982), under 'Monstre'.

[28] Gilbert Lascault, *Le Monstre dans l'art occidental* (Paris: Klincksieck, 1973), pp. 378–87. On monsters, see also Jeffrey Jerome Cohen (ed.), *Monster Theory: Reading Culture* (Minneapolis and London: University of Minnesota Press, 1996).

[29] Michel Leiris, *Le Point cardinal*, 1927, in *Mots sans mémoire* (Paris: Gallimard, 1969), pp. 35–6: 'Alors je vis l'Ingénue qui . . . m'indiquait d'une main obscène le porche de ses cuisses . . . Je me rappelais seulement un bond, une ascension rapide et cette chute vertigineuse à travers les replis d'une matrice dont les méandres indéfiniment multipliés m'avaient conduit jusqu'ici.' My translation.

[30] Green, *Gods of the Celts*, p. 225.

[31] Joanne McMahon and Jack Roberts, *The Sheela-na-Gigs of Ireland and Britain: The Divine Hag of the Christian Celts, an Illustrated Guide* (Cork: Mercier Press, 2000), p. 82.

[32] Ross, 'Divine hag of the pagan Celts', p. 146.

[33] Anne Ross, *Pagan Celtic Britain: Studies in Iconography and Tradition*

(London: Routledge & Kegan Paul; New York: Columbia University Press, 1967), p. 233.

[34] On this well-established feature of Celtic mythology, see Proinsias Mac Cana, *Celtic Mythology* (London: Chancellor, 1996), pp. 82–94.

[35] Although the tales included in the *Mabinogi* have survived in rather late manuscripts (between *c.*1225 and *c.*1425), most of them were composed much earlier. See A. O. H. Jarman and Gwilym Rees Hughes, *A Guide to Welsh Literature*, 6 vols (Swansea: Davies, 1976), vol. 1, pp. 190–1.

[36] See, for example, Green, *Celtic Goddesses*, p. 57.

[37] Ibid., p. 63.

[38] Chevalier and Gheerbrant, *Dictionnaire des symboles*, under 'Virginité'.

[39] See also Jane Cartwright's discussion of virgin foot-holders in this volume.

[40] Green, *Celtic Goddesses*, p. 62.

[41] Mac Cana, *Celtic Mythology*, p. 132.

[42] That is, 'the people, tribe or nation of Ana'; MacKillop, *Dictionary of Celtic Mythology*, under 'Ana'.

[43] Green, *Celtic Goddesses*, pp. 196–202, considers the issue of 'the goddess and saint' and argues that the figure is at the interface of paganism and Christianity. Mac Cana goes further, claiming that 'it is clear beyond question that the saint has usurped the role of the goddess and much of her mythological tradition' (*Celtic Mythology*, p. 34). In their *Les Fêtes celtiques* (Rennes: Éditions Ouest-France Université, 1995), Françoise Le Roux and Christian-J. Guyonvarch express the same opinion at the end of the subchapter devoted to St Brigid's feast: 'To conclude, the very temporary feast of Saint Brigid has been substituted for *Imbolc*. It is quite logical to assume that the Christian celebration is the continuation of the pagan one: the very name of Saint Brigid already allows us to deduce that *Imbolc* was under the patronage of the major Irish female divinity Brigit. The nominal similarity must have widely contributed to the transfer. A close formal concordance of the purification and lustration rites has ensued' (pp. 91–2). My translation.

[44] See, for instance, MacKillop's *Dictionary of Celtic Mythology*, 'IMBOLC . . . Old Irish name for a seasonal feast of pre-Christian origin fixed at 1 February on the Gregorian calendar . . . From earliest times, Imbolc was associated with Brigit, the fire-goddess, and after Christianization with St Brigid of Kildare, eventually becoming known as St Brigid's Day. The saint, it should be pointed out, was often seen as the patroness of sheep, the pastoral economy, and fertility in general.'

[45] Ross, 'Divine hag of the pagan Celts', p. 161.

[46] Miranda J. Green, *Dictionary of Celtic Myth and Legend* (London: Thames and Hudson, 1992), p. 97.

[47] Namely the goddess that is the personification of the power and authority of a kingdom. The motif is widespread and has been used, for example, by Chaucer in his *Wife of Bath's Tale*.

[48] Myles Dillon, *The Cycles of the Kings* (London: Geoffrey Cumberlege; New York: Oxford University Press, 1946), p. 39.

[49] See, for instance, MacKillop, *Dictionary of Celtic Mythology*, p. 62.

[50] The MS known under the title of *The Book of Taliesin* must have been transcribed during the last quarter of the thirteenth century. It contains a miscellaneous collection of poems, probably compiled in the thirteenth century, and ascribed to the late sixth-century bard Taliesin. Taliesin became a folktale figure; see, for example, *Hanes Taliesin*, 'The story of Taliesin'; for details, see Jarman and Rees Hughes, *A Guide to Welsh Literature*, pp. 106–110.

[51] Its main recension was apparently compiled in the eleventh century from two ninth-century versions; Robert Welch (ed.), *The Oxford Companion to Irish Literature* (Oxford: Clarendon Press, 1996), p. 562.

[52] The *geis* was a ritual prohibition or proscription placed upon heroes or other important personages in Irish narratives. See MacKillop, *Dictionary of Celtic Mythology*, p. 361 (under *Togail Bruidne Da Derga*). On the taboo known as *geis*, see *Dictionary of Celtic Mythology*, p. 221 (under *geis*).

[53] Lisa M. Bitel, *Land of Women: Tales of Sex and Gender in Early Ireland* (Ithaca, NY: Cornell University Press, 1996), p. 210. Ross adopts an even more explicit rendering: 'her pudenda reached to her knees'; 'Divine hag of the pagan Celts', p. 147.

[54] McMahon and Roberts, *Sheela-na-Gigs of Ireland and Britain*, p. 70.

[55] Stock, 'Hag of Castle Hautdesert'.

[56] Kelly, *Sheela-na-Gigs*, p. 45.

[57] Bede, *A History of the English Church and People*, trans. Leo Sherley-Price (Harmondsworth: Penguin, 1955), pp. 86–7.

[58] H. R. Ellis Davidson, *Viking and Norse Mythology* (London: Chancellor, 1996), p. 124.

[59] McMahon and Roberts, *Sheela-na-Gigs of Ireland and Britain*, p. 75.

[60] Green, *Celtic Goddesses*, p. 188.

[61] David Williams, *Deformed Discourse: The Function of the Monster in Medieval Thought and Literature* (Exeter: University of Exeter Press, 1996), p. 3.

[62] Cited ibid., p. 5.

[63] See Pseudo-Dionysius, *The Celestial Hierarchy*, in Denys le pseudo-Aréopagite, *Œuvres complètes*, trans. Maurice de Candillac (Paris: Aubier-Montaigne, 1943), ch. 2.

[64] Pseudo-Dionysius, *The Celestial Hierarchy*. English translation in Williams, *Deformed Discourse*, pp. 11–12.

[65] Jacques Lacan, *Le Séminaire, livre XX, Encore*, ed. Jacques-Alain Miller (Paris: Seuil, 1975); 'Encore: Seminar XX: God and the *jouissance* of the woman' (1972–3), trans. Jacqueline Rose, in Juliet Mitchell and Rose (eds), *Feminine Sexuality: Jacques Lacan and the* école freudienne (London: Macmillan, 1982), pp. 137–48.

[66] Williams, *Deformed Discourse*, p. 6.

[67] See Kappler, *Monstres, démons et merveilles*, p. 197.

[68] Weir and Jerman, *Images of Lust*, p. 36.

⁶⁹ See, for instance, Frank Horvat and Michel Pastoureau, *Figures romanes* (Paris: Seuil, 2001).

⁷⁰ Ibid., p. 34.

⁷¹ Ibid., p. 35.

⁷² Williams, *Deformed Discourse*, pp. 316–17.

⁷³ Michael Camille, *Image on the Edge: The Margins of Medieval Art* (London: Reaktion, 1992).

⁷⁴ Mikhail Bakhtin, *Rabelais and his World*, trans. Hélène Iswolsky (Cambridge, MA: MIT Press, 1968).

⁷⁵ Michael Camille, 'Gothic signs and the surplus: the kiss on the cathedral', *Yale French Studies*, 88 (1991), 151–70.

⁷⁶ Camille, 'Gothic signs', 151.

⁷⁷ Andersen, *Witch on the Wall*, p. 120, mentions several examples. He also provides a description of the sheelas, of their gestures and attitudes, in a catalogue at the end of his book ('Catalogue and maps', pp. 139–58). The description of the sheela of Kiltinane church (Co. Tipperary), for instance, reads: 'Standing posture, with knees widely splayed, and one hand (the "upper" hand) raised to the head. Turnip-shaped head set on a thin neck, flat breasts. The "lower" hand is very large, with fingers spreading fan-wise towards the slit of pudenda very clearly shown' (n. 88, p. 149).

⁷⁸ Green, *Gods of the Celts*, p. 212.

⁷⁹ In *Witch on the Wall*, Andersen devotes interesting paragraphs to those Baubo statuettes; pp. 133–4.

⁸⁰ Tertullian, *De cultu feminarum* (*The Appearance of Women*), bk 1, ch. 2; cited in Alcuin Blamires with Karen Pratt and C. W. Marx (eds), *Woman Defamed and Woman Defended: An Anthology of Medieval Texts* (Oxford: Clarendon Press, 1992), p. 51.

⁸¹ Sarah Salih, *Versions of Virginity in Late Medieval England* (Cambridge: Brewer, 2001), pp. 74–98.

⁸² Margaret R. Miles, *Carnal Knowing: Female Nakedness and Religious Meaning in the Christian West* (Boston: Beacon Press, 1989), p. 2.

⁸³ Salih, *Versions of Virginity*, p. 85.

⁸⁴ On this issue, see Weir and Jerman, *Images of Lust*. They explain that one of the aims of their contribution to what has been written on the sheelas is to show that 'they are Christian carvings, part of an iconography aimed at castigating the sins of the flesh, and that they were only one element in the attack on lust, luxury and fornication' (pp. 15–17).

⁸⁵ Salih, *Versions of Virginity*, pp. 85–7.

⁸⁶ Luce Irigaray, 'Così fan tutti', in *This Sex which is Not One*, trans. Catherine Porter (Ithaca, NY: Cornell University Press, 1985), pp. 86–105 (pp. 90–1).

4

Virginity and Chastity Tests in Medieval Welsh Prose

JANE CARTWRIGHT

According to a Middle Welsh proverb: 'E gont a del yw frovi hwyr e daw yw friodi' (A tried and tested cunt marries late).[1] This saying not only highlights the importance of virginity in medieval Welsh society, but also implies, in a rather threatening tone, that the value of a young girl entering the marriage market was considered to be significantly impaired – even irrevocably damaged – if she had already lost her virginity. Officially, early medieval Welsh law recognized nine different kinds of marital union (including gift by kin, rape and elopement), and in each case sexual intercourse rather than a marriage ceremony marked the *rite de passage* necessary for a *morwyn* (maiden) to become a *gwraig* (wife).[2] The most respectable form of union seems to have been *uniad o rodd cenedl* when a girl was given to a man by her kin, and she was, of course, expected to be a virgin – pure, inviolate and not yet pregnant. While the most in-depth treatment of medieval chastity tests to date – Kathleen Coyne Kelly's *Performing Virginity and Testing Chastity in the Middle Ages* – discusses 'a wide assortment of texts in English, French, German, and Latin', it does not provide much detail on the Welsh material.[3] While there is a clear overlap in some of the material, in particular the medical texts, my work focuses on the legal as well as mythological and theoretical implications and functions of the chastity test.

In the above proverb the verb *profi* (*frovi*) implies that the girl who encounters difficulty in finding a marriage partner is sexually experienced, but the literal meaning of *profi* is to test. Numerous medieval texts (in Welsh as in other languages) refer to various means of verifying virginity or testing chastity. The girl could be subjected to a physical examination; she could be given a potion or medicinal drink; made to wear a chastity-testing object; subjected to an ordeal; or her chastity could become the subject of a prophecy.[4] Since virginity, ultimately an invisible entity, was difficult to locate in the body, it was often depicted metaphorically in legendary material and visualized as an object – a flower, a clean white shirt, an untainted mirror.[5] The testing of female virginity and chastity is a common literary motif,[6] and, as one might expect, this popular misogynist theme is not confined to the Christian west or to the medieval period. Here the aim is to examine a selection of tests which occur in Middle Welsh texts, some of which are native and original, others of which are vernacular translations into Middle Welsh. The range of texts studied is diverse and, whilst some texts are specific to Wales, for example the legal texts, and may be seen to represent a distinctively Welsh culture, others, such as the medical texts, reflect much broader ideas and practices current in the medieval and even classical periods. The aim, therefore, is to shed light upon the mental landscape of medieval Wales and its broader context (geographical and temporal) which both facilitated the generation of the texts discussed and was influenced and reinforced by the concepts expressed in writing. The chapter moves thematically across this landscape visiting a variety of nodes within its discursive structure. The objective is to elucidate the wider terrain rather than imposing one, inevitably simplistic, interpretation upon the signific-ance of virginity and chastity tests within the medieval Welsh dis-course. At the same time it is recognized that the meanings (be they literal or metaphorical) and uses (be they real or ideal) of the tests can begin to be elucidated, albeit as elements within a complex and multiple discourse which ranges from moral to economic concerns and may even be seen to contain an undertow of subversion.

The tests demonstrate not only the desires to uncover whether a woman is a virgin and to control female sexuality, but also the tendency to doubt a woman's word. Even the paragon of all virgins, the Blessed Virgin Mary, has her physical virginity put to the test in the apocryphal infancy gospels. *Buched Meir* (the Life of the Virgin Mary) was translated or adapted into Welsh sometime before the end of the thirteenth century, and relates how Mary and Joseph's chastity was subjected to doubt. They were required to drink the bitter waters of the temple and turn around seven times; had they lied, they would have risked sudden death.[7] Joseph, who had been suspected of raping Mary, is vindicated and the crowd fall at Mary's feet 'y erchi madeueint ydi am eu dryctyp' (to request forgiveness from her for their suspicions). Later in the *buchedd* Mary, having just given birth to Jesus in a cave, comes under suspicion again when the midwife Salome, famously also represented in the Middle English N-Town and Chester mystery cycles, notices that there is no blood or afterbirth. She subjects the Virgin to a physical examination with unexpected results: her hand, which dares to probe the Virgin's body, withers and becomes deformed.[8] The apocrypha confirm Mary's virginity *in partu* and *post partum*, and all who doubt her purity are punished accordingly. In the Middle Welsh Life of St Collen, the saint is given a lily by the pope which had previously regenerated from a withered stem in front of the pagans as proof that the Virgin had borne a son.[9] The lily, used frequently as a symbol of Mary's purity and often depicted in medieval annunciation scenes, here furnishes miraculous confirmation of Mary's unique physical condition – pregnant but paradoxically still a virgin, fertile but untainted by original sin. While the Marian virginity-tests humiliate the accusers and vindicate the virgin, in other medieval sources it is often the accused who is subjected to public ridicule, and the women who pass the tests are few and far between.

The Fourth Branch of the Mabinogi: Aranrhod and Goewin

Virginity and the power associated with virginity are of primary importance to the events of the *Fourth Branch of the Mabinogi*. Math son of Mathonwy, lord of Gwynedd, has an unusual affliction:

> Ac yn yr oes honno, Math uab Mathonwy ny bydei uyw, namyn tra uei y deudroet y[m]mlyc croth morwyn, onyt kynwryf ryuel a'y llesteirei.[10]

> And at that time Math son of Mathonwy might not live save while his two feet were in the fold of a maiden's lap, unless the turmoil of war prevented him.[11]

Goewin ferch Pebin acts as his virgin foot-holder, but her beauty attracts the unwanted attention of Gilfaethwy (Math's nephew). Gwydion (Gilfaethwy's brother) hatches a cunning plan in order to remove Math from his court at Caer Dathyl and arrange for Gilfaethwy to sleep with Goewin in Math's bed. Her handmaidens are driven from the chamber and she is brutally raped.

Although rape, at least in the early period, was considered to be one of the nine forms of legal union, it was also regarded as a punishable offence for which a number of fines were payable, including *amobr*, which was payable to the virgin's territorial lord/king.[12] The lord, to a certain extent, appears to have been responsible for defending the virginity of the maids who lived within his territory, and *amobr* was paid to the lord whenever a virgin was raped, given to a man by her kin or whenever the girl herself committed a sexual act which was deemed inappropriate. In the case of sexual promiscuity, *amobr* appears to have been extracted from the girl's family until she was declared a common prostitute. In 1336, for example, three women were declared prostitutes in Bromfield and were given white rods symbolic of their sexual transgressions: 'so that their kinsfolk would not henceforth be troubled for *amobr*'.[13] According to Robert Rees Davies, the Marcher lords in particular were keen on exploiting the financial benefits of *amobr*. By the fourteenth century *amobr* 'had deteriorated into a sordid pretext for increasing the lord's revenue', and it was not abolished by the English crown until the sixteenth century.[14]

In the magical world of the *Mabinogi* no fines are levied, although Gwydion and Gilfaethwy are punished for their crime. Math uses his magic wand to transform the brothers into animals and, for a period of three years, they reproduce; each year they are transformed into different animals and bring forth offspring. As Roberta Valente points out, the punishment fits the crime: since they have committed a sexual assault, they are punished sexually.[15] Math, Goewin's lord, has failed to protect her virginity, but now he acts honourably towards her and makes her his wife. She is thus saved from the humiliation of becoming Gilfaethwy's wife, and rescued from her ambivalent position in society. Following the rape Goewin can no longer be classified as a *morwyn* (virgin), but nor is she anyone's *gwraig* (wife): ' "Arglwyd", heb y Goewyn, "keis uorwyn a uo is dy draet weithon. Gwreic wyf i." '[16] ('Lord', said Goewin, 'seek now a maiden to be under thy feet. I am a woman.')[17]

In this unusual case, not only is Math responsible for protecting the virgins in his territory; his sovereignty is completely dependent upon the physical purity of one of the maidens of his realm. The protective role played by Math's virginal foot-holder may be compared to the role of the king's foot-holder in the Welsh laws of court. According to *Llyfr Iorwerth*, the *troedyavc* (foot-holder) was responsible for offering protection to the king, and would hold the king's feet in his lap, with his back to the fire, until the king retired to his chamber.[18] While the courtly foot-holder's power is associated with his privileged position within the court, Goewin's power is associated exclusively with her virginity. The notion that a virgin (or even a chaste wife) possesses supernatural powers is a common motif in folk literature as well as hagiography.[19] The virgin is frequently attributed with protective powers or healing properties. For instance, in the Life of Melangell, the Welsh patron saint of hares, a hare takes refuge under Melangell's skirt and the pursuing hounds, presumably aware that Melangell's body radiates sanctity, cower and refuse to go near the animal. Brochwel Ysgithrog witnesses the scene and offers Melangell lands upon which she founds a sanctuary and nunnery.[20] Although other Welsh saints offer protection to animals, it is undoubtedly significant that the hare seeks protection under Melangell's skirt: the power of her virginity protects the creature, since feminine sanctity and virginity are inextricably linked.

In the case of Goewin, when the maid loses her virginity she also loses her protective powers. Math has to seek another virgin to hold his feet and thus protect his realm. Gwydion, having served his penance, is consulted and suggests that Math choose Aranrhod. Rather than emphasize his own relationship with Aranrhod (she is his sister), he focuses on Math's familial relationship with her (she is his niece).[21] When asked to confirm that she is a virgin Aranrhod gives Math an ambiguous answer: 'I know not but that I am'. Since Math's life hangs in the balance, he subjects Aranrhod to a virginity test:

> Yna y kymerth ynteu yr hutlath a'y chamu. 'Camha di dros honn,' heb ef, 'ac ot wyt uorwyn, mi a ednebydaf.' Yna y camawd hitheu dros yr hutlath, ac ar y cam hwnnw, adaw mab brasuelyn mawr a oruc. Sef a wnaeth y mab, dodi diaspat uchel. Yn ol diaspat y mab, kyrchu y drws a oruc hi, ac ar hynny adaw y ryw bethan ohonei. A chyn cael o neb guelet yr eil olwc arnaw, Guydyon a'y kymerth, ac a droes llen o bali yn y gylch, ac a'e cudywad. Sef y cudyawd, y mywn llaw gist is traed y wely.[22]

> Then he took the magic wand and bent it. 'Step over this,' said he, 'and if thou art a maiden, I shall know.' Then she stepped over the magic wand, and with that step she dropped a fine boy-child with rich yellow hair. The boy uttered a loud cry. After the boy's cry she made for the door, and

thereupon dropped a small something, and before anyone could get a second glimpse of it, Gwydion took it and wrapped a sheet of silk around it, and hid it. The place where he hid it was inside a small chest at the foot of his bed.[23]

The wand, quite obviously a phallic symbol, demonstrates not only that Aranrhod is not a virgin, but that she has also concealed two pregnancies. Math has already used his wand to punish Gwydion and Gilfaethwy for their sexual misconduct; now he employs the wand again to determine whether or not Aranrhod is a virgin. Her failure to pass the test results in her public humiliation and she flees the room ashamed, perhaps expecting to be punished for being a *twyllforwyn* (false virgin).

Stith Thompson and John Arnott MacCulloch record erroneously that the virginity test in the *Mabinogi* involves passing *under* a rod; the fact that Aranrhod steps over the wand, and, in the process, opens her legs as she straddles the phallic symbol, is important to the sexual imagery of the test.[24] Thomas Gwynn Jones proposes a connection between the virginity test and the folk custom of *priodas coes ysgub* – an informal marriage ceremony which involved stepping over a broom handle. He suggests that there is a linguistic connection between the Welsh word for wand (*llath*) and the legal term for a marriage which involved elopement or abduction without the consent of the girl's kin (*llathlud*): 'one wonders whether the element *llath*, "wand, staff" in the term *llathlud* in the Welsh Law, may refer to the practice of stepping over a rod, especially a bent rod as a chastity test in the tale of Math'.[25] The white rod, as we have seen, was also symbolic of sexual transgression: it was given to sexually promiscuous women and, according to some law texts, a silver rod was given to the king when a virgin in his territory was raped.[26] In the *Fourth Branch of the Mabinogi* Math's wand reveals publicly that Aranrhod's reputation is no better than a prostitute's. She is scorned by her brother Gwydion who reminds her that on only one occasion can a maid lose her virginity: 'ni'th elwir bellach byth yn uorwyn' (Never again shalt thou be called maiden!).[27]

According to the Welsh law of women, the girl's close family, her *cyfnesefiaid* – that is, her parents, brothers and sisters – may be called upon to vouch for her physical purity, especially, as we shall see below, if she were found to be a *twyllforwyn* (false virgin) on her wedding night. In medieval Wales there was a close bond between brother and sister. The girl's legal status in society was closely linked to that of her brother and the fines payable for insulting a girl (*sarhaed*) or murdering her (*galanas*) were equivalent to half of her brother's *sarhaed* and *galanas*. Gwydion is thus an obvious candidate to vouch for his sister's virginity. However, as Christopher McAll notes in his discussion of the false virgin:

> Obviously if the *cyfnesefiaid* are to be reliable witnesses in such a case, it is essential that they should have had the opportunity of observing the behaviour of the girl from close quarters over a considerable period of time, or at least, from the age of twelve onwards.[28]

First impressions might lead one to assume that Gwydion offers his sister to Math in an attempt to trick him and thus take revenge for the punishment inflicted upon him and Gilfaethwy. Nevertheless, it is also possible that his sister became pregnant during his three years absence, and that he genuinely believed her to be a virgin. He certainly seems disappointed by her actions and rears her youngest son in order to remind her permanently of her shame and humiliation.

According to a legal triad in *Llyfr Cyfnerth*, a pregnant woman wishing to identify the father of her child should swear an oath in front of a priest and vow that she will give birth to a serpent if she lies about the paternity of the child.[29] Whilst it is possible that the oath was meant to be taken literally, it is more likely that the woman in question was intended to fear an abnormal or premature birth. Despite the lack of textual references to contraception and abortion in Welsh sources, these must have been real issues which concerned the Welsh community. The virginity test in the *Mabinogi* appears to act almost as an abortifacient – dispelling any 'foreign bodies' from the female body tested. Medieval medical recipes designed to increase the flow of menstrual blood and clean out the womb may in fact have acted as abortifacients.[30]

Aranrhod's 'culpability' makes her a more interesting and credible character than Goewin, Math's virgin foot-holder. While Goewin disappears from the legend, and no further mention is made of whether Math succeeds in finding another virgin to replace her, Aranrhod remains one of the main characters. By foregrounding Aranrhod and developing the analysis of her character the author is, at least implicitly, acknowledging the greater interest in transgression and the social reality of such behaviour. Such a weighting of the narrative structure opens up a potentially subversive space and therefore lends the legend literary complexity. Ultimately, however, the message implicit in this branch of the *Mabinogi* is that virginity and fertility were not personal, private matters, for they were of extreme importance to the kin group as a whole.

Twyllforwyndod: 'false' virginity and the Welsh law texts

If a young woman was discovered to be a false virgin on her wedding night, that is, if she had misled her partner into believing that she was a virgin and he discovered that she was not, then the Welsh laws recommended that the girl be subjected to a public shaming ritual in which the wedding guests were called into the room and the girl's nightshirt was severed to reveal her genitalia:

> Os hitheu ny mynn y diheura6, lladher y chrys yn guu6ch a'e gwerdyr, a roder dinawet bl6yd yn y lla6 g6edy ira6 y losg6rn. Ac o geill y gynhal, kymeret yn lle y ran o'r argyfreu. Ac ony eill y kynhal, bit heb dim.

> If she does not wish to be vindicated, let her shift be cut off as high as her genitals and let a year-old steer with its tail greased be put into her hand. And if she can hold it, let her take it in place of her share of the *argyfrau.* And if she cannot hold it, let her have nothing.[31]

Since she had deceived her husband as to her sexual inexperience, the laws prescribed that she be punished by means of sexual humiliation. Another version of the law texts suggests that candles should be lighted and 'her shift cut before her as high as her pubes, and behind her as high as her buttocks'.[32] Once again it is clear that to medieval Welsh society (at least in theory) a girl's sexual and reproductive organs were not considered to be private parts, but were very much of concern both to her own kin group and to her husband's family. If the girl had already entered into sexual relations then there was a chance, of course, that she could be pregnant with another man's child.

The laws do not shed any light on how the girl's partner is to detect *twyllforwyndod*. Presumably he was expected to doubt her purity if she did not bleed when they first had intercourse. This would explain why the *neithiorwyr* (wedding guests) were called into the bedroom: to examine the sheets and thus act as witnesses to the husband's accusations. Yet, as Kelly has argued, the hymen is largely a social construct and although the presence of hymeneal blood was taken as one of the important signs of virginity in the Middle Ages, it was also acknowledged that not all virgins bleed when they first experience sexual intercourse.[33] The fact that a girl's physical intactness may be damaged accidentally during sport or a physical examination is also explicitly acknowledged in the work of the early church fathers.[34] In a relocation of virginity from the individual body to the community, the Welsh laws point out that it is difficult to determine whether a woman is a virgin or not once her body has reached physical maturity. For this reason, an opportunity was given to the girl's close family to defend her honour and argue that she was a virgin prior to her wedding night. If the *cyfnesefiaid* were unwilling to vouch for her virginity then the girl was ostracized by her kin and rejected by her partner. She forfeited her right to her *cowyll* (payment for her virginity) which was usually promised to the girl by her husband on their wedding night.[35] Nor was she entitled to *agweddi* or *argyfrau*, the usual payments required when a couple separated within the first seven years of marriage.[36] Instead the girl was given a year-old steer if she could hold on to its tail, which had been deliberately greased to make it slippery. This derisory form of compensation was obviously meant to mock rather than reward the *twyllforwyn*. The same kind of punishment was also meted out to the deserted mistress who had voluntarily entered into a clandestine relationship with a man and then been rejected. As Nerys W. Patterson has argued, there is a strong element of burlesque in the treatment of the false virgin and the deserted mistress and the symbolism implicit in grasping a bullock's greased tail is overtly sexual.[37]

According to the letter of Welsh law, women could not inherit land. Although there were exceptions to this rule, it seems that generally the principal attributes a Welsh woman brought with her to a marriage were her status, beauty and reputation. Her kindred were expected to contribute moveable goods in the form of a dowry (*argyfrau*), but were not legally bound to contribute wealth in the form of lands. In this respect, a woman's body (her physical purity and fertility) was perhaps her most important contribution to the marital contract, a contract which depended primarily on sexual union. One could argue that the virginity of the bride was even more important to medieval Welsh society than it was to a society which allowed women to inherit land and wealth in the absence of male heirs.[38] The law texts may be seen as reflecting a set of ideals laid down by the society which produced them.

The extent to which these ideals reflect social reality is an extremely complex problem. As Davies points out: 'They were written by law-men for law-men and are thereby more concerned to display the subtlety of legal argument rather than to provide an insight into actual social situations.'[39] Dafydd Jenkins has shown that although the law texts were continuously rewritten and adapted, they persisted in preserving archaic elements, and it is extremely difficult to use the Welsh texts to date specific practices or punishments.[40] The law texts describe an elaborate, burlesque punishment for the false virgin, but whether Welsh women who deceived their husbands were actually punished in this way is not clear. Although it is not known to what extent female virginity and chastity were put to the test in medieval Wales and whether false virgins were punished as recommended in the Welsh law texts, a similar form of punishment involving public exposure of the 'private' parts crops up elsewhere in legendary material.

Tegau Eurfron and the three chastity tests

Numerous medieval legends, usually associated with King Arthur's court, describe a magical chastity-testing mantle which will not fit false virgins or women who have been unfaithful to their husbands. When placed on an unchaste wife the mantle rises up above the woman's genitalia and exposes to all those present the nature of her sin. If the wife has only thought unchaste thoughts then the mantle will merely crinkle to reveal a toe. However, in the vast majority of different versions of this legend the mantle rises well above the pudenda, usually to the neck. All of the noblewomen at Arthur's court (except one – in Welsh tradition, Tegau Eurfron) are humiliated in a burlesque ritual which is similar to the treatment of the false virgin in the Welsh law texts. The mantle resembles a garment that has been cut with shears or scissors in an incomplete thirteenth-century German poem and a fifteenth-century Scottish ballad, 'The Boy and the Mantle'.[41] In the anonymous twelfth-century *Lai du Cort Mantel* and Ulrich von Zatzikhoven's *Lanzelet* a brooch on the mantle bursts open and the ladies' buttocks are also revealed for comic effect.[42] Other versions of the legend, including Robert Biket's twelfth-century French *Lai du Cor* and Heinrich von dem Türlîn's thirteenth-century German *Diu Crône*, refer to a chastity-testing horn or goblet from which no cuckold can drink without spilling his beverage.[43] As Kelly has noted, the women are rarely punished for their infidelity, since the test has a tendency to rebound on the men: it is frequently the men who have insisted on the test who are humiliated, not the women.[44] Many of the medieval European versions of the legend locate the chastity tests in Wales: in *Lai du Cor, Lai du Cort Mantel, Le Livre de Caradoc* and *Huth Merlin* the chastity tests take place at Arthur's court at Caerleon (the location of Arthur's court in Geoffrey of Monmouth's influential *Historia Regum Britanniae*); in *Lanzelet* the tests occur at 'Kardigan' (Aberteifi) and at the end of the *Lai du Cort Mantle* the author states that Caradoc left the mantle at an abbey in Wales where it had recently been discovered. Nevertheless, there is no extant medieval Welsh version of the legend.

A summarized Welsh version of *Chwedl Tegau Eurfron* is preserved in an eighteenth-century manuscript in the hand of Gwallter Mechain.[45] In the Welsh legend Arthur's sister (the wife of Urien Rheged) sends three magical chastity-testing objects to the court: (i) a mantle which could not be worn by an adulterous wife, since it would crinkle around her neck, (ii) a drinking horn which would stick to the lips of a cuckold and (iii) pork chops which would choke any husband who had been deceived by his wife.[46] None of the women of the court dare to try on the mantle except Tegau Eurfron, and her husband is the only knight to succeed in drinking from the horn and eating the chops. Even Gwenhwyfar, Arthur's queen, refuses to try on the mantle and attempts to discourage Arthur from drinking from the horn. Her noncommittal response to Arthur's request for assurance is reminiscent of Aranrhod's ambiguous affirmation of her virginity: 'Fe ofynnodd y brenhin Arthur iw frenhines Gwenhwyfar, a allai fe yfed? Hithau a attebodd, "Gwnewch o's mynnwch." '[47] (King Arthur asked his queen Gwenhwyfar if he could drink. She answered, 'Do so if you wish.')

Although the Welsh legend of Tegau Eurfron is preserved in a late manuscript, a version of the tale involving a chastity-testing mantle was certainly current in late medieval Wales. Numerous Welsh poets from the fourteenth and fifteenth centuries refer to Tegau Eurfron (Tegau of the golden breast) and she is frequently used as a paragon in Welsh courtly love poetry and formal praise poetry.[48] The element *Teg* in her name (meaning pretty) provided the poets with plenty of opportunity to emphasize the beauty of the women they were praising and the combination *Teg/Tegau* was also convenient for the purposes of the Welsh *cynghanedd*.[49] Dafydd ap Gwilym (*fl.* 1315/20–1350/70) compares his lover Morfudd to Tegau and on another occasion when complaining that Dyddgu has refused his affections he refers to her as 'ail Degau' (a second Tegau).[50] Other poets, including Tudur Penllyn, Lewys Glyn Cothi and Dafydd ab Edmwnd, refer to Tegau's mantle, and Guto'r Glyn (c.1435–c.1493) praises his patron's wife's chastity by suggesting that Gwenhwyfar, the wife of Siôn Edwart from Chirk, could quite confidently wear Tegau's mantle since it would adequately reach the floor.[51] Thus it seems that Tegau Eurfron, a character belonging to myth (where a wife's chastity could be tested with magical objects), was employed by medieval poets and compared to real Welsh women. The aim here was not to doubt the wife's chastity or humiliate any of the real women present, but rather to flatter and praise their fidelity. The chastity-testing objects could quite easily have been used for comic effect in Welsh erotic or satirical poetry, but I have not yet come across any examples which refer to Tegau's mantle in this context.[52]

Tegau's chastity is contrasted with Gwenhwyfar's (Guinevere's) infidelity in the Welsh triads, for in Aberystwyth, NLW MS Peniarth 47, the triad 'Teir Aniweir Wreic Ynys Prydein' (Three unfaithful wives of the island of Britain) follows hard on the heels of 'Teir Diweirwreic Ynys Prydein' (Three faithful or chaste wives of the island of Britain).[53] The two women represent extremes of sexual behaviour which correspond to the Eve/Mary dichotomy that permeated medieval discourse. However, while Tegau is named as one of the three faithful wives of the island of Britain, Gwenhwyfar's reputation excels all three unfaithful wives, since 'she shamed a better man than any of the others'. The triads appear to have acted as mnemonic aids to professional storytellers in Wales and they often preserve remnants of medieval tales that are no longer extant. Tegau's reputation as a model of chastity in medieval Wales is here confirmed, although no extant Middle Welsh tale relates her legend. Nor are there extant stories relating how Hemthryd daughter of Mabon (who is named in the same triad) became known as the paragon of female chastity, and excelled even Tegau Eurfron's reputation.[54]

The chastity-testing mantle is included in some of the lists which describe the magical properties of the Thirteen Treasures of the island of Britain.[55] Here Tegau's mantle detects cases of false virginity as well as adultery, although the former is not specifically mentioned in Gwallter Mechain's eighteenth-century summary of *Chwedl Tegau Eurfron*. Many of the other treasures listed are otherworldly objects capable of testing a man's courage, his social standing, or other attributes considered important in the idealized world of medieval chivalry. The Coat of Padarn Beisrydd, for example, would fit a well-born man, but would go nowhere near a churl. The treasures represent a medieval male fantasy; just as a nobleman might have wished for a magical mantle that would make him invisible on the battlefield (the mantle called *Llen Arthur*), so he might also have desired a magical mantle that would reveal to him whether his wife had been faithful to him during his absence. Although it is perhaps impossible to prove that the tale is of Celtic provenance, it is quite obvious that the central motif – the magical chastity-testing object that could automatically read a woman's body – was extremely popular in many different cultures over a wide period of time. Whilst it is possible to discern lines of transmission and affiliation between many of the continental versions of the tale, it is also possible that a motif as popular and comically rewarding as the chastity-testing mantle could occur in other guises in other genres completely independently.[56]

The humour in the tale works on various levels: it is bawdy, visual and slapstick, but it is also quite subtle in its criticisms and may be read in more than one way. On one level it functions as a misogynist warning to all husbands that they should not trust their wives and a sharp reminder to all 'loose' women that they will be publicly humiliated if their sexual deceptions are uncovered (as in the Welsh laws regarding the false virgin). Male fidelity is never an issue and the virtuous wife, symbolized by Tegau Eurfron, is a rarity. Gwenhwyfar/ Guinevere, as R. Howard Bloch points out, 'far from an exception, is the figure of everywoman [and] the vehicle of universal guilt'.[57] Yet the hundreds of ladies who fail the test and the cuckolds who are ridiculed for expecting better of them all belong to the upper classes, and the humour is all the more effective since it mocks the privileged and satirizes Arthurian chivalric ideals. Thérèse Saint-Paul argues that the humour in the tale is used for conservative purposes. Through the medium of laughter the story both acknowledges and reinforces the desired norms of social behaviour: 'a satire of the abnormal which thereby reinforces the norms'.[58] Kelly is also of the opinion that the test simultaneously upholds and undermines medieval ideas of chivalry. The testing object

> functions metonymically here, pointing as it does to a breakdown of societal norms. Both women and men have transgressed their (assigned) roles . . . The scene in which men choose to ignore or nullify the results of

the chastity ordeal effectively functions to deny the knowledge of such a failure in the homosocial system.[59]

As in the *Fourth Branch of the Mabinogi*, when the perceived norms of society are subverted, chaos and disorder result and one of the symptoms of a dysfunctional society is seen to be sexual deception by women. Exactly how to identify that deception was not only a pre-occupation of legendary material, but was also an issue that cropped up in medical and scientific treatises.

Virginity and the medical texts

In his *Historia* Herodotus (*c*.490–25 BC) describes how King Pheros, who had been blind for ten years, received an oracle informing him that he would regain his sight if he washed his eyes in the urine of a faithful woman who had never slept with any man other than her husband. Eventually he found a woman who cured him and married her.[60] It is possible that the woman Herodotus had in mind was meant to be a virgin, and that her physical purity lent special healing powers to her urine. Certainly uroscopy, the analysis of a patient's urine, was one of the most common methods of diagnosing illness in both the classical and the medieval periods. According to Galenic theory, an imbalance in the four humours led to physical illness and this imbalance could be detected in the urine and subsequently corrected. Medieval medical treatises – including the Middle Welsh texts – were heavily dependent upon classical medical theory. As Morfydd E. Owen has shown, although some of the Welsh texts are associated with the native physicians of Myddfai, medieval Welsh medical lore is very much a part of wider European medicinal inheritance.[61]

Welsh treatises on urosocopy refer to using various kinds of urine to heal afflictions as well as to identify the causes of disease. Cardiff, Central Library, MS 3.242, for example, refers to using human urine to heal a wound and a mixture of ram's urine and breast milk to heal deafness; it does not, however, note any afflictions which can be cured by washing in a virgin's urine.[62] Urine analysis could be employed not only to detect illness but also to identify pregnancy, determine the length of pregnancy and differentiate between a sexually active woman and a genuine virgin. In Aberystwyth, NLW MS Mostyn 88, a small hand sketched in the margin occurs three times as though pointing to particularly important or interesting sections of the text: on one occasion the example given is a means of verifying virginity, the second, pregnancy, and the third indicator highlights the range of different colours of urine and emphasizes that the liquid should be collected in a clean glass receptacle, allowed to settle and held up to the sun's rays for examination.[63] The colour of the virgin's urine is likened to an unripened apple:

> Dwr morwyn ieuangk lan a ddyly uod ual aual heb adduedu. Ac o hynny dwr du las ual lliw plwm a arwyddoka gleindyd morwyndod.[64]

> The urine of a pure, young virgin should be like an unripened apple. And silvery black urine, similar in colour to lead, signifies purity of virginity.

The choice of colour here (black) is somewhat unexpected, since other medical texts state that a virgin's urine should be white in colour.[65] The Welsh urine test is perhaps meant to indicate that the virgin's urine should be silver or translucent, rather than cloudy. Mostyn 88 (like *De secretis mulierum*) also confirms that the presence of seed in the bottom of the urine may be taken as a sign of intercourse between a man and a woman: 'a ddengys daruod i choreptio sef yw hynny torri i morwyndod'[66] (which demonstrates that she has been corrupted, that is that her virginity has been broken). According to the Welsh text, bloody urine in which the blood had coagulated like milk indicated that the woman was with child, and subsequently her urine would alter as her pregnancy progressed.[67] Thus, the colour and appearance of urine could be used to determine whether or not a girl was telling the truth about her sexual (in)experience.

Another recipe for verifying virginity, which also involves urine, is found in one of the medical texts associated with the physicians of Myddfai. According to *Llyfr Coch Hergest*:

> Or mynny wybot g6ahan r6ng g6reic a mor6yn. nad uaen muchud y my6n d6fyr. a dyro idi oe yuet. ac os g6reic byd yn diannot hi a y bissa6. os mor6yn, nyt a m6y no chynt.[68]

> If you wish to differentiate between a [sexually active] woman and a virgin sharpen jet stone into water and give it her to drink. And if she is a woman she will go and urinate immediately. If she is a virgin she will not wish to go [and urinate] any more than usual.

Although this diagnostic appears strange at first, it is in fact completely consistent with medieval medical theory concerning virginity and the female body. When examined in the context of other medical treatises and lapidaries it confirms medieval concepts relating to virginity and sheds light on medieval views regarding female anatomy.

An almost identical virginity test is found in a lapidary by Albertus Magnus of Cologne (c.1190–1280).[69] The influence of this text on the Welsh material is apparent, although it does not necessarily follow that the *Mineralia* was the direct source for the Welsh test. The *Llyfr Coch* fails to mention that jet stone can be used to relieve labour pains or that it can provoke menstruation in women when burnt between their legs. Fumigation using various substances was commonly prescribed for women suffering from retention of the menses and it was also recommended for women who abstained from sexual intercourse. Suffocation of the womb was considered to be the curse of chastity; since, according to Galenic theory, women as well as men produced seed, it was not considered healthy for a woman to retain her seed indefinitely. Though sexual intercourse was usually believed to be healthy and necessary for the proper functioning of the human body, fumigation could release pent-up menstruation or female seed without damaging a woman's virginity. [70]

Various medieval physicians, including Gilbertus Anglicus, Nicholas of Florence and William of Saliceto, refer to fumigation as a means for testing virginity.[71] Jet stone, coal, cockle or dock are burnt between the girl's legs and if she smells or tastes the fumes then she is supposed to be sexually experienced, whereas if she is a virgin she should not be able to sense the smoke. Virginity tests involving fumigation are more difficult to understand than those involving urine-provoking beverages, since surely only the girl herself could verify whether or not she could taste the substance. It is not known whether the medical tests for virginity were actually carried out, but Albertus Magnus implies that they were and that the properties of jet were known *from experience*.[72] Why jet stone in particular is included in the recipes is unclear.

While tests involving jet could involve fumigation as well as preparing a drink for the virgin, both methods can be shown to rely on an acceptance of the paradigm that proposed an inverse similarity of the male and female genital organs. In the medieval period it was generally accepted that the male body was the norm and that the female body was an inferior version of the male body. Most texts include diagrams of the male body in their discussions on general issues such as bleeding. While, for example, the male body is illustrated in a section on *gwaedu* (bleeding) in Mostyn 88, no diagrams of the female body are extant in Welsh medical texts. The female body was considered to be similar to the male body in almost all respects, but with inverted genitals, almost like a wax impression of the male genitals.[73] No mention is made of the clitoris, since this did not correspond to any part of the male body;[74] and no attempt is made to differentiate between the openings of the female urethra and vagina. Because men appeared to have one opening through which sperm and urine passed, it was believed that women passed urine and menstrual blood through the same hole.

Urine, then, was believed to pass through the uterus, and the uterus of a virgin was believed to be smaller than that of a sexually experienced woman. According to Soranus, the uterus would become larger during sexual intercourse just as the penis would elongate.[75] A virgin's vagina would be tighter than that of an experienced woman and it would take longer for her to urinate. Nicholas of Florence differentiates between the way in which a virgin urinates and the way in which a woman passes water:

> The urine of a virgin is thin and clear because the passages of the womb and vulva are narrow, so nothing descends into the urine except what is subtle, neither thickening nor muddying it. Because of this, a virgin urinates more delicately and for a longer period of time than does a woman who has been corrupted.[76]

Thus, if a virgin was given a drink containing fragments of jet stone (as in the Welsh test), it would not automatically pass through her, whereas the more experienced woman, with a larger urethra and slacker 'entrance' to her body, would pass water more easily. It was probably assumed that the fragments of jet (like seed) would 'muddy' the urine and alter its appearance. In the case of fumigation with jet the fumes would pass through an experienced woman's genitals, but would not penetrate the tight vagina of a virgin. As Kelly has shown, the female body was believed to be closed but not sealed; in other words, even the body of a virgin possessed passages which were permeable, since menstrual blood and urine had to be emitted without defloration.[77] First blood, which is often taken as a sign of virginity, is variously described as being due to the destruction of a venous membrane or to the veins in the sides of the vagina bursting on penetration. While recipes for faking virginity as well as verifying virginity are occasionally found in medieval medical tests,[78] the Welsh texts, though including numerous recipes relating to fertility, promoting sperm, urine and menses, do not, as far as I am aware, describe any means of *faking* virginity. The tests could plausibly have been censored, but it is more likely that these particular recipes were never included. Identifying virginity appears to have been considered more important than faking it.

Although it was extremely important that a girl be a virgin on her 'wedding' night, she was not expected to remain a virgin: in the eyes of secular society fertility – and in particular the ability to produce male heirs – was perhaps even more important than virginity. As one might expect, the Welsh medical texts pay more attention to fertility and pregnancy than they do to virginity. Fertility, chastity and piety were all considered to be important characteristics for women within marriage. Many of the virginity tests, particularly those found in legendary material, double up as chastity tests aimed at revealing whether married women have had adulterous affairs. Male chastity, however, is not tested. Virginity also was considered to be primarily a female attribute and, perhaps since it was both precious and em-powering, perpetual virginity does not seem to have been frequently encouraged in medieval Wales. In Wales, *amobr* was extracted, presumably from the parents. Although *amobr* may not have been enforced uniformly all over Wales throughout the whole of the medieval period, court rolls and ministers' accounts reveal that it made considerable sums of money for certain territorial lords.[79] Thus, virginity was an economic as well as a moral concern, and little wonder that few lords were willing to donate lands and provide long-term financial assistance for nunneries where women could remain perpetual virgins. Whilst numerous monasteries for men were founded in medieval Wales, only three small and economically unstable houses for women appear to have existed.[80] Virginity was an important commodity in the medieval marriage market, but not a personal treasure to be withdrawn and safeguarded from society indefinitely.

Notes

This is based on the final chapter of my Ph.D. thesis, 'Y Forwyn Fair, Santesau a Lleianod: Agweddau ar Wyryfdod a Diweirdeb yng Nghymru'r Oesoedd

Canol' (unpublished doctoral thesis, University of Wales, Cardiff, 1996). I am grateful to Professor Sioned Davies and Dr Marged Haycock for their helpful comments and suggestions concerning the original Welsh chapter in my thesis.

[1] Aberystwyth, NLW, MS Peniarth 17, fols 30–1 (second half of the thirteenth century). Translations from Middle Welsh are my own unless otherwise stated. A more literal translation of this would be as follows: 'The cunt which comes to be tested marries late.'

[2] On the nine legal unions see T. M. Charles-Edwards, 'Nau Kynywedi Teithiauc', in Dafydd Jenkins and Morfydd E. Owen (eds), *The Welsh Law of Women* (Cardiff: University of Wales Press, 1980), pp. 23–39. On *gwraig briod* in the eyes of the Church see Christopher McAll, 'The normal paradigms of a woman's life in the Irish and Welsh law texts', in Jenkins and Owen (eds), *Welsh Law of Women*, pp. 7–22 (pp. 16–17).

[3] Kathleen Coyne Kelly, *Performing Virginity and Testing Chastity in the Middle Ages* (London and New York: Routledge, 2000), p. 11.

[4] Gerald of Wales, for instance, refers to the art of scapulimancy, prophesying whether a woman was chaste or not by using a ram's shoulder-blade; Gerald of Wales, *The Journey through Wales/The Description of Wales*, trans. Lewis Thorpe (Harmondsworth: Penguin, 1978), pp. 145–6.

[5] For other examples of this motif see Cartwright, 'Y Forwyn Fair', pp. 177–81, and Kelly, *Performing Virginity*, pp. 8–9 63–74.

[6] See Stith Thompson, *Motif-Index of Folk-Literature*, 6 vols (Bloomington: Indiana University Press, 1932–6), vol. 3, pp. 312–16.

[7] The test is similar to that in Numbers 5:16–31 which involves testing a wife's fidelity.

[8] Mary Williams, 'Buched Meir Wyry', *Revue Celtique*, 33 (1912), 207–38 (218, 220).

[9] Sabine Baring-Gould and John Fisher, *Lives of the British Saints*, 4 vols (London: Cymmrodorion, 1907–13), vol. 4, pp. 376–7.

[10] *Math Uab Mathonwy Pedwaredd Gainc y Mabinogi*, ed. Ian Hughes (Aberystwyth: Adran y Gymraeg, Prifysgol Cymru, Aberystwyth, 2000), p. 1.

[11] *The Mabinogion*, trans. Gwyn Jones and Thomas Jones (London: Everyman, 1949; new revised edition 1993), p. 47.

[12] On rape see Jenkins and Owen (eds), *Welsh Law of Women*, pp. 49, 86–8, 139, 155, 177.

[13] Robert Rees Davies, *Lordship and Society in the March of Wales 1282–1400* (Oxford: Clarendon Press, 1978), p. 137, n. 25.

[14] Ibid., 137–8, and Davies, 'The twilight of Welsh law, 1284–1536', *History*, 51 (1966), 143–64 (155).

[15] Roberta Louise Valente, 'Merched y Mabinogi: women and the thematic structure of the four branches' (unpublished doctoral thesis, Cornell University, 1986), pp. 252–3.

[16] *Math*, p. 5.

[17] *Mabinogion*, p. 52.
[18] *Llyfr Iorwerth*, ed. Aled Rhys Wiliam (Cardiff: University of Wales Press, 1960), p. 18. On the Welsh laws of court see T. M. Charles-Edwards, Morfydd E. Owen and Paul Russell (eds), *The Welsh King and his Court* (Cardiff: University of Wales Press, 2000).
[19] See Thompson, *Motif-Index*, vol. 3, pp. 314–15.
[20] For the Life of Melangell see Huw Pryce, 'A new edition of the *Historia Divae Monacellae*', *Montgomeryshire Collections*, 82 (1994), 23–40. On the female saints of Wales and the importance of virginity in Welsh hagiography see Jane Cartwright, 'Dead virgins: feminine sanctity in medieval Wales', *Medium Ævum*, 71 (2002), 1–28.
[21] See *Math*, p. 7; *Mabinogion*, p. 54.
[22] *Math*, pp. 7–8.
[23] *Mabinogion*, p. 54. The 'small something' is an undeveloped child, which I take to mean a foetus.
[24] John Arnott MacCulloch, *Celtic Mythology* (London: Constable & Co., 1918), p. 96; Thompson, *Motif-Index*, vol. 3, p. 314; Kelly, *Performing Virginity*, p. 66.
[25] Thomas Gwynn Jones, *Welsh Folklore and Folk Custom* (London: Methuen, 1930), p. 185. Jenkins and Owen, on the other hand, take the element *llath* to mean 'stealth' as in *lladrad* (theft) (*Welsh Law of Women*, p. 208). For a detailed discussion of *llathrud* see Charles-Edwards, 'Nau Kynywedi Teithiauc', in *Welsh Law of Women*, pp. 30–2.
[26] Morfydd E. Owen, 'Shame and reparation: women's place in the kin', in Jenkins and Owen (eds), *Welsh Law of Women*, pp. 40–68 (p. 43, n. 13). See also pp. 142–3.
[27] *Math*, p. 8; *Mabinogion*, p. 55.
[28] McAll, 'The normal paradigms of a woman's life', p. 9.
[29] Arthur W. Wade-Evans, *Medieval Welsh Law* (Oxford: Clarendon Press, 1909), p. 129.
[30] Danielle Jacquart and Claude Thomasset, *Sexuality and Medicine in the Middle Ages*, trans. Matthew Adamson (Cambridge: Polity Press, 1988), p. 92. One of the Latin recipes in the Welsh medical text found in *Llyfr Coch Hergest* could perhaps be interpreted in this way; see Oxford, Jesus College, MS 111, col. 953 (*Llyfr Coch Hergest*). *Le Plus Ancien Texte des Meddygon Myddveu*, ed. Pol Diverres (Paris: Maurice le Dault, 1913), p. 132.
[31] Jenkins and Owen (eds), *Welsh Law of Women*, pp. 166–7.
[32] Wade-Evans, *Medieval Welsh Law*, p. 276.
[33] Kelly, *Performing Virginity*, esp. pp. 9–13, 28.
[34] See, for instance, Augustine, *Concerning the City of God Against the Pagans*, trans. Henry Bettenson (Harmondsworth: Penguin, 1972), bk 1, ch. 18 (p. 28).
[35] On *cowyll* see Dafydd Jenkins, 'Property interests in the classical Welsh law of women', in Jenkins and Owen (eds), *Welsh Law of Women*, pp. 76–8, and the definition of the term given on p. 196.
[36] *Agweddi* refers to the matrimonial property that a woman could take with

her if she and her husband separated within seven years (the amount depended upon her status); *argyfrau* refers to the property which she brought to the husband's household and may be translated, according to Jenkins and Owen, as dowry (ibid., pp. 79–85, and the glossary, pp. 187–8, 191).

[37] Nerys W. Patterson, 'Honour and shame in medieval Welsh society', *Studia Celtica*, 16–17 (1981/2), 73–103 (80).

[38] Nevertheless, the rules were flouted and in many areas women did succeed in owning or sharing lands; see, for instance, Anthony David Carr, *Medieval Anglesey* (Llangefni: Anglesey Antiquarian Society, 1982), pp. 156–61.

[39] R. R. Davies, 'The status of women and the practice of marriage in late-medieval Wales', in Jenkins and Owen (eds), *Welsh Law of Women*, pp. 93–114 (p. 93).

[40] Dafydd Jenkins, *Cyfraith Hywel: Rhagarweiniad i Gyfraith Gynhenid Cymru'r Oesoedd Canol* (Llandysul: Gwasg Gomer, 1970), p. 9.

[41] O. Warnatsch, 'Der Mantel, Bruchstück eines Lanzeletrones des H. von dem Türlîn (nebst einer Abhandlung über die Sage vom Trinkhorn und Mantel und die Quelle der Krone', in K. Weinhold (ed.), *Germanische Abhandlungen*, vol. 2 (Breslau: Koebner, 1883). For 'The Boy and the Mantle' see *English and Scottish Ballads*, ed. Francis James Child (London: Samson Low, 1861), pp. 3–16.

[42] F. A. Wulff, 'Le conte du mantel, texte français des dernières années du XIIe siècle', *Romania*, 14 (1885), 343–80; Ulrich von Zatzikhoven, *Lanzelet*, ed. Kenneth Grant Tremayne Webster and Roger Sherman Loomis (New York: Columbia University Press, 1951).

[43] *The Anglo-Norman Text of Le Lai du Cor*, ed. C. T. Erickson, Anglo-Norman Text Society, 24 (Oxford: Blackwell, 1973); *Diu Crône*, ed. G. H. F. Scholl (Stuttgart: Litterarischer Verein, 1852). Thérèse Saint-Paul, 'The magical mantle, the drinking horn and the chastity test: a study of a "tale" in Arthurian Celtic literature' (unpublished doctoral thesis, University of Edinburgh, 1987), provides a comprehensive survey of all known versions of the chastity-testing horn/mantle motif and summarizes more than forty versions of the tale.

[44] Kelly, *Performing Virginity*, pp. 76–9. One exception to this rule is an Irish poem, thought to have been compiled in the fifteenth century, found in the *Duanaire Finn* (Book of the Lays of Fionn); *Duanaire Finn*, ed. Gerard Murphy, Irish Texts Society, 28 (London: Simpkin Marchall, 1933), pp. 330–5.

[45] Aberystwyth, NLW, MS 2288. Graham C. G. Thomas, 'Chwedlau Tegau Eurfron a Thristfardd Bardd Urien Rheged', *Bulletin of the Board of Celtic Studies*, 24 (1970), 1–9.

[46] The continental versions of the tale refer only to either a chastity-testing horn or a mantle. It is fitting that Welsh culture, which placed great emphasis on triadic narrative structure, should produce a tale which comprised three different tests.

[47] Thomas, 'Chwedlau Tegau Eurfron', p. 1.

[48] See, for example, *Gwaith Dafydd ap Gwilym*, ed. Thomas Parry (Cardiff: University of Wales Press, 1979), pp. 140, 144, 151, 175, 252, 292. She is also referred to in the poet's prose: *Yr Areithiau Pros*, ed. D. Gwenallt Jones (Cardiff: University of Wales Press, 1934), pp. 30, 65.

[49] A complicated system of 'sound-chiming', involving repetition of consonants and internal rhyme, found in strict-metre Welsh poetry; see *The New Companion to the Literature of Wales*, ed. Meic Stephens (Cardiff: University of Wales Press, 1998), pp. 139–40.

[50] *Gwaith Dafydd ap Gwilym*, pp. 140, 252; *Dafydd ap Gwilym: His Poems*, trans. Gwyn Thomas (Cardiff: University of Wales Press, 2001), pp. 110, 185: 'one like Tegau'.

[51] *Gwaith Tudur Penllyn ac Ieuan ap Tudur Penllyn*, ed. Thomas Roberts (Cardiff: University of Wales Press, 1958), p. 14; *Gwaith Lewys Glyn Cothi*, ed. Dafydd Johnston (Cardiff: University of Wales Press, 1995), p. 362; *Gwaith Dafydd ab Edmwnd*, ed. Thomas Roberts (Bangor: Welsh MSS Society, 1914), p. 66; *Gwaith Guto'r Glyn*, ed. Ifor Williams and John Llywelyn Williams (Cardiff: University of Wales Press, 1961), p. 270.

[52] On Welsh erotic and satirical poetry see *Canu Maswedd yr Oesoedd Canol/Medieval Welsh Erotic Poetry*, ed. Dafydd Johnston (Cardiff: Tafol, 1991) and *Gwaith Prydydd Breuan, Rhys ap Dafydd ab Einion, Hywel Ystorm, a Cherddi Dychan Dienw o Lyfr Coch Hergest*, ed. Huw M. Edwards (Aberystwyth: Centre for Advanced Welsh and Celtic Studies, 2000).

[53] *Trioedd Ynys Prydein*, ed. and trans. Rachel Bromwich (Cardiff: University of Wales Press, 1978), pp. 174, 200.

[54] *Trioedd*, p. 174. Tegau is not listed in another version of the triad found in the White Book of Rhydderch *c*.1350, although Hemythryd (=Emerchet?) is referred to in this earlier text (here made Mabon's wife rather than his daughter).

[55] *Trioedd*, pp. 241–2. The mantle is listed as one of the treasures in the following manuscripts: Aberystwyth, NLW, MSS Peniarth 51 (*c*.1460), Peniarth 60 (*c*.1500), Peniarth 77 (*c*.1576), Mostyn 159 (1586–7) and London, BL, MS Add 15, 047 (1575–76). See also P. C. Bartrum, 'Tri Thlws ar Ddeg Ynys Brydain', *Études celtiques*, 10 (1962/3), 434–77.

[56] See, for example, Nicolaus Alemannus' notes on Procopius' *Arcana* (*c*.500–*c*.562): T. W., 'Influence of medieval upon Welsh literature', *Archaeologia Cambrensis*, ser. 3, 9 (1863), 7–40 (16–17).

[57] R. Howard Bloch, *Medieval Misogyny and the Invention of Western Romantic Love* (Chicago: University of Chicago Press, 1991), pp. 96–7.

[58] Saint-Paul, 'Magical mantle', p. 24.

[59] Kelly, *Performing Virginity*, pp. 78–9.

[60] Herodotus, *The Histories*, trans. Aubrey de Sélincourt (Harmondsworth: Penguin, 1972), p. 170.

[61] See Morfydd E. Owen, 'Meddygon Myddfai: a preliminary survey of some medieval medical writing in Welsh', *Studia Celtica*, 10 (1975/6), 210–33.

[62] Cardiff, Central Library, MS 3.242 (= Hafod 16); Ida B. Jones, 'Hafod 16 (A mediaeval Welsh medical treatise)', *Études celtiques*, 7 (1955/6), 46–75, 270–339 (curing wounds with urine, 296–8) and Ida B. Jones, 'Hafod 16 (*suite*)' and 'Hafod 16 (*suite et fin*)', *Études celtiques*, 8 (1958/9), 66–97, 346–93 (cure for deafness, 66).

[63] Aberystwyth, MS Mostyn 88 (NLW, MS 3026, *c.*1488–9), fols 31, cols a and b, 33, col. a. The manuscript is in the hand of Gutun Owain.

[64] Aberystwyth, Mostyn 88, fol. 31, col. b. A more literal translation of 'du las' is 'blue black'.

[65] See, for example, the *De secretis mulierum*, trans. Helen Rodnite Lemay (Albany, NY: State University of New York Press, 1992), pp. 128–9.

[66] Aberystwyth, Mostyn 88, fol. 31, col. b.

[67] Ibid., col. a.

[68] Oxford, Jesus College, MS 111, col. 938; *Le plus ancien texte*, ed. Diverres, p. 60.

[69] Albertus Magnus, *Book of Minerals*, trans. Dorothy Wycoff (Oxford: Clarendon Press, 1967), p. 93.

[70] Laurinda S. Dixon, 'The curse of chastity: the marginalization of women in medieval art and medicine', in Robert R. Edwards and Vickie Ziegler (eds), *Matrons and Marginal Women in Medieval Society* (Woodbridge: Boydell, 1995), pp. 49–74; Kelly, *Performing Virginity*, pp. 22–32. See Jonathan Hughes in this volume for further discussion.

[71] Esther Lastique and Helen Rodnite Lemay, 'A medieval physician's guide to virginity', in Joyce E. Salisbury (ed.), *Sex in the Middle Ages: A Book of Essays* (New York: Garland, 1991), pp. 56–82 (pp. 63, 72); Kelly, *Performing Virginity*, pp. 29–31.

[72] The idea that there is a relationship between jet and virginity testing is found in classical writings as early as the first century CE, for instance, Pliny, *Natural History*, ed. and trans. David Edward Eichholz (London: Heinemann, 1962), p. 115.

[73] See Jacquart and Thomasset, *Sexuality and Medicine*, p. 37.

[74] It was not until the sixteenth century that an accurate description of the clitoris appeared, associating it with particular sensitivity in women. See also Jacquart and Thomasset's comments on Albert the Great; ibid., p. 46.

[75] *Soranus' Gynecology*, trans. Owsei Temkin (Baltimore: Johns Hopkins University Press, 1956), p. 15.

[76] Lastique and Lemay, 'A medieval physician's guide', p. 61.

[77] Kelly, *Performing Virginity*, pp. 26–9.

[78] See Helen Rodnite Lemay, 'William of Saliceto on human sexuality', *Viator*, 12 (1981), 165–81 (176); John F. Benton, 'Trotula, women's problems and the professionalization of medicine in the Middle Ages', *Bulletin of the History of Medicine*, 59 (1985), 30–53; Joan Cadden, 'Medieval, scientific and medical views of sexuality: questions of propriety', *Mediaevalia et Humanistica*, NS, 14 (1986), 157–71 (164).

[79] In 1334 the surveyor of Denbigh calculated the return on *amobr* at £41

annually and in 1395 in Kidwelly it was calculated at £21. 6*s.* 8*d.*; see Davies, *Lordship and Society*, pp. 137–8.

[80] There were Cistercian houses for women at Llanllugan and Llanllŷr as well as a Benedictine priory at Usk. I examine why there may have been so few houses for religious women in Wales in 'The desire to corrupt: convent and community in medieval Wales', in Diane Watt (ed.), *Medieval Women in their Communities* (Cardiff: University of Wales Press, 1997), pp. 20–48.

5

Four Virgins' Tales: Sex and Power in Medieval Law

KIM M. PHILLIPS

Medieval virginity is in vogue, judging by a number of recent titles.[1] This sexuality *manqué*, which is really a sexual identity unto itself (the virgin is defined by sexuality as much as the common woman or the sodomite), is enduringly fascinating to theological and feminist historians alike. Sexuality, too, is as chic a historical field as exists at present, and sexualities are social constructions.[2] The practices, identities and even the desires associated with sexuality are produced by their unique cultural context. They are also therefore political constructions, in the term's broadest sense of signifying relationships of power. Regulation and restriction are indeed inextricable from sexualities' formation, through the prescription of licit and illicit forms of sexual behaviour. For women in the medieval period (as in many others), the ideal of premarital virginity formed a key part of the control and appropriation of female sexuality.

Most medieval scholarship on virginity has focused on its place in devotional life, particularly with regard to women and female figures such as virgin martyrs.[3] An increasingly sophisticated range of recent studies has demonstrated the great variety of meanings, practices and experiences of virginity in medieval Christianity. The importance of virginity in secular life remains relatively little explored, yet premarital virginity was fundamental to shaping the identity of the lay maiden.[4] Some of the subtleties which have been identified in holy virginity seem lacking in the lay variety. For example, while Sarah Salih has shown that 'one is not born, but rather becomes, a virgin', so that even a lustful wife and mother such as Margery Kempe could reclaim a virginal state,[5] secular models were less flexible. In the latter, virginity was something a woman possessed but was not intrinsic to her, and once 'lost' was irretrievable. Also complex was the relationship between holy virginity and power or autonomy, with some recent works noting that the apparently 'transgressive' female virgin (transgressive in rejecting the traditional feminine roles of wife and mother) was also deeply conformist in choosing a role praised by patristic writers from Tertullian onward, creating a 'paradox' at the centre of female virginity.[6] Study of lay virginity challenges the notion of the autonomous virgin, forcing us to confront the fathers, mothers, communities, manorial lords and judges who took an interest in a maiden's virginity and sought ways to punish or compensate for its loss.

This article examines the tales of four young English virgins who lived from the late thirteenth to mid-fifteenth centuries, encoded in the records of common, canon, manorial and borough law. Power, money and the female body form a nexus of interlocking concerns in social groups including (in these examples) the lower nobility, well-off and less prosperous peasantry and landholding towndwellers. The aim is not to exhaust any one of the topics, but to demonstrate the potential of medieval legal texts for explorations of the gendered forms of power encoded in the country's legal institutions, and the inscriptions of such power upon the young virgin's body.

Rose

Rose, daughter of Nicholas le Savage, appeals John de Clifford of rape and breach of the king's peace, that in the vill of Irchester in Northampton[shire] in a certain croft which belonged to her father and which lies near the house of Nicholas her father, when Rose went into the croft westwards towards the church at sunrise, there came the aforesaid John together with other unknown men wickedly and in felony aforethought and took Rose in his two arms forcibly and against the will of Rose and put her on a dappled [?] palfrey and brought her by the aforesaid unknown felons to a certain vill which is called Middleton in Oxford[shire]. And when they came there, he and the other unknown felons took her and brought her to the door of his hall, which faces north and south and the door of the aforesaid hall opens westwards, and there he made her get down and, together with the other unknown felons, he took her in his arms and led her to his bed and there made her to be divested of a miniver robe in which she was dressed. And when she was disrobed he took her in his two arms and made her sleep with him in the same bed and there held her all naked and slept with her on the right side of the bed. And moreover he held Rose's hands with his left hand and raped her virginity so that Rose departed all bloody from John etc. And afterwards, when Rose wanted to escape from the hands of John, the same John took Rose and imprisoned her in a certain upper room in the aforesaid house, and there shut her up securely imprisoned from Sunday after the Feast of St Hilary in the eighth year of the reign of King Edward until Martinmas in the tenth year of the same king's reign. On this day she escaped at dawn through a certain stone window from the aforesaid upper room. And she quickly raised the hue and cry and instantly sued against him by writ of the lord king at the lord king's court.[7]

Common law was not much interested in female virginity, except in some cases of its forceful theft.[8] Then it allowed the woman the right to bring an appeal of felony against her attacker, through the strict procedure of first raising the hue and cry, procuring a writ by which she alleged the occurrence of the crime in formal legal terms and appearing before the king's justices at Westminster or during their progress through the provinces.[9] It was lucky for Rose that when she tumbled out of John de Clifford's window on 11 November 1282 the court of King's Bench was set up for its Michaelmas term in Oxford. Having raised the hue and cry and swiftly procured a writ, Rose had time to prosecute her case before the justices packed up and moved on, probably by 25 November.[10]

It was essential that Rose herself go before the justices,[11] but it is unlikely that she went alone. Certainly, in order to present her case according to the phrasing which was demanded in felony hearings, she would have had to seek advice from a lawyer, a *narrator*, attached to the court, and either learn her lines from him, or employ him to present her case.[12] The version preserved is no verbatim reporting of the tale, but a court clerk's synthesis and Latin translation of the material presented throughout the hearing, which became the possession of the chief justice as a reference aid for later trials.[13] Any notion that the *conte* represents Rose's individual voice should therefore be discounted. It is also instructive to note the procedure followed: the plaintiff or their *narrator* would present the *conte* or *narratio*, the defendant would make a formal defence and the plaintiff would present a replication of their original *conte*, which might then be followed by further rejoinders from the defendant and plaintiff.[14] The record contains numerous pedantic details which cast an illusion of precision and comprehensiveness, but these were supplied at the advice of the *narrator* or perhaps in response to the justice's questions (the dappled palfrey, the orientation of Clifford's hall and placement of its door, the side of the bed on which the sexual rape occurred). Inclusion of such apparently irrelevant details was no doubt designed to test the consistency of Rose's story, during the repetition of the *conte* or in later cross-examination.

In fact, the tale is not comprehensive but contains significant silences and puzzles. The journey from Irchester in Northamptonshire to Middleton Stoney in Oxfordshire (some 37 miles as the crow flies and considerably further by road) probably took at least a day, yet there is no sign that Rose cried out at passers-by, despite passing through numerous settlements. She was held prisoner in Clifford's house for twenty-one months, and (given her miniver gown and the property said to belong to her father) was probably of lower noble or franklin status, yet there is no indication that her family attempted to trace her. It is not the validity of Rose's appeal which concerns me, but the existence of gaps in the tale. These remind us that Rose, or her legal counsel, has consciously constructed a narrative, and that the clerk has only recorded the details he perceives to be germane.

One detail is clearly crucial. Describing the rape, the clerk stumbles into repetition: Clifford made Rose undress and slept with her; he held her there naked and slept with her on the right side of the bed; 'and moreover he held Rose's hands with his left hand and raped her virginity [*rapuit ei virginitatem*] so that the aforesaid Rose departed all bloody from the aforesaid John'. The repetitions may reflect the slight variations in the *conte* as it was reiterated, or the cross-examining process – 'Were you a virgin?' or 'Did he rape your virginity?' In either case, it was a detail the narrator and the clerk used to enhance the validity of the *conte*.

In 1282 one did not need to claim violated virginity to be considered a victim of rape. *Raptus* and its variants in Latin, French and English mean, essentially, 'seizing', 'taking', 'carrying off by force', so it is helpful when considering medieval common-law on rape to ask 'what' is being seized and 'from whom?'[15] From the late thirteenth century to the end of the medieval period legal opinion tended to conflate sexual rape with abduction more than had previously been the case, and the series of statutes of rapes beginning in 1275 reflected this conflation. They also progressively involved parties beyond the raped woman herself by allowing the king and, by 1382, male members of the victim's family, to bring the case before the courts.[16] During the fourteenth and fifteenth centuries, then, English law reflected a strong cultural sense that *raptus* involved the seizure, and possibly sexual assault, of a woman (whether maid, wife or widow) to the detriment of her father, husband or other male relative. This view was probably influenced by the rise of Parliament as a legislative body, and the influence of male lay elites both there and in the courts of the realm.[17] The older view – that *raptus* was primarily a crime of violence and sexual assault for which only the wronged woman could lay charges – endured, however, and continued to influence the treatment of rape cases in the royal courts. English common-legal views on rape varied synchronically as well as over time.

The importance of virginity as a determining factor was one element which twelfth- and thirteenth-century commentators were superficially agreed upon (the woman need not have been a virgin), yet dispute is evident below the surface of discussion. Of the major treatises, *Glanvill* (*c*.1187–9) and *Fleta* (late thirteenth century) emphasize sexual violence, while *Britton* (*c*.1291–2) adds that rape is a felony whether the woman be a virgin or not.[18] Bracton's treatise (*c*.1218–29) offers by far the lengthiest analysis, and is revealing. It speaks of the appeal called the 'rape of virgins' (*de raptu virginum*), demanding castration as punishment 'that there be member for member, for when a virgin is defiled she loses her member', going on to assert that rapes of married women, widows, nuns, matrons, concubines or prostitutes, were less serious, yet nonetheless rapes, and concluding that 'to defile a virgin and to lie with one defiled [are different deeds]'.[19] Similarly, in *Placita Corone*, a mid- to late thirteenth-century guide to pleading in the royal courts, the appeal of *raptus* includes mention of the victim's loss of virginity.[20] The attitudes indicated in Bracton are taken further and expressed more bluntly in *The Mirror of Justices* (early fourteenth century), not a legal treatise but a discussion of points of law by an interested layman. It is a work justifiably dismissed by legal historians, because its inaccuracies of interpretation,[21] but those same errors make it interesting to the cultural historian. The author makes no attempt to resolve his confusion. 'Rape is committed in two manners: it is either of things or of women', he asserts, and is anxious to distinguish between *stuprum* ('the felonious taking away of a woman's maidenhood'), fornication, adultery, incest and rape ('strictly speaking the abduction of a woman with intent to marry her').[22] Note that this passage closely echoes the twelfth-century canon-legal scholar Gratian's discussion of *raptus*.[23] Yet later passages state that an appeal of rape must include the phrase 'and took away her virginity', and 'it is an abuse that rape is extended to women who are no maids'.[24] The author also hopelessly confuses felony with mortal sin, which makes his understanding legally erroneous but historically interesting, as it hints at the complexity of sexual morality which a contemporary could bring to his or her interpretation of the law. Apart from anything else, it seems he had encountered Gratian's canon-legal definition of *raptus* or an account of it, and saw no confusion in employing this in a discussion of common law.

While common law and interested commentators strained to get a fix on a definition of rape, the underlying attitudes revealed in treatises and statutes help make sense of the narratives which emerge from individual cases. The case of Rose, daughter of Nicholas le Savage, came before the royal court during a period of transition in concepts of rape. Only she could bring the appeal, and the crime was primarily one of sexual violation, yet abduction was an important factor in her *raptus* and it was useful to stress this in her *conte*. Perhaps more useful still was to stress the loss of her virginity. The verb *rapere* could and often did take an intransitive form in rape cases, but in this and other cases it was transitive, 'rapuit ei virginitatem'. If *raptus* was a crime in which violent seizure took place, it was useful to identify the object which had been stolen. As Bracton and the author of *The Mirror of Justices* were more comfortable identifying rape where something tangible was stolen, so the justices who sat in judgement on the case found this a detail which strengthened her tale.

The architects and practitioners of English common-law drew on a wide range of traditions, including pre-conquest English laws which emphasized sexual assault and made little of virginal status, Roman law which stressed abduction (and from which *raptus* and its variants were taken), and canon law which was most concerned with the violation of virgins.[25] This web of meanings helps to explain apparent confusions, and allows us to place the *narratores*, justices and clerks of the court within a broader framework of cultural meanings. Of the three justices of the King's Bench in 1282, Ralph of Hengham, himself a noted legal scholar, received his education through the Church, and Walter of Wimborne was a clerk in orders.[26] The loss of virginity, like abduction in the minds of those who helped to shape parliamentary statutes, was an offence they could comprehend. The sexual rape of a sexually experienced woman was more problematic: what was seized in the latter instance, and from whom? The notoriously low rate of convictions for *raptus* throughout the period has often been noted.[27] Judges were reluctant to impose penalties of life or limb, but forcing payment of compensation for loss of virginity seemed more reasonable. This is what happened to Rose. Although her case was at first thrown out on a technicality (the usual fate of rape appeals), the crown took up the case and, following the jurors' indictment, John was found guilty and ordered to pay £10 compensation.[28] Scattered evidence from a range of other legal sources indicates that premarital virginity was commonly believed to have a value which could be matched in money, and fathers, mothers and communities were concerned to enforce compensation even when the courts were not.

Isabella

> Deposition of John Russell of Bootham in the suburbs of York.
> To the fourth and fifth articles the deponent says that he has heard the said Sir John Collom say that Robert Chew deflowered the said Isabella Alan, his kinswoman, and thus deflowered he left her twenty marks from his own purse to spend.[29]

In 1453 John Russell was called before the York consistory court to give testimony concerning the disputed marriage of Agnes Cosyn and Robert Chew. With a number of other deponents, Russell drew the court's attention to a previous sexual encounter between Chew and Isabella Alan, who was related to Agnes Cosyn in the third or fourth degree. By the canonical laws on valid marriage that previous encounter created a bond of affinity between Chew and Cosyn – made them, in effect, related to one another. If the court could establish a sexual relationship between Chew and Alan, his marriage to Agnes Cosyn would be invalid.[30] Where other witnesses, including John Collom, vicar of the local church of Garton-in-the-Wolds, simply asserted that Chew had known Isabella Alan carnally, John Russell's fuller deposition includes a fascinating detail: Robert Chew had given Isabella the sum of 20 marks from his purse, because by him she had lost her virginity (*deflorata est*).

It is therefore quite by chance that record of this payment survives. Had Cosyn and Chew's marriage not been contested, Isabella Alan's defloration and compensation would probably have gone unnoticed by the church and by future historians. While church courts were concerned with sexual morality and regularly compelled men and women to appear before local deacons or the bishop on charges of fornication, adultery, prostitution or pimping, defloration as such was not generally pursued.[31] The only occasions when the ecclesiastical courts (as opposed to canon-legal scholars) paid much attention to virginity or its loss were in some cases of women attempting to procure annulments of marriage on the grounds of their husbands' impotence, such as in a 1378 case from Ely where a woman offered her body for inspection to demonstrate that though married she was still a virgin.[32] Living in a remote village in the Yorkshire wolds, away from the prying eyes of diocesan officials, Isabella's deflowering would in the normal run of things have attracted little interest.

Financial compensation to women for premarital loss of virginity is a matter, if not hidden, at least veiled from medieval English history. It belongs less to the legal than to the more informal realm of familial or community policing of sexual behaviour.[33] It was (unsurprisingly) a gender-specific form of sexual control: the deflowering of maidens required financial redress, though loss of male virginity did not. The payments no doubt helped to make up for the damage to the young woman's eligibility for respectable marriage by providing her with an attractive dowry.

The widespread existence of such a system is glimpsed through common-law records on rape. The notable failure of victims to appear before justices to pursue appeals of rape was due in part to the practice of settling the matter out of court through private reparations, and sometimes this factor is recorded. 'The jurors testify that [Agnes Mason and Adam Turner] have come to an agreement'; 'afterwards [Alice Stanchard] confessed . . . that Thomas, Simon's son, had undertaken to make amends to her for it'.[34] Other legal records offer occasional glimpses, such as a fifteenth-century petition to Chancery made by Robert Trenender, brazier of Bristol, and Isabel his wife, asserting that Philip Rychard had defiled their daughter and had failed to pay the damages set by ward arbitrators: 'unto hyr maryage a pype and halfe of wodd or els betwyxe yis and wyttsontyde twenty pounde of mony'. Further examples will probably emerge over time, as historians chance upon them.[35] Robert Mannyng of Brunne, composing his confessor's manual 150 years before Robert Chew made reparations to Isabella Alan, clearly articulated the necessity for rapists to compensate their impoverished victims:

> ȝyf þou rauysshe a maydyn poure
> Þou art holde to here socoure,
> And þat shal be at here wyl
> For as she wyle, þou shalt fulfyl.
> For þou hast do here a tresun:
> Þou hast stole here warysun [gift or treasure].[36]

Mannyng leaves no doubt about the money/body nexus of virginity; a maiden's virginity was not only a spiritual but also a firmly material treasure. In Chew and Rychard's cases, theft of premarital virginity was an extremely expensive transgression for these men of probably middling status. The 20 marks (£13. 6s. 8d.) Chew paid was nearly three times the £5 annual income that Sir John Fortescue in the 1470s reckoned 'a fair living for a yeoman' which might also be earned by a skilled craftsman, and was well above even the minimum contemporary income for a gentleman (£10 per annum).[37] Philip Rychard, possibly a dyer or (more likely given the size of the payment) a merchant trading in dyes, was required to pay out a still heftier toll. Yet mid-fifteenth-century dowries of 10, 20 and 25 marks exchanged between families of well-off peasant status indicate that Chew and Rychard paid sums which would have constituted substantial but not abnormal-sized dowries in such a middling social group.[38] Isabella and the unnamed Trenender daughter hardly match the 'poor maidens' of Mannyng's text. Those poorer girls, with less to lose by way of social standing, were driven to seek recourse of law through appeals of rape to secure their compensation. The size of their payments is usually not recorded, but in 1202 one woman received half a mark and in 1242 another received 4 marks – considerably less than the payments made to women with the family clout to pursue the matter out of court.[39] These smaller sums better resemble the bequests which comfortable burghers made towards the dowries of 'poure madyns' in the mid- and later fifteenth century. Olive Dade of Norwich in 1516 left 10s. apiece to the marriages of ten 'honest maides', John Carre, former mayor of York, in his 1487 will left 40s. each to fifteen poor maidens for their marriages, and Sir Richard Newton of Somerset in 1448 left 5 marks in total to five poor maids 'in recompense that y have don in synnes of flesshe'.[40] Newton's guilty conscience came too late for his paramours, but his remorseful bequest befits a moral culture in which defloration required reparations. While the outcome of deflowering daughters of lowest status families remains invisible, what the girls of middling and low-middling social levels had in common was that their virgin anatomies had attained the status of currency: items of exchange in which families had a strong interest, assessable for monetary value, to be saved up and spent in the marriage bed.

Matilda

Illey. Nothing is presented. But in fact Matilda, daughter of Matilda Kettle, has been deflowered and as they have not presented it the vill is in mercy (fine, 12d.).[41]

In May 1293 on the manor of Halesowen, Matilda Kettle and the jury of the vill who had neglected to report her misdemeanour were each fined 12 pence upon the report that she had been deflowered (*deflorata est*).[42] Although the record does not use the customary term for the transgression – 'leyrwite' – it is clear that this was the fault meant. Leyrwite was a fine for villein female fornication (a 'fine for lying down'), usually imposed on young unmarried women, and was among the many dues which lords could impose upon their servile tenants.[43] At Hales, seigneurial power to levy the fine was enshrined in the 1214 deed by which King John granted the manor to the bishop of Winchester.[44] Leyrwite does not appear in the records of all medieval manors, and where it does it was levied erratically.[45] The late thirteenth- and fourteenth-century lords of Hales – abbots of the Premonstratensian abbey of Halesowen – enforced 117 amercements for leyrwite from 1270 to 1348, but only nine from 1349 to 1386.[46] This fits well with what other historians have noted about the sharp decline in leyrwite amercements in the post-plague era, connected to the general move towards free status by the peasantry in the improved economic conditions which then prevailed.[47]

Answers to why manorial lords exerted their right to punish certain women's premarital fornication through fines, and why at certain times and not others, remain somewhat elusive. Tim North has offered the most developed interpretation, arguing that as leyrwite amercements frequently followed the conviction and fine for immorality in ecclesiastical courts, they therefore represented reimbursement to the lord for the alienation of his property.[48] This strongly materialistic account is modified by L. R. Poos and R. M. Smith's observation that leyrwite in Halesowen and childwite in Redgrave were disproportionately levied on daughters of the poorer families, indicating a degree of moral zeal on the part of the better-off villagers who tended to make up presentment juries.[49] Zvi Razi reads leyrwite as evidence for illegitimacy rates.[50] Other interpretations are brief: Jean Scammell and Eleanor Searle pass over the topic fleetingly in the course of their lengthy debates on merchet;[51] Barbara Hanawalt, P. J. P. Goldberg and Judith M. Bennett glance at the subject while considering premarital village sex from a social-historical perspective;[52] and E. D. Jones's useful findings do not lead him to clear conclusions, though he doubts that the fine had a primarily economic function.[53] I wish to offer a new hypothesis, based on forty-eight instances of leyrwite at Hales from 1270 to 1307 – a time of social unrest and peasant resistance on the manor. Many, perhaps even most, of the recorded leyrwite amercements of this period were used punitively by the abbot and canons of Hales as an instrument of shame and subjugation to subdue rebellious tenant families.

In 1293 Matilda Kettle was identified as 'daughter of Matilda Kettle' because her father Roger Kettle had died eleven years earlier. The circumstances of his death were among the most shocking that historians interested in pre-1381 peasant resistance have found.[54] Kettle, though a villein, was no lowly peasant. As a frequent pledge for other villagers, member of local juries, holder of tenancies possibly amounting to 20 acres and possessor of livestock and horses, he was of considerable wealth and standing relative to other tenants.[55] Yet rather than seeking a life of respectability and acquiescence Kettle was the abbey's most dangerous firebrand. His name appears repeatedly in the rolls from 1271 (the rolls begin in 1270) until the year of his death, 1282, in many instances of what Jim Scott, an observer of present-day peasant societies, has usefully labelled 'everyday resistance'.[56] Examples include his persistent refusal to pay a required heriot,[57] taking his corn to a mill other than the abbot's to be ground,[58] and consistent refusal to attend the manor court, especially in 1279–80. Each transgression suggests that Kettle's rebellion was against the dues and powers he was subject to as a man who, though comfortably off and locally important, was of indubitably servile status.

It was through more public forms of resistance, however, that Kettle riled the abbot to a degree which would prove fatal. Peasant insurgency was rife in Halesowen through the thirteenth century, from the time the manor was given to the Premonstratensians in 1218. The abbot and canons proved hard landlords. By the end of the century rents were twice as high as they had been earlier in the century, entry fines had also doubled, labour services in some cases had increased by a third, tenants were obliged to grind their corn at the abbot's mill (more expensive than alternatives), the lord exerted firm control over the manorial land market and imposed seigneurial dues such as merchet and heriot at exorbitant rates.[59] The tenants reacted not only with traditional forms of passive or 'everyday' resistance, but also by pursuing their grievances in the royal courts.[60] Attempting to quell the unrest once and for all, in 1279 the abbey ordered Kettle (evidently the ringleader) to pay the enormous sum of 100s. for 'unjustly' impleading the abbot in the king's court. As a final insult, the abbot loftily pronounced that he would 'put aside his indignation' at Kettle's waywardness and condescend to allow him to hold his land according to the judgement of the case: that is, as a villein tenant, subject to all the duties befitting his servile status.[61]

As Kettle did not pay and continued to resist authority, the abbey resorted to draconian measures in 1282.[62] Roger Kettle, John Thedrich and an unnamed man were seized, beaten and put in the stocks for a day and a night. Thedrich's wife Alice, pregnant with twins, was severely beaten, went into premature labour, and both she and the twins died. Roger Kettle died within a month as a result of his mal-treatment. In 1285 the abbot appealed to the royal court against his tenants, and was rewarded by the court's finding that 'the tenants are villeins forever'. Refusing to be crushed utterly, Hales tenants finally brought charges against their landlords in 1292 for the events of 1282–3, but they lost their case as the abbey was found to be wielding just force against rebellious tenants.[63] In 1293 Matilda Kettle, daughter of Roger and Matilda Kettle, along with Julian Thedrich, daughter of John and Alice Thedrich, and five other young women, were fined for leyrwite by the manor court.

The 1293 leyrwite amercements of Matilda Kettle and Julian Thedrich could be purely coincidental with the broader context of resistance. But examination of the activities of women fined for fornication and of their families, from 1270 to 1307, suggests other-wise. Of the forty-eight women fined for leyrwite examined here, only twenty-seven may with confidence be identified with a particular family (the other twenty-one are named by place of residence rather than surname). Of those identifiable women, I have traced instances of resistance on the part of members of their immediate families and (in a few cases) themselves in twenty-one instances.[64] Daughters and sisters of the Belgambe, Simon, Balle, de Bruera, Burry, Bond, Dunn and de Fraxino families, to name only some of the restive tenants, shared with the Kettle and Thedrich daughters the distinction of amercement for leyrwite, mostly after the suppression of 1292. Moreover, leyrwites are clustered in the years 1279–81 (thirteen amercements), 1293 (seven) and 1301–4 (thirteen), with only scattered examples in other years. The third grouping is not obviously linked to the uprising, but the clusters in 1279–81 and 1293 fit with the moments at which the struggles between lord and tenants reached their peak. Investigation of other manors will be necessary to establish whether the use of leyrwite to punish rebellion went beyond Hales, but it is notable that among the five manors of Spalding Priory almost 50 per cent of leyrwite fines came from one manor, Sutton, which happened to be the most mutinous and difficult to control of all the priory's holdings.[65]

Leyrwite emerges, in late thirteenth-century Halesowen at least, as a means of asserting seigneurial control over an insurgent population. This was probably not its only or universal function, yet it was a potent tool for the task, both as a means of stigmatizing those at fault through public shame, and as a powerful reminder of their servile status. But who was meant to feel the impact of such stigma: the women themselves, or their families? Probably both. Young women were involved in the uprising against the abbey – running away from the manor, fined for verbal abuse of the abbot and joining in with other women in burning the lord's hedges, and on one occasion knocking down the bailiff's gallows.[66]

But the connection of leyrwite amercees with rebel families, and the evidence that in some cases it was the woman's father, mother or brother who was fined for her defloration, clearly demonstrate that a daughter's loss of virginity was a shame borne by the whole family.[67] Even if readers are unconvinced by the theory of 'everyday resistance', it is noteworthy that the families of many of the women fined for leyrwite from 1270 to 1307 were not, in contrast to Poos and Smith's findings, of 'poor' status, but sometimes the daughters of well-off, influential men of the manorial elite. The singling out of wealthy daughters was unusual at Hales over a longer period: according to Razi's findings, 58 per cent of leyrwite fines from 1270 to 1348 were levied upon poor daughters, 31 per cent on 'middling', and only 7 per cent on 'rich'.[68] If it was a fine more usually imposed upon poor villein tenants, on this and other manors, its imposition on the daughters of the village elite was probably meant as a particularly demeaning gesture, shaming the family of the recipient through association with lowly status and assertion of servility, as well as through sexual disgrace.

Mariota

> Know men present and future that I, Mariota, daughter of Ellen formerly wife of Paul the Goldsmith of York, in my free power and virginity, have given, conceded, and by this my present charter confirmed, to Jeremy Lorfeuer, citizen of York, and Agnes his wife, all my land with its buildings and other appurtenances in Fossgate in York.[69]

In 1286 or 1287 Mariota, the daughter and heir of a dead York goldsmith, granted to Jeremy and Agnes Lorfeuer real property which she had of the gift of her mother, Ellen.[70] As an heiress who was still unmarried, she possessed and by this deed asserted her right to transfer property at her own will. The phrase 'in my free power and virginity' (*in mea libera potestate et virginitate*) is a strong avowal of her legal powers as an unmarried woman. To use Cordelia Beattie's phrase concerning medieval single women, she takes up the 'subject position' of the virgin, a position which buttresses her legal authority.[71]

This last of my four virgins' tales, representing a use of virginity within English borough-law (though not confined to that code), is certainly the most positive. Where the tales of Rose le Savage, Isabella Alan and Matilda Kettle all deal with the loss of virginal identity, Mariota Goldsmith's deed records the legal usefulness of the unmarried state. More broadly, Mariota's charter would seem to fit well within medievalists' traditional perception of virginity as an empowering state for women, though the empowerment is legal and financial rather than the heightened spiritual freedom of virgins usually discussed.

Such usages of virginity as a legal identity function in the same way as deeds made by widows asserting their rights to act in their 'pure', 'free' or 'lawful' widowhood.[72] A year or two before Mariota made her deed, in the neighbouring parish of St Edward in Walmgate, Ellen, daughter of Reginald le Grant, granted all her land in Walmgate in her 'lawful virginity and power' to Gaudin the goldsmith.[73] In contrast to the empowering assertion of virginity, two daughters of Ralph de

Bootham of York after marriage referred to transactions they had undertaken while 'in girlish years' or under the age of majority,[74] in documents which demonstrate the non-binding nature of legal actions taken by under-age girls.[75]

Some manor court rolls show virginal identity used in authorizing land transactions in a range of periods and places. The Halesowen court rolls of October 1293 record that Quenilda, one of three daughters and heirs of Orme of Hill, had previously quitclaimed her share of the inheritance to her sisters 'in her virginity' in return for six cattle and a mare for her dowry.[76] Also in that turbulent year an enquiry found that Agnes Thedrich had surrendered her whole estate to the abbot, while 'in her virginity', and that William Thedrich her husband was required to pay an entry fine to take up the land.[77] On the manor of Wakefield in November 1307 the jurors in a land dispute between tenants swore that Maude de Fugheleston, heir to the land, had come to the manor court and surrendered the land 'in her free virginity'.[78]

It is just possible that women were more likely to use the legitimating identity of virgin when they were engaged in transferring real property rather than chattels. Evidence from wills complicates this picture, however. Of the twenty-two York women from 1391 to 1491 who appear to have been single women – never to have married – when making their wills, twenty of the women leave no real property, only chattels and relatively modest sums of money.[79] Alice Langthorn made her will in 1465, declaring herself to be 'Alice Langthorn daughter of William Langthorn, late citizen and merchant of the city of York', and making her will 'in my pure virginity', and among other bequests left half a messuage of land which she had inherited from her father to one Richard Peverson.[80] On the other hand, Matilda Pede in 1452 left a burgage plot in Helmsley with its appurtenances to William Snaweshill, along with bequests of clothing to various female beneficiaries, and describes herself simply as 'daughter of Gerard Pede'.[81] And Agnes Kilburn, who in her 1477 will identified herself not as anyone's daughter but as 'puella', left no real property. Her numerous bequests, mostly to other women, include quantities of cloth. This and the mention of her servant, Katherine Fribus, suggest that she was not a young maiden but an older single woman in the cloth business.[82] *Puella* here signifies virginity rather than youth. In Norwich in 1504 Katherine Gardener made her will as a *puella*, including a bequest of land, but three other Norwich women whose English wills describe them as 'maid' leave money and chattels only.[83] A will was, however, a religious as well as a worldly document, and claiming a virginal identity there would probably have had implications of spiritual purity.

The example of Mariota and the language employed in her deed thus bring us back to holy virginity. The phrase 'in my free power and virginity', and others, such as Alice Langthorn's 'pure virginity', would catch the eye of any scholar of sacred virginity, with their implications of the powers and freedoms associated with the purity of that estate. They remind us also that divisions between sacred and profane were blurred in medieval contexts. Those scribes and clerks who produced secular documents would hardly have been unaware of the special estate accorded female virgins in a devotional context, and may have translated that into legal powers of ownership and transference. Similarly, the authors of saints' lives and works praising perpetual chastity could hardly have been unaware of the powerful messages on virginity and its loss which pervaded legal documents. The kinds of questions which studying legal records raises about possession and control of virginity, and about the bluntly material value sometimes accorded maidens' premarital purity, might in turn be put to use in new readings of religious literature. We know better now, as a result of many-layered recent readings, than to view lay or religious virgins as either powerful or powerless in their estate, but it may be instructive to reconsider questions of whose interests were served by removing active earthly sex from the lives of holy women.

Notes

I am indebted to several people for their help in the research for this article, in particular Cordelia Beattie and Jeremy Goldberg for generously directing me to several of the examples discussed, to Louise Wheatley for her help with the York Merchant Adventurers' Hall archives, to the Borthwick Institute and Norfolk Record Office for access to documents or provision of copies, and to Martin Jones as ever for critical reading.

[1] Cindy L. Carlson and Angela Jane Weisl (eds), *Constructions of Widowhood and Virginity in the Middle Ages* (Basingstoke: Macmillan, 1999); Kathleen Coyne Kelly and Marina Leslie (eds), *Menacing Virgins: Representing Virginity in the Middle Ages and Renaissance* (London: Associated University Presses, 1999); Kathleen Coyne Kelly, *Performing Virginity and Testing Chastity in the Middle Ages* (London: Routledge, 2000); Sarah

Salih, *Versions of Virginity in Late Medieval England* (Cambridge: Brewer, 2001); Jocelyn Wogan-Browne, *Saints' Lives and Women's Literary Culture, c.1150–1300: Virginity and its Authorizations* (Oxford: Oxford University Press, 2001).

2 For the state of scholarship on the history of sexualities see Robert A. Nye, 'Introduction', in Nye (ed.), *Sexuality* (Oxford: Oxford University Press, 1999), pp. 3–18, and Kim M. Phillips and Barry Reay, 'Introduction: sexualities in history', in Phillips and Reay (eds), *Sexualities in History: A Reader* (New York: Routledge, 2002), pp. 1–23.

3 Masculinity and virginity were not mutually exclusive concepts – see essays by John Arnold and Joanna Huntington in this collection; Kelly, *Performing Virginity*, pp. 91–118 and Kelly, 'Menaced masculinity and imperiled virginity in Malory's *Morte Darthur*', in Kelly and Leslie (eds), *Menacing Virgins*, pp. 97–114 – but it is undeniable that virginity was more often a feminized than a masculinized virtue; Kelly and Leslie, 'Introduction: the epistemology of virginity', in Kelly and Leslie (eds), *Menacing Virgins*, pp. 15–25 (p. 16).

4 See my *Medieval Maidens: Young Women and Gender in England, 1270–1540* (Manchester: Manchester University Press, 2003).

5 Salih, *Versions of Virginity*, pp. 1, 166–241; see also Wogan-Browne, *Saints' Lives*, pp. 123–50.

6 Cindy L. Carlson and Angela Jane Weisl, 'Introduction: constructions of widowhood and virginity', in Carlson and Weisl (eds), *Constructions of Widowhood and Virginity*, pp. 1–21, esp. pp. 6, 12, 19–20; Kelly and Leslie, 'Introduction', pp. 16–18.

7 *Select Cases in the Court of King's Bench* (henceforth *SCCKB*), ed. George Osborne Sayles, 6 vols, Selden Society, 55, 57, 58, 74, 76, 82 (London: Quaritch, 1936–65), vol. 1, pp. 101–2. To save space I have condensed the text: for a full transcript see the edition cited.

8 Of the many works dealing with medieval English laws on rape, the best starting points are two recent articles by Henry Ansgar Kelly, 'Statutes of rapes and alleged ravishers of wives: a context for the charges against Thomas Malory, knight', *Viator*, 28 (1997), 361–419, and 'Meanings and uses of *raptus* in Chaucer's time', *Studies in the Age of Chaucer*, 20 (1998), 101–65, and Corinne Saunders's lucid survey in *Rape and Ravishment in the Literature of Medieval England* (Cambridge: Brewer, 2001), ch. 1.

9 Technically, a woman could bring an appeal of felony in only two instances – her own rape or the death of her husband in her arms – though court records show that in fact women occasionally brought other appeals; Sayles, 'Introduction', in *SCCKB*, vol. 3, pp. lxxii–lxxiv.

10 Sayles, 'Introduction', in *SCCKB*, vol. 2, pp. lxxiii–lxxvii. Michaelmas term always began on 6 October and usually ran until 25 November.

11 Sayles, 'Introduction', in *SCCKB*, vol. 2, p. lxxxiii.

12 On the early use of attorneys or *narratores* see Sayles, 'Introduction', in *SCCKB*, vol. 1, pp. xci–cviii.

13 Sayles, 'Introduction', in *SCCKB*, vol. 1, pp. lxxix–lxxxii, cxvi–cxxiv; vol. 2, pp. cviii–cxv. Rose probably reported her case to the court or to her *narrator* in English, which then needed to be translated into the French used at court before the clerk produced his Latin fair copy.

14 G. J. Turner and Theodore F. T. Plucknett, 'Introduction', in *Brevia Placitata*, ed. Turner and Plucknett, Selden Society, 66 (London: Quaritch, 1951), pp. xv–cxlvii (p. xv); Elsie Shanks, 'General introduction' and S. F. C. Milsom, 'Legal introduction', in *Novae Narrationes*, ed. Shanks and Milsom, Selden Society, 80 (London: Quaritch, 1963), pp. ix–xxiv, xxv–ccxiv (pp. ix, xxv); John Hamilton Baker, *An Introduction to English Legal History*, 3rd edn (London: Butterworths, 1990), pp. 90–2. On the matter of voices in rape narratives see Barbara A. Hanawalt, *'Of Good and Ill Repute': Gender and Social Control in Medieval England* (New York: Oxford University Press, 1998), pp. 124–41.

15 Contemporary French terms include *ravir*, *rap*, *ravissement*, and Middle English included *rape* and *reve* (past tense *reft* or *rafte*). See James A. Brundage, 'Rape and seduction in the medieval canon law', in Vern L. Bullough and Brundage (eds), *Sexual Practices and the Medieval Church* (Buffalo, NY: Prometheus, 1982), pp. 141–8; Kathryn Gravdal, *Ravishing Maidens: Writing Rape in Medieval French Literature and Law* (Philadelphia: University of Pennsylvania Press, 1991), pp. 4–5; Kelly, 'Meanings and uses of *raptus*'. In this discussion I use 'rape' in its medieval sense of *raptus*, rather than the modern sense of sex without consent.

16 For the statutes see first Kelly, 'Statutes of rapes', then the works of those whose views he revises: J. B. Post, 'Ravishment of women and the Statutes of Westminster', in J. H. Baker (ed.), *Legal Records and the Historian* (London: Royal Historical Society, 1978), pp. 150–64; Post, 'Sir Thomas West and the Statute of Rapes, 1382', *Bulletin of the Institute for Historical Research*, 53 (1980), 24–30; E. W. Ives, ' "Agaynst taking awaye of women": the inception and operation of the Abduction Act of 1487', in Ives, R. J. Knecht and J. J. Scarisbrick (eds), *Wealth and Power in Tudor England* (London: Athlone, 1978), pp. 21–44.

17 I explore this idea in 'Written on the body: reading rape from the twelfth to fifteenth centuries', in Noël James Menuge (ed.), *Medieval Women and the Law* (Woodbridge: Boydell, 2000), and still feel it has validity although I would step back slightly from the clear chronology of changing perceptions mapped there. Medieval rape had multiple meanings, and to an extent these changed over time, but the variations were probably more layered than sequential.

18 *The Treatise on the Laws and Customs of the Realm of England Commonly Called Glanvill*, ed. George Derek Gordon Hall, 2nd edn, with material by Michael Clanchy (Oxford: Clarendon Press, 1993), p. 175; *Fleta*, ed. H. G. Richardson and G. O. Sayles, Selden Society, 72 (London: Quaritch, 1953), vol. 2, pp. 88–9; *Britton*, ed. Francis Morgan Nichols, 2 vols (Oxford: Clarendon Press, 1865; repr. Holmes Beach: Gaunt, 1983), vol. 1, pp. 17, 55, 115.

[19] Henry de Bracton, *On the Laws and Customs of England*, ed. George E. Woodbine and trans. Samuel E. Thorne, 4 vols (Cambridge, MA: Belknap, 1968), vol. 2, pp. 344–5, 403, 414–18.

[20] *Placita Corone*, ed. J. M. Kaye, Selden Society, supplementary ser., 4 (London: Quaritch, 1966), pp. 7–8, 29.

[21] See for example Kelly, 'Statutes of rapes', pp. 384–6.

[22] *The Mirror of Justices*, ed. W. J. Whittaker, Selden Society, 7 (London: Quaritch, 1895), pp. 28–9.

[23] See Saunders, *Rape and Ravishment*, pp. 77–8.

[24] *Mirror of Justices*, pp. 59, 141, 172.

[25] Saunders, *Rape and Ravishment*, chs 1 and 2.

[26] Sayles, 'Introduction', in *SCCKB*, vol. 1, pp. xliv–xlv, liii, lv.

[27] See for example Ruth Kittel, 'Rape in thirteenth-century England: a study of the common-law courts', in D. Kelly Weisberg (ed.), *Women and the Law: A Social Historical Perspective*, 2 vols (Cambridge, MA: Schenkman, 1982), vol. 2, pp. 101–15; Post, 'Ravishment of women', pp. 152–6.

[28] See Kelly, 'Statute of rapes', pp. 382–3, and Post, 'Ravishment of women', p. 155, for debate over whether payment would have been made in this way before the statute of 1275.

[29] York, Borthwick Institute for Historical Research (henceforth BIHR), Cause Paper (henceforth CP) F 189.

[30] R. H. Helmholz, *Marriage Litigation in Medieval England* (Cambridge: Cambridge University Press, 1974), p. 78.

[31] Richard M. Wunderli, *London Church Courts and Society on the Eve of the Reformation* (Cambridge, MA: Mediaeval Academy of America, 1981), pp. 81–102. Although canon law was concerned with rape in theory, in practice rape cases in England were usually brought before royal rather than ecclesiastical courts; Wunderli, *London Church Courts*, p. 91.

[32] Helmholz, *Marriage Litigation*, pp. 88–9.

[33] A more formalized system perhaps operated in fourteenth-century Parisian episcopal courts where a handful of records indicate that women demanded compensation for dowry or child maintenance in cases where their seducers or lovers would not marry them; see Jean-Philippe Lévy, 'L'officialité de Paris et les questions familiales à la fin du XIVe siècle', in *Études d'histoire du droit canonique dédiées à Gabriel le Bras*, 2 vols (Paris: Sirey, 1965), vol. 2, pp. 1265–94 (p. 1283). I owe this reference to Peter Biller.

[34] *The Roll of the Shropshire Eyre of 1256*, ed. Alan Harding, Selden Society, 96 (London: Quaritch, 1980), p. 258; *Rolls of the Justices in Eyre being the Rolls of Pleas and Assizes for Lincolnshire, 1218–19*, ed. Doris Mary Stenton, Selden Society, 53 (London: Quaritch, 1934), pp. 579–80. Ruth Kittel found 18 instances of out-of-court settlements in 142 thirteenth-century rape cases; 'Rape in thirteenth-century England', pp. 107–8; see also Roger D. Groot, 'The crime of rape *temp.* Richard I and John', *Journal of Legal History*, 9 (1988), 324–34; Post, 'Ravishment of women', pp. 152–3.

35 Public Record Office, C1 45/24. Hanawalt has also found a London case in which a man was ordered to pay the large sum of £40 to the city chamberlain to keep in trust until his young victim came of age ('Whose story was this?', p. 133).

36 Robert Mannyng of Brunne, *Handlyng Synne*, ed. Idelle Sullens (Binghamton, NY: Medieval and Renaissance Texts and Studies, 1983), ll. 2185–90.

37 Christopher Dyer, *Standards of Living in the Later Middle Ages: Social Change in England c.1200–1520* (Cambridge: Cambridge University Press, 1989), pp. 31–2.

38 P. J. P. Goldberg, *Women, Work, and Life Cycle in a Medieval Economy: Women in York and Yorkshire, c.1300–1520* (Oxford: Oxford University Press, 1992), pp. 245–6; Mavis E. Mate, *Daughters, Wives and Widows after the Black Death: Women in Sussex, 1350–1535* (Woodbridge: Boydell, 1998), pp. 25–6.

39 Kittel, 'Rape in thirteenth-century England', p. 108.

40 Norwich, Norfolk Record Office, Will of Olive Dade, 1516; Goldberg, *Women, Work, and Life Cycle*, pp. 156–7.

41 *Court Rolls of the Manor of Hales, 1270–1307* (henceforth *Hales Court Rolls*), ed. John Amphlett, Sydney Graves Hamilton and R. A. Wilson, 3 vols, Worcestershire Historical Society (Oxford: Parker, 1910–33), vol. 1, p. 231.

42 A marginal note in the record, 'Misericordia 12*d*.', indicates that Matilda, as well as her fellow villagers, was required to pay a fine; *Hales Court Rolls*, vol. 1, p. 231, n. 2.

43 For origins of leyrwite see Jean Scammell, 'Freedom and marriage in medieval England', *Economic History Review*, 2nd ser., 27 (1974), 523–37 (526–7).

44 For the deed see Amphlett, 'Introduction', in *Hales Court Rolls*, vol. 1, pp. xi–xii.

45 Tim North, 'Legerwite in the thirteenth and fourteenth centuries', *Past and Present*, 111 (1986), 3–16 (14–15); E. D. Jones, 'The medieval leyrwite: a historical note on female fornication', *English Historical Review*, 107 (1992), 945–53 (946, table 1).

46 Zvi Razi, *Life, Marriage and Death in a Medieval Parish: Economy, Society and Demography in Halesowen 1270–1400* (Cambridge: Cambridge University Press, 1980), pp. 64–71, 138–9.

47 North, 'Legerwite', 15; Jones, 'Medieval leyrwite', 946–9.

48 North, 'Legerwite'.

49 L. R. Poos and R. M. Smith, ' "Legal windows onto historical populations"? Recent research on demography and the manor court in medieval England', *Law and History Review*, 2 (1984), 128–52 (149–50).

50 Razi, *Life, Marriage and Death*, pp. 64–71, 138–9.

51 Scammell, 'Freedom and marriage', pp. 526–7; Eleanor Searle, 'Freedom and marriage in medieval England: an alternative hypothesis', *Economic*

History Review, 2nd ser., 29 (1976), 482–6 (483); Jean Scammell, 'Wife-rents and merchet', *Economic History Review*, 2nd ser., 29 (1976), 487–90 (488). The remainder of the debate, in *Past and Present*, 82 (1979), 3–43, and 99 (1983), 123–60, focuses on merchet.

52   Barbara A. Hanawalt, *The Ties that Bound: Peasant Families in Medieval England* (New York: Oxford University Press, 1986), pp. 194–6; Judith M. Bennett, *Women in the Medieval English Countryside: Gender and Household in Brigstock before the Plague* (New York: Oxford University Press, 1987), p. 96; Goldberg, *Women, Work, and Life Cycle*, pp. 208–9, 250.

53   Jones, 'Medieval leyrwite', 953. His suggestion that the high numbers of amercements recorded at Sutton might indicate brothel activity seems unlikely.

54   Cited by Zvi Razi in 'Family, land and the village community in later medieval England', *Past and Present*, 93 (1981), 3–36 (15–16); Razi, 'The struggles between the abbots of Halesowen and their tenants in the thirteenth and fourteenth centuries', in T. H. Aston et al. (eds), *Social Relations and Ideas: Essays in Honour of R. H. Hilton* (Cambridge: Cambridge University Press, 1983), pp. 151–67 (pp. 161–2); Peter Franklin, 'Politics in manorial court rolls: the tactics, social composition, and aims of a pre-1381 peasant movement', in Zvi Razi and Richard Smith (eds), *Medieval Society and the Manor Court* (Oxford: Clarendon Press, 1996), pp. 162–98 (p. 188).

55   Razi, 'Struggles', pp. 161–2.

56   Jim Scott, 'Everyday forms of peasant resistance', *Journal of Peasant Studies*, 13/2 (1986), 5–35.

57   *Hales Court Rolls*, vol. 1, pp. 52, 55.

58   Ibid., p. 136.

59   Razi, 'Struggles', pp. 154–8.

60   For what follows ibid., pp. 160–3.

61   *Hales Court Rolls*, vol. 1, pp. 119–20.

62   That Kettle paid no money is apparent from a September 1282 entry, in which his wife Alice is let off half the overall fine but is ordered to pay the remainder. She paid 9*s.* 4*d.*, leaving 40*s.* 8*d.* outstanding. By this time it is clear that Roger Kettle was dead; *Hales Court Rolls*, vol. 1, p. 215.

63   Razi, 'Struggles', pp. 162–3; also Razi, 'The Toronto School's reconstitution of medieval peasant society: a critical view', *Past and Present*, 85 (1979), 141–57 (154–5).

64   It is not possible to list these exhaustively here, but see for example *Hales Court Rolls*, vol. 1, pp. 49–50, for an occasion of group passive resistance; pp. 4, 6, 45, 86, 109, 113, 131, 148, 152, 184, 204, for John Simon's misdeeds (he was related to leyrwite amercees Julian and Matilda Simon); and p. 246 for Richard de Bruera burning down the lord's mill in October 1293, six months after his sister Margery's leyrwite amercement. These examples could be multiplied many times.

[65] Jones, 'Medieval leyrwite', 946, table 1, and 950–1.

[66] *Hales Court Rolls*, vol. 1, pp. 116–17, 121, 122, 232, 245, 247, 257, 261, 270–1, 325, 348.

[67] Ibid., pp. 120, 161, 381–2, 501.

[68] Razi, *Life, Marriage and Death*, p. 67, table 12.

[69] York Merchant Adventurers' Hall (henceforth YMAH), Fossgate Deed 1.

[70] The deed's contents are calendared in David M. Smith, *A Guide to the Archives of the Company of Merchant Adventurers of York*, Borthwick Texts and Calendars, 16 (York: University of York, 1990), pp. 57–8.

[71] Cordelia Beattie, 'Meanings of singleness: the single woman in late medieval England' (unpublished doctoral thesis, University of York, 2001), esp. part 2. A clear statement of married and widowed women's rights is in Caroline M. Barron, 'The "golden age" of women in medieval London', *Reading Medieval Studies*, 15 (1989), 35–58.

[72] See for example *Ancient Deeds Belonging to the Corporation of Bath, XIII–XVI Centuries*, ed. C. W. Shickle (Bath: Bath Records Society, 1921), pp. 5, 26, 28, 55, 71–2, 85–6, 95, 120, 127, 129.

[73] YMAH, St Edward Walmgate Deed 10, calendared in Smith, *Company of Merchant Adventurers*, p. 111.

[74] Under borough customs girls entered their majority at ages ranging from 12 to 16; Mary Bateson (ed.), *Borough Customs*, 2 vols, Selden Society, 18, 21 (London: Quaritch, 1904–6), vol. 2, pp. 158–9.

[75] YMAH, Testamentary Business 1 (Receipt and acquittance of Margaret d. of Ralph of Bootham, 1285), and Walmgate Quitclaim 3 (Ellen d. of Ralph de Bootham, 1290); Smith, *Company of Merchant Adventurers*, pp. 105, 135.

[76] *Hales Court Rolls*, vol. 1, p. 255.

[77] Ibid., pp. 261–2.

[78] *Court Rolls of the Manor of Wakefield*, ed. William Percy Baildon, Yorkshire Archaeological Society, 36 (Leeds, 1906), vol. 2, p. 60.

[79] My perception that they have never married is because twenty-one of the women refer to themselves as 'daughter of' rather than 'wife' or 'formerly wife of', and make no mention of children of their own. The remaining woman calls herself 'puella', which may mean 'young maiden' or simply 'virgin'. For the wills, see BIHR, PR 1, fol. 45; Probate Register (henceforth PR) 2, fols 13, 155, 247v, 407v, 414v, 557v, 637; PR 3, fols 35, 535, 543, 563; PR 4, fols 3, 32, 147v, 175; PR 4c, fol. 149; PR 5, fols 18, 168, 171, 393v.

[80] BIHR, PR 4c, fol. 149.

[81] BIHR, PR 2, fol. 247v.

[82] BIHR, PR 5, fol. 18.

[83] Norwich Norfolk Record Office, Wills of Katherine Gardener 'puella' (1504), Olive Dade 'maide' (1516), Rose Wellys 'mayde' (1532) and Christian Worlich 'mayde' (1538).

6

The Labour of Continence: Masculinity and Clerical Virginity

JOHN H. ARNOLD

G erald of Wales tells us:

> Linen grows out of the earth green, but it is rooted up, dried, trimmed, boiled, twisted, and after much long work the white colour is produced. Thus for our flesh to arrive at the virtue and beauty of chastity, it must fast and pray and keep watch, and must labour at continence and dry up inborn enticements, that it might ascend to that dignity of virtue which we desire. Linen is twisted moreover so that it will not easily come apart, and therefore not only are the lusts of the flesh to be restrained, but all memory of them eradicated from the innermost heart.[1]

If we are interested in medieval concepts of male chastity and virginity, Gerald's *Jewel of the Church* is a good place to begin. Written as an instructional and exhortatory work for the Welsh clergy in the late twelfth century, the *Jewel* collates a large amount of material – canonical commentary, biblical glossing, *exempla* – during a period when the sexual mores of ecclesiastical men were a topic of particular concern. The increasing emphasis on the miraculous nature of the eucharist, and the concomitant necessity for purity amongst its clerical confectors, combined with the longer standing drive against clerical marriage and concubinage to render the sexuality of churchmen a matter of extreme importance within twelfth- and thirteenth-century ecclesiastical discourse.[2] Indeed, Gerald spends about a quarter of the

Jewel discussing chastity. If we place the *Jewel* together with stories contained in Jacobus de Voragine's *Golden Legend* and Caesarius of Heisterbach's *Dialogue on Miracles*, we have a pretty good snapshot of popular narrative materials within western Christendom during this period.

Gerald's metaphor, borrowed from a commentary by Bede on the book of Exodus, presents what is in some ways a reassuring picture of male chastity. By working on the body through prescribed and well-established strategies – asceticism, turning to God, self-monitoring – a man can achieve control of sexual desire and eventually ascend to the whiteness of purity. Continence is an act of labour, one that follows a hard but familiar path. However, as we will see, this is not the full story, either in medieval culture in general or even the *Jewel* in particular. Gerald's metaphor sketches two arenas of labour, the body and the 'innermost heart', but the relationship between this pair is unclear. Furthermore, in using the image of linen, chastity is figured as a *production*, rather than an innate quality revealed or attained. What is the nature of this chastity? How does it fit with medieval conceptions of masculinity? Male purity was problematic, not least in what to call it. As Maud McInerney asks mockingly, 'what, after all, is a male virgin?'[3] It is far from clear how virginity could be distinguished from chastity for medieval men. There is no clear marker: no hymen (however culturally constructed or imaginary) to be breached, no pregnancy to be avoided.[4] If the signs of purity were problematic for women, they were equally so for men. And if virginity implied (as various writers argued) freedom from sex not only in the body but in the mind, the tendency for the penis to become erect and even on occasion to ejaculate without, one might argue, any clear command on the part of its owner caused further problems.[5] But this is not to argue that male virginity did not exist, or was unrepresentable in the medieval period. It is precisely the efforts of medieval authors to overcome these problems of signification and, more importantly, to negotiate the implications they had for masculinity, that make the male virgin an interesting figure. In what follows, for the sake of simplicity I will initially use the term 'chastity' to cover 'virginity' also, but will later suggest a particular way in which we might distinguish between the two, and perhaps provide an answer to McInerney's question.[6]

The most extended discussion to date of male virginity in the later Middle Ages is provided by Kathleen Coyne Kelly.[7] Kelly presents two key arguments about male virginity: that, in contrast to female virginity, it is not investigated but 'assayed' – that is, it is not a mystery to be uncovered, but a taken-for-granted element which needs testing; and that whereas female virginity had, in the Middle Ages, some clear narrative tropes for its representation, male virginity is bound up with a more fluid and elusive masculinity, one that refuses to make the male body into an *object* – or, alternatively, represents the endangered male body as feminized – thus preserving the subject-position and mystique of masculinity in general.[8] Kelly's analysis shares some factors with wider contemporary critiques of masculinity: for example, within film theory, Steve Neale's suggestion that whereas femininity is positioned as something demanding investigation, masculinity is narrativized as an individual test against an implicitly known ideal.[9] However, as Leon Hunt has argued, this distinction may be too neat: in certain kinds of heroic cinema, 'masculinity may well be investigated *by* being tested'.[10] That is, we may be better served in our analyses of gender if we do not believe too readily the fictions of authority and stability that masculinity overtly tells about itself, but consider more carefully the ways in which its production through narrative representation may indicate a more complex picture.

In any case, Kelly's analysis of male virginity, although intriguing and critically productive, needs supplementing with further analysis of the evidence. Her account makes use of a very broad chronological range of material: here, I will focus chiefly on western Christendom from the late twelfth to the late thirteenth century, not least because I suspect that one step we need to take in our studies of masculinity is to be more attuned to its specific variations in different times and places. So what can we say about male virginity, from the material provided by the *Jewel*, the *Golden Legend* and the *Dialogue*?

In considering the stories of male chastity I would suggest that, contrary to Kelly's analysis, one can identify four basic narrative patterns, two of which relate to the powers and actions of the self, and two of which focus on outside intervention. The first, and perhaps most familiar, pattern is lust overcome and chastity protected by bodily chastisement. Gerald of Wales, for example, tells us of St Benedict who, when tempted by visions of women sent by the devil, threw himself into a briar patch until lust was defeated; of St Ammonius who pierced his body with a red-hot iron; of a hermit called Godric, from Gerald's own time, who in his efforts to conquer lust tried fasting, Benedict's briar-patch method and, finally, the old faithful: sitting in freezing water.[11] The *Golden Legend* similarly relates

Benedict's use of the briar patch, noting that 'from that time on he no longer felt the temptation of the flesh', and has freezing water as the method used by St Bernard in his youth.[12] In these narratives, the struggle with lust is part of a general mode of ascetic struggle with the world; we are presented essentially with a dramatization and extension of male monastic identity and its attempts to discipline the body.[13] As in Gerald's linen metaphor, the body is disciplined through physical punishment, and thus the will triumphs over somatic desires. Although the means of discipline presumably require a degree of commitment on the part of the ascetic, the relationship they indicate between body and will is reassuringly hierarchical. The body can be tamed through pain in a methodical fashion, and the tools with which this is achieved are potentially available to all.

The second pattern, following a familiar progression from the former emphasis on bodily chastisement, is the direct exercise of will over the self.[14] There are some examples of this kind involving saints, but they tend to the undramatic: St Christopher, for example, rebuffing through the power of prayer two women sent to seduce him; or St Alexis who, on his wedding night, gave his bride a lengthy lecture on the benefits of virginity and then left her. There is the more famous story of St Bernard discouraging a hostess from entering his bed at night by crying out 'Thieves! Thieves!' to wake the household – but the dramatic element of the story is focused more on the mistress than on Bernard.[15] There is a general assumption that saints possess will, and the stories demonstrate that will rather than dramatize it; and thus it is in these narratives that we see Kelly's concept of virginity 'assayed'. More interesting are the narratives in the *Jewel* which concern less saintly men. Gerald notes the examples of Louis VII of France and an archdeacon of Louvain, both of whom were prescribed the use of a prostitute by doctors to combat illness caused by a lack of sex. Both men stoutly refused the treatment, and subsequently died chaste.[16] We further hear of a monk who arranged an illicit rendezvous with a girl in an orchard. They went in amongst the trees until they reached a point where the girl declared that 'no one will see us here except God'; not the wisest words, as this then prompted the monk to think the better of it and leave her.[17] A more dramatic narrative is presented by Caesarius, who tells of a novice in his monastery called Richwin, who was in love with a nun. She writes to him, promising that she will give herself to him if he quits the monastic life. Richwin wrestles with his conscience for some time, before throwing himself to the ground in his cell, with his feet poking out of the door, and crying 'Unless, devil, thou drag me away by the feet I will never follow thee!' Thus his will triumphs and lust is banished.[18] In the slippage between the internal world of the will and the external drama that Richwin enacts, we may simply be seeing a familiarly medieval solution to the narrative problem of representing interiority. But by turning an internal struggle into an external ritual, masculinity is also dramatized rather than simply asserted. Although Richwin projects the force of desire onto the devil, his battle reminds the reader that body and will are in a struggle, and the drama of the story depends upon the suppressed narrative path: that Richwin loses and leaves his cell. Masculinity here is tried, but through being tried, the relationship between body and will is investigated; or, perhaps we might say, the nature, power and extent of the will is placed under question, and dramatized through being refigured as a struggle between the will and the body.

Our third trope is what one might call narratives of revelation: linked, perhaps, to the exercise of will, but frequently involving outside intervention. For example, Caesarius tells of a lazy monk called Thomas who was tempted from his labours by a demon in the form of a girl. She led him away from his work on the pretext of taking him to visit his parents. When he asked her why she was leading him off the track into the woods she disappeared, revealing her diabolical nature; Thomas then realized that he was in danger of temptation.[19] Gerald of Wales provides further stories: a good man had arranged an assignation with a hostess. When she arrived, he was asleep, and dreaming that a toad was swallowing his hand. He awakes to find the women holding his hand, and so sends her away realizing his fault. In similar vein, a monk who had arranged to meet a girl has a preparatory nap and dreams of the fires of hell, which upon awakening leads him to repentance.[20] In the *Golden Legend*, these moments of revelation are linked more closely with the object of desire: St Josaphat is said to have been courted by a woman who offers to convert to Christianity if he sleeps with her but once. Josaphat has a dream wherein he is shown heaven and hell, and awakes to find that 'the beauty of that maiden and the others seemed to him more fetid than dung'.[21] St Anthony, having overcome 'the spirit of fornication', was permitted to see the devil in the form of a black child prostrate and conquered before him; Anthony remarked that 'having seen you in all your ugliness, I will fear you no longer'.[22] In these tales, the object of desire is essentially devilish or linked to damnation, and it is this revelation – implicitly allowed through God's grace – that saves our male protagonists.[23] The implications of revelation are intriguing: bestowed by God, they obviously bespeak his favour; but the failure of the men to notice what is happening unaided implies a certain lack in their masculine identity. This lack, of course, makes much more sense in a medieval context, where the need to humble oneself before God is a central concept of religious identity; but it nonetheless undermines elements of masculine discernment and self-government. Intriguing, too, is the content of revelation: for men to turn away properly from lust, the object of desire must be revealed as *undesirable* – a toad, a demon, dung. If beauty is revealed as ugliness, is desire in any sense being controlled, or simply redirected? Whilst these tales bless their male protagonists with the Almighty's favour, they do not easily underwrite a stable or authoritative *masculinity*.

Finally, our fourth trope: temptation overcome by divine physical intervention. Here, for example, is a tale shared by Caesarius and Gerald of a nun courted by a monk: she tries to sneak out of her convent at night to meet him, but finds her way barred by crucifixes. In one version, she then returns with an axe to smash the obstacle, but finds the tool miraculously stuck to her shoulder, shocking her into repentance. In the other, she prays to the Virgin Mary to remove the crosses. Mary, however, smacks her across the jaw so hard that she is knocked out – but wakes repentant.[24] The narrative focus here is on the woman, but it is presented as a tale of male chastity preserved. We find in the *Golden Legend* how St Eusebius is similarly protected from an amorous woman by his guardian angels physically preventing her from reaching him.[25] But there are other, more profound, kinds of physical intervention: for example, the *Golden Legend* also recounts how Master Reginald, a Parisian canon lawyer, decided to join the Dominicans in old age. He had a vision of the Virgin Mary who granted him a gift, anointing his body into monastic asceticism thus: 'at the loins she said "May your loins be girt with the cincture of chastity"' and so on for his other members.[26] Elsewhere the *Golden Legend* reminds us that the power of Mary's chastity 'penetrated all who looked upon her', removing their desires. [27] This reworking of the flesh is nothing, however, compared to the most radical interventions. Caesarius again: a monk called Bernard at Clairvaux was troubled by lust. He then dreamt that he was being pursued by a man, dressed like an executioner, carrying a long knife, accompanied by a black dog. Eventually his pursuer caught and castrated him, feeding his balls to the hound.

The monk awoke to find himself physically intact, but permanently freed from lust.[28] Gerald tells a similar tale, of a monk called Eliah who built a monastery for women. He found himself seized with desire for his charges, and took himself into the wilderness to fast. Angels found him there and removed his problem by castrating him – again, metaphysically rather than physically. Gerald asserts that a similar experience came to Abbot Hugh of Lincoln in his own time.[29] As Jacqueline Murray has noted about such stories, the Church had been quite clear since the Council of Nicaea in 325 CE that actual, physical castration was not a suitable treatment for lust.[30] Illustrating this, the *Golden Legend* tells how a young man on pilgrimage committed the sin of fornication. The devil appeared to him in the guise of St James the Apostle, and persuaded him to castrate himself and then commit suicide. The man was saved by the real James, but it is clear that actual self-mutilation is not praiseworthy.[31] However, the image of castration – castration as a gift, as an act of mercy – metaphorically encodes a particular freedom from desire.

The roots of these stories of mystical castration lie in the early Church, drawing scriptural authority from Matthew 19:12 ('there are eunuchs who castrate themselves on account of the kingdom of heaven') and developed in a number of early accounts of male holiness and purity.[32] Stories of castration freeing men from sexual desire are provided by Cassian and Gregory the Great, while Origen – who castrated himself in order to teach Christianity to men and women alike without impediment – supplied a powerful example, one that gave some comfort to Peter Abelard after his involuntary gelding.[33] Cassian, in propounding his six stages of chastity, contextualizes this gift of castration: the sixth and highest stage involves complete freedom from sexual desire, even in the unconscious mind. Lust is finally made absent. As Michel Foucault notes, discussing Cassian's disciplinary progression, 'Since this is a supranatural phenomenon, only a supranatural power can give us this freedom, spiritual grace.' It is, Foucault suggests, 'a blessing one may hope for but not attain'.[34] Here, again, we meet a disjunction from Gerald's initial, reassuring metaphor for working upon the body: the gift of castration, whilst bespeaking God's favour, effectively abandons the project of controlling the body in favour of freedom *from* the body. However, if this freedom is ultimately achievable only via supranatural means, an exceptional holiness effectively displaces the project of masculine self-control and, indeed, implies that masculinity is in itself inevitably imperfect.

So what further can we say about these narratives of virginity and chastity? First, although the gendering of virginity identified by Kelly can be noted, it is not absolute. One can find examples of these kinds of stories told about women as well as men: for example, the *Golden Legend*'s account of St Justina has various demons in the guise of handsome young men jumping into bed with her and her resisting temptation through will-power;[35] Caesarius tells of a noble matron inflamed by lust who jumps into a river until her desires depart, much like St Bernard.[36] Gerald relates the story of a priest who sleeps in the same room as his daughter-in-law and is tempted by her presence; however, when he places his hand on her breast she cries out 'Thieves! Thieves!' to wake the household, again like St Bernard.[37] Gerald also notes a nun who is seized by lust when she catches sight of a passing cleric. She battles her desire with her will, and when asleep has a vision of the cleric revealed to be a demon – so she cuts him in half with a scythe, which awakens her from her dream.[38] Here we have a story of both revelation and will-power. So women's virginity can, on occasion, also be narrated much like male virginity, as a test of will-power and bodily control. And men can, on occasion, be disempowered and threatened as much as women. Caesarius tells the story of a knight who joined the cloister, but was pursued by his wife. She attempts to seduce him back into the world, and actually has him abducted for this purpose, following a pattern not dissimilar to some rape narratives.[39] The *Golden Legend*'s story of an unnamed youth, tortured by the Emperor Decius, who whilst tied up bites out his own tongue and spits it in the face of the woman sent to seduce him, narrates the male body vulnerable and displayed.[40] If, as R. Howard Bloch has argued, a female virgin can be violated simply through the sight of her body, one can again find a male parallel: Odo of Cluny's life of St Gerald relates how, after death, his corpse insisted on keeping its hands covering his breast and genitalia, 'anxious to preserve the modesty of chastity'.[41] The narratives, implications and meanings of male and female virgins are not as clear-cut as some writers have tried to suggest. This is not to argue that gender is not a feature in the representation of virginity, but it ought to draw us back from generalizing in too broad and bold a manner about what happens to the gendering of virginity in the Middle Ages.[42]

Following on from this, there is a tension in the stories of male virginity between lust as an external force – frequently identified as a conflation of women and demons – and lust as an internal, immanent presence. The former can lead to the most appallingly misogynistic stories, but most are less clear-cut. Gerald's story told above, of the woman who fends off the priest by crying out 'Thieves! Thieves!', makes it clear that the fault lies with the priest, not the daughter-in-law; and Gerald indicates, when relating various stories of priests being tempted by the sight of women, that the fault lies as much with the men as with the women.[43] In fact, in opposition to the common claim that women are the bearers of uncontrolled desire in medieval discourse, it is quite clear that men are similarly afflicted, and afflicted most of all when they are young.[44] Gerald notes that it is more praiseworthy if men restrain themselves from lust when they are young, because it is much harder then, and he quotes (probably apocryphally) Isidore of Seville as saying that if one embraces chastity only in old age, when lust has departed, one is not actually practising continence.[45] Gerald also cites Jerome and Augustine on how hard chastity is, because of the *innate* bodily desire residing in human beings; Gerald's answer is that we must still struggle, and he emphasizes that men possess *will* as well as bodies.[46]

But if will-power is the answer, how are we to read the narratives of external intervention discussed above? As noted, there are different models here: one emphasizing self-control, the other narrating miraculous aid; and Gerald, at least, presents these in what modern analyses of masculinity might assume to be reverse importance. That is, he tells first about bodily chastisement, then about self-control, and then – apparently as the highest order – external intervention, such as miraculous castration. The answer to this conundrum – of whether will matters or not – is that there are two kinds of continence, which we might perhaps at this point distinguish as chastity and virginity. The former is about the *control* of lust, achieved through the exercise of will, but perhaps aided by bodily chastisement when in the grip of youth; note, for example, that it was when St Bernard was young that he resorted to sitting in freezing water, whereas his later adventures fending off women are in his maturity, and he uses will-power alone. The tension in this model – and what qualifies it as masculinity *investigated* rather than simply tested – is that will-power is always liable to failure. It is a struggle, not a given. Although he argues that lust is strongest in youth, Gerald also notes that he has seen many priests who have remained 'spotlessly continent (or at least . . . without scandal)' suddenly in maturity or even old age committing 'sins of lust' and having children.[47] Combating lust with will is a very long war, and you need lose the battle only once to fail in the fight.

In contrast, what we might call male virginity is a different state: lust made absent. This is the import of the stories of divine intervention: they rank more highly than exercise of will, first because they indicate the bestowal of God's grace, and second because they present a fantasy of transcendence. In Gerald's opening metaphor of working linen, the path from chastity to virginity is a continuum. But a little later on Gerald notes that 'abstinence from such sweet and enjoyable pleasures by certain elect ones (who have happily exchanged vile and temporary pleasures for precious eternal ones) can procure fellowship with the angels'.[48] This is the state for only a blessed few, those who have lost all desire and have transcended human pleasure. Furthermore, as we have seen, when Gerald comes to narrate such a state, he turns to external intervention: the gift of metaphysical castration, which alters the being. Virginity that is not a divine gift is not truly virginity because it might yet fail.

Analyses of medieval male sexuality have tended to underwrite certain notions about masculinity and control, both medieval and modern. For example, Pierre Payer's examination of theological and canonical discussions of sex argues that, particularly in the late twelfth and early thirteenth centuries, the 'bridling of desire' is based upon an image of the dominance of reason over concupiscence: 'the active feature is that of dominion, rule, lordship, domination'.[49] Thus the struggle between the body and the will is figured within the language of a particular kind of masculinity, related to medieval political notions of hierarchy and dominion. Whilst helpful in explaining abstract and normative ideas of sexuality and masculinity, an analysis of masculinity in action – for example, within narrative – may complicate the picture. In a few exceptional cases, such as that of St Bernard, one is presented with an assumed masculine virtue that is assayed (to use Kelly's term) rather than investigated. But in many of the narratives of male chastity, we are presented with a masculinity that is investigated – that is, placed under question as to its nature, extent and stability – *through* being tested. Gerald's plethora of stories about continence maps a variety of responses, and consciously admits to a degree of confusion over what, precisely, is shown.[50]

At the furthest end of the scale, and somewhat exploding the opposition of external threat and immanent fault, Gerald reports verbatim a letter from Hildebert, bishop of Le Mans, replying to a consultation from a local abbot about an afflicted monk. This monk, it appears, experienced sexual desire and ejaculation when prostrate for prayer (but not, curiously enough, when in bed at night); specifically, Hildebert tells us in rather shocked tones, the monk experiences masturbation as by another *man*'s hand. The bishop's response is confused: he allows that this might well be an attack by Satan, and suggests prayers; but he also prescribes a certain kind of medical treatment, rubbing a concoction onto the monk's genitalia. Hildebert then expresses doubt about the abbot's claim that the monk is a virgin, suggesting that, given what the man is experiencing, this might no longer be an applicable title. Furthermore, Hildebert says, he finds it difficult to conceive of the monk carrying *no* culpability in the matter, given how far it progresses (that is, to ejaculation), and suggests that the man should also be asked to examine his conscience and try bodily chastisement.[51] Here we have every trope about male chastity mixed together into a somewhat confusing mélange. There is instability here, a masculinity that is assaulted but also culpable, and a chastity that may be shored up by external intervention but also by inner self-control.

One might suggest that the problem for masculinity – what renders it unstable or uneasy – is the body: that, as Murray has suggested, male embodiment can be as problematic for masculine identity as female embodiment has been considered for women.[52] Certainly part of the problem is the body: Gerald tells us as much in the *Jewel* when he admits that Jerome, amongst others, wrote that 'It is beyond nature not to make use of that you were born with, and to destroy the very core of your self.'[53] Bodies could undoubtedly be threatening, moving against the conscious will, harbouring desires that threatened the serenity of the inner man. Perhaps, however, we might say that bodies present the basis for the essential drama of masculinity – the field of battle, which permits the exercise of valour. If Dyan Elliott is correct in suggesting that female virginity gains its value because it contradicts the assumed tendency of women to lust – that female virginity is, of its nature, rare, fragile and miraculous – we might say that in contrast, male chastity sets a difficult but achievable task wherein a man can set about being a (holy) man by following a disciplinary programme. In short, female virginity is fantasized as an extraordinary ontology, whereas male chastity dramatizes a form of male agency.[54]

However, there is another element to this. The relationship between body, will and desire is not so simply affirmed in every narrative that we have examined. If bodies pose a soluble problem for male subjects, the *desire* within men is a more uneasy element. The 'solution' posed by the gift of mystical castration is a curious one: not only is it (and the virginity it implies) limited to an extraordinary and elect few, it is also based upon a conflicted idea of desire and embodiment. To have desire removed by external agency short-circuits the drama of masculine control; there is no lordship or dominion here, only a kind of manumission from the corporeal. Furthermore, it is unclear whether medieval commentators truly believed castration to supply physiological freedom from sexual appetite. The point of Origen's castration was to avoid scandal rather than remove desire – the latter, in any case, Origen said it failed to do.[55] Was desire rooted in the body, or elsewhere? If bodies were part of the problem, minds were also a factor; and arguably the more important one. Many of the stories of threatened chastity concern men who have *thought* of women rather than encountered them in corporeal reality; and it is unclear whether the desire engendered from the imagination sprang from outside (as an act by the devil) or was more truly immanent. In many cases, the two intertwine, as interior and spontaneous thoughts and desires on the part of a man spur the devil to reflect them back in magnified form.[56]

Kelly has suggested that, in contrast to female virgins, male virginity lacks any particular kind of threat; in a parallel fashion, McInerney argues that, whereas for women, chastity is the preservation of the sealed body, with men it 'appears to have to do . . . with keeping what is inside in, with the retention of seed'.[57] I would argue, however, that there is a threat to male virginity, and it lies in the problematic and permeable relationship between 'inside' and 'outside'. Desire lurks within, located in an amorphous and shadowy interiority, that can at certain points be identified with the body, but at other points dances away into the shadows of the mind. But desire becomes most dangerous when it meets an exterior element with which it can resonate and which amplifies it: the sight or presence of a woman. And yet these triggers for desire may also be imagined, not real. So male virgins do have to keep the 'outside out' – but with a rather uncertain notion of what constitutes 'outside' and where the boundaries of 'in' and 'out' are located. If one drama of masculinity is the exercise of the will over the body, masculinity's ever-present collapse is also founded on the will, and its limits.

Gerald's metaphor of the worked linen would presumably have been a reasonably comforting one for his clerical audience, finding their feet in this new world of male chastity and self-control. It promises progression, a plan, a reassuring teleology. But Gerald (like Jacobus and Caesarius) was writing under the shadow of a longer cultural tradition, using narratives passed down within Christian discourse over several centuries. The ghosts of the early Church haunted the high Middle Ages in these stories, bringing with them confused and conflicting ideas about purity and selfhood, forged in very different times and contexts.[58] And these tensions had effects not only within narrative, but also on real men in their lived experiences. When a bishop, in 1300, came to admonish Benedictine monks on chastity and good conduct, he reminded them that they should guard themselves against the company of women (forbidding them the cloister, the refectory, dormitory and infirmary). Why? Not because the women would attempt to tie them up and seduce them, but because it was from women that sprang 'temptation, perverse thoughts, and shameful fantasies'.[59] The exclusion of women from the lives of men was misogynist, certainly; but it was rooted in the failures of masculinity, in the failure of the male *will*. The labour of continence was beyond many, and male virgins – those ascendant, angelic beings – were undoubtedly, as McInerney puts it, 'as rare as hen's teeth'.[60] Most men would have to settle for twisting the yarn of male selfhood indefinitely; and as any textile historian knows, linen dirties and decays over time.

Notes

My thanks to Jacqueline Murray, Anke Bernau and Sarah Salih for thoughts, comments and suggestions for this article.

[1] 'Bissus enim de terra oritur viridis, sed eruta siccatur, tunditur, coquitur torquetur, et magno longoque exercitio ad candidum perduciter colorem. Sic caro nostra ut ad virtutem decoremque perveniat castitatis necesse est jejunet, oret, vigilet, et omni continentia laboret et delectationes ingenitas siccet, ut ad eam dignitatem virtutis quam desideramus ascendat. Retorquetur autem bissus ne facile solvatur, cum non solum carnis luxuria restringitur, sed tota ejus memoria ab intimo corde eradicatur'; Gerald of Wales, *Gemma Ecclesiastica*, distinctione II, chapter 1 (II/1), in *Giraldus Cambrensis Opera*, ed. J. S. Brewer, Rolls Series, 21 (London: Longman, 1862), vol. 2, p. 173 (henceforth *Gemma*). An English translation is provided in Gerald of Wales, *The Jewel of the Church: A Translation of* Gemma Ecclesiastica *by Giraldus Cambrensis*, ed. and trans. John J. Hagen (Leiden: Brill, 1979), p. 134 (henceforth *Jewel*). My translation differs from Hagen's somewhat, but I will provide references in the notes to both Latin and English versions.

2 See Dyan Elliott, *Fallen Bodies: Pollution, Sexuality and Demonology in the Middle Ages* (Philadelphia: University of Pennsylvania Press, 1999), p. 22; Jo Ann McNamara, 'The *Herrenfrage*: the restructuring of the gender system, 1050–1150', in Clare A. Lees (ed.), *Medieval Masculinities: Regarding Men in the Middle Ages* (Minneapolis: University of Minnesota Press, 1994), pp. 3–29. Gerald frames his lengthy discussion of continence with an emphasis on the eucharist and the need for clerical purity; *Gemma*, II, proem, p. 168, and II/1, p. 170; *Jewel*, pp. 127, 131. Legislation against clerical marriage and concubinage had been framed in the eleventh century, but anxiety about these issues was reaching a new pitch of insistence in the mid- to late twelfth century; see Henry Charles Lea, *A History of Sacerdotal Celibacy in the Christian Church*, 2 vols (London: Williams & Norgate, 1907), vol. 1, pp. 385–407; Jo Ann McNamara, 'Chaste marriage and clerical celibacy', in Vern L. Bullough and James A. Brundage (eds), *Sexual Practices and the Medieval Church* (Buffalo, NY: Prometheus Books, 1982), pp. 22–33.

3 Maud Burnett McInerney, 'Rhetoric, power and integrity in the passion of the virgin martyr', in Kathleen Coyne Kelly and Marina Leslie (eds), *Menacing Virgins: Representing Virginity in the Middle Ages and Renaissance* (London: Associated University Presses, 1999), pp. 50–70 (p. 57).

4 On the complexities of feminine virginity, see Sarah Salih, *Versions of Virginity in Late Medieval England* (Cambridge: Brewer, 2001).

5 For discussion, see Elliott, *Fallen Bodies*, pp. 14–34.

6 See also McInerney's assessment that, for many medieval writers, 'virginity' and 'chastity' are used interchangeably when applied to men; 'Rhetoric, power, and integrity', p. 58.

7 Kathleen Coyne Kelly, *Performing Virginity and Testing Chastity in the Middle Ages* (London: Routledge, 2000), pp. 91–118.

8 Ibid., pp. 93–101, 118.

9 Steve Neale, 'Masculinity as spectacle: reflections on men and mainstream cinema', *Screen*, 24 (1983), 2–16 (16).

10 Leon Hunt, 'What are big boys made of? *Spartacus*, *El Cid*, and the male epic', in Pat Kirkham and Janet Thumim (eds), *You Tarzan: Masculinity, Movies, and Men* (London: Lawrence & Wishart, 1993), pp. 65–83 (p. 65).

11 Gerald, *Gemma*, II/10, pp. 213–15; *Jewel*, pp. 163–4.

12 Jacobus de Voragine, *The Golden Legend*, trans. W. G. Ryan, 2 vols (Princeton: Princeton University Press, 1993), vol. 1, p. 187; vol. 2, p. 99.

13 For an analysis of the broader context of monastic discipline of selfhood, see Talal Asad, 'On ritual and discipline in medieval Christian monasticism', *Economy and Society*, 16 (1987), 159–203.

14 Gerald of Wales notes the division himself, explaining that having presented examples of continence based on external aids, such as briar patches, he is now going to discuss triumphs through what he calls 'interior virtue divinely inspired'; *Gemma*, II/11, p. 216; *Jewel*, pp. 165–6.

[15] Jacobus, *Golden Legend*, vol. 2, p. 13; vol. 1, p. 371; vol. 2, p. 99. See similarly Gerald, *Gemma*, II/11, p. 222; *Jewel*, p. 169; the source of the story is William of St Thierry's Life of Bernard. In the *Golden Legend*, Bernard survives another night-time encounter with an amorous lass by the simple expedient of rolling over in bed and ignoring her until she goes away; vol. 2, p. 99.

[16] Gerald, *Gemma*, II/11, pp. 216–18; *Jewel*, pp. 166–7.

[17] Gerald, *Gemma*, II/11, p. 225; *Jewel*, p. 172.

[18] Caesarius Heisterbacensis, *Dialogus miraculorum*, ed. Joseph Strange, 2 vols (Cologne, 1851), IV/94 (vol. 1, pp. 260–1). English translation in Caesarius of Heisterbach, *The Dialogue on Miracles*, trans. H. von E. Scott and C. C. Swinton Bland, 2 vols (London: Routledge, 1929), vol. 1, pp. 297–8.

[19] Caesarius, *Dialogus miraculorum*, V/51.

[20] Gerald, *Gemma*, II/11, pp. 222, 223–4; *Jewel*, pp. 170, 172.

[21] Jacobus, *Golden Legend*, vol. 2, pp. 365–6.

[22] Ibid., vol. 1, p. 93.

[23] See also the story of a man being seduced by a devil in the shape of a woman. St Bernard, dressed as a pilgrim, arrives and asks the woman a series of questions, which result in her unmasking as a demon. As the text notes, a very similar story is told with regard to St Andrew: Jacobus, *Golden Legend*, vol. 2, pp. 113–14.

[24] Caesarius, *Dialogus miraculorum*, VII/33; *Dialogue*, vol. 1, pp. 501–2; Gerald, *Gemma*, II/11, pp. 224–5; *Jewel*, p. 171.

[25] Jacobus, *Golden Legend*, vol. 2, p. 30.

[26] Ibid., vol. 2, pp. 49–50.

[27] Ibid., vol. 1, p. 149.

[28] Caesarius, *Dialogus miraculorum*, IV/97; *Dialogue*, vol. 1, pp. 302–3. Note that the English translation bowdlerizes the story, omitting the dog.

[29] Gerald, *Gemma*, II/17, pp. 245–7; *Jewel*, pp. 187–8.

[30] Jacqueline Murray, 'Mystical castration: some reflections on Peter Abelard, Hugh of Lincoln and sexual control', in Murray (ed.), *Conflicted Identities and Multiple Masculinities: Men in the Medieval West* (New York: Garland, 1999), pp. 73–91 (p. 74).

[31] Jacobus, *Golden Legend*, vol. 2, p. 8.

[32] For the general background, see Jacqueline Murray, 'Supernatural castration: a response to masculine sexual anxiety in the Middle Ages', unpublished conference paper delivered at The Queer Middle Ages Conference, CUNY Graduate Center, New York, NY, October 1997. My thanks to the author for sharing this material with me. See also Matthew S. Kuefler, 'Castration and eunuchism in the Middle Ages', in Vern L. Bullough and James A. Brundage (eds), *Handbook of Medieval Sexuality* (New York: Garland, 1996), pp. 279–306.

[33] See Murray, 'Supernatural castration' and 'Mystical castration'; Elliott, *Fallen Bodies*, p. 16.

[34] Michel Foucault, 'The battle for chastity', in *Ethics, Subjectivity, and Truth: Essential Works of Foucault*, vol. 1, ed. Paul Rabinow (New York: New

Press, 1997), pp. 185–97 (p. 193). This essay – an extract from Foucault's unpublished fourth volume to his *History of Sexuality* – was originally published in Philippe Ariès and André Béjin (eds), *Western Sexuality* (Oxford: Blackwell, 1985); the more recent edition is to be preferred, as it contains a retranslation and some additional material.

[35] Jacobus, *Golden Legend*, vol. 2, p. 193–5.

[36] Caesarius, *Dialogus miraculorum*, IV/102; *Dialogue*, vol. 1, pp. 310–11.

[37] Gerald, *Gemma*, II/17, p. 248; *Jewel*, p. 189. One could note that for the priest to have a daughter-in-law implies a lack of prior chastity; as Gerald's general comments and exhortations about the relatively *recent* demand for clerical celibacy make clear, however, this was perhaps more a reflection of common reality than an implicit further condemnation.

[38] Gerald, *Gemma*, II/11, pp. 222–3; *Jewel*, p. 170.

[39] Caesarius, *Dialogus miraculorum*, IV/93; *Dialogue*, vol. 1, pp. 295–6.

[40] Jacobus, *Golden Legend*, vol. 1, pp. 84–5. This *contra* Kelly, who strenuously attempts to read the narrative as shifting attention away from the male virgin to his female tormentor; see *Performing Virginity*, pp. 96–7. One could usefully contrast this tale with the torments suffered by St Christina. Amongst other indignities, she has her tongue cut out, which she too then spits at her torturer; *Golden Legend*, vol. 1, p. 387. My thanks to Sarah Salih on this point.

[41] R. Howard Bloch, *Medieval Misogyny and the Invention of Western Romantic Love* (Chicago: University of Chicago Press, 1991), p. 100: 'a virgin seen is no longer a virgin'. Odo of Cluny is quoted in Jane Tibbetts Schulenberg, 'Saints and sex, *ca.*500–1100: striding down the nettled path of life', in Joyce E. Salisbury (ed.), *Sex in the Middle Ages: A Book of Essays* (New York: Garland, 1991), pp. 203–31 (p. 226).

[42] As, I would suggest, is ultimately the case in Jo Ann McNamara's undeniably important and imaginative '*Herrenfrage*', and 'An unresolved syllogism: the search for a Christian gender system', in Murray (ed.), *Conflicted Identities*, pp. 1–24.

[43] Gerald, *Gemma*, II/16, pp. 239–42; *Jewel*, pp. 182–4.

[44] See for example Alain de Lille's warning: 'When you are young, come close to a raging fire more readily than to a young woman': *The Art of Preaching*, trans. Gillian R. Evans (Kalamazoo: Cistercian Publications, 1981), p. 35.

[45] Gerald, *Gemma*, II/8, pp. 199–200; *Jewel*, pp. 153–4.

[46] Gerald, *Gemma*, II/9, p. 208; *Jewel*, p. 160.

[47] Gerald, *Gemma*, II/23, p. 279; *Jewel*, p. 211.

[48] Gerald, *Gemma*, II/2, p. 177; *Jewel*, p. 137.

[49] Pierre J. Payer, *The Bridling of Desire: Views of Sex in the Later Middle Ages* (Toronto: University of Toronto Press, 1993), p. 134.

[50] See, for example, the complicated story told about a cleric who spurns the love of a woman and is punished by falling hopelessly in love with another woman who rejects him in turn. The man enters a monastery, but suffers from unrequited desire for the rest of his days without relief. Having related

the story in great detail, Gerald seems uncertain about what it is supposed to show (as it appears to contradict most of what he has been saying about chastity and self-control): 'there are many things in this story to be wondered at', he says, and suggests that the cleric's punishment was divinely inflicted 'either as a punishment or as purification', which certainly leaves the interpretative options open; *Gemma*, II/13, pp. 228–31; *Jewel*, pp. 174–6.

51 Gerald, *Gemma*, II/14, pp. 232–5; *Jewel*, pp. 177–9.

52 Jacqueline Murray, '"The law of sin that is in my members": the problem of male embodiment', in Samantha J. E. Riches and Sarah Salih (eds), *Gender and Holiness: Men, Women and Saints in Late Medieval Europe* (London: Routledge, 2002), pp. 9–22. My thanks, once again, to the author for pre-publication access.

53 'Ultra naturam est non exercere quod natus sis, et interficere in te radicem tuam'; Gerald, *Gemma*, II/9, p. 208; *Jewel*, p. 160.

54 Elliott, *Fallen Bodies*, p. 47.

55 See Yves Ferroul, 'Abelard's blissful castration', in Jeffrey Jerome Cohen and Bonnie Wheeler (eds), *Becoming Male in the Middle Ages* (New York: Garland, 1997), pp. 129–49.

56 See Elliott's discussion of Augustine's theories about sexual fantasies: *Fallen Bodies*, p. 19.

57 Kelly, *Performing Virginity*, p. 95; McInerney, 'Rhetoric, power, and integrity', p. 58.

58 For these contexts, see Peter Brown, *The Body and Society: Men, Women and Sexual Renunciation in Early Christianity* (New York: Columbia University Press, 1988).

59 Statutes of Bishop Ralph of Walpole, 1300, in *Ely Chapter Ordinances and Visitation Records, 1241–1515*, ed. Seiriol J. A. Evans, *Camden Miscellany* 17, Camden Record Society, 3rd ser., 64 (London, 1940), pp. 10–11.

60 McInerney, 'Rhetoric, power, and integrity', p. 58.

7

Edward the Celibate, Edward the Saint: Virginity in the Construction of Edward the Confessor

JOANNA HUNTINGTON

'The theory that Edward's childlessness was due to deliberate abstention from sexual relations lacks authority, plausibility, and diagnostic value.'[1] In his important work on Edward the Confessor, Frank Barlow rejects the possibility that Edward was a virgin. Indeed, for Barlow, virginity is an irritation:

> not only is the story of Edward's virginity without good authority, it is also implausible, and, far from helping us to understand the situation and events, merely obscures. It is a typical example of that irrationality and ignorant credulity with which the eleventh century abounds.[2]

This chapter, however, is concerned not with the 'real' Edward, but with a shift in the portrayal of Edward the Celibate, which played a crucial part in the creation of Edward the Saint. Later medieval constructions of Edward provided models of kingship and legitimization of the contemporary royal dynasty via its association with the saintly Edward.[3] In the early stages of his cult, however, Edward's sanctity was not fixed, but took different forms which reflected and consolidated the concerns of his biographers. Just as there are 'multiple masculinities', so too there are multiple virginities, some of which are seen in Edward's *vitae*.[4] That one version of his virginity eventually triumphed over the others contributes to our emerging understanding of twelfth-century perceptions of saintly virginity. I suggest, therefore, that tracing Edward's virginity, far from obfuscating, not only helps us better to understand the nature of Edward's early cult, but also offers useful insights into twelfth-century paradigms and deployments of virginity.

Edward's purported virginity is referred to in several sources, but is chiefly a product of his *vitae* and the documents of his canonization process. The early Latin *vitae* will be considered here: the main focus will be Osbert of Clare's *Vita beati Eadwardi regis Anglorum*,[5] with reference to the eleventh-century anonymous *Vita Ædwardi regis qui apud Westmonasterium requiescit*[6] and Aelred of Rievaulx's *Vita S. Edwardi regis et confessoris*.[7] The development of the story of Edward's virginity, states Barlow, 'is not in doubt . . . Osbert of Clare took three themes from [*Vita Æd.*]: God's choice of Edward as king before his birth, Edward's life-long chastity, and his miracles, and on the basis of these constructed a fully realized saint's life.'[8] I suggest that this model of the development of the story of Edward's chastity needs amending.

The anonymous work is an intriguing and much-studied text.[9] There is still debate as to the date and process of the *vita*'s composition: it has been variously suggested that it was written in two stages, the first part in 1065–6 and the second part in 1067,[10] as a single piece in 1068–70,[11] or as a single piece but earlier, perhaps in 1066–7.[12] Overall, Barlow's model of the two-stage composition is the most convincing. The *Vita Æd.* essentially concerns itself with the interests of the king's wife Edith. In the first section, according to Barlow's editorial division, Edward is almost marginalized, and the real heroes are Edith, her father Godwin and her brothers. The second part focuses on Edward and his religious life.

The second *vita* was written *c.*1138 by Osbert of Clare, prior of Westminster.[13] This version is partially based on the latter section of the anonymous work, but downplays the earlier work's emphasis on Edith and her kin, and portrays Edward as saintly. Osbert's *Vita beati Ead.* supported the unsuccessful bid for Edward's canonization in *c.*1138–9. Having given a copy of his *vita* to the papal legate, Alberic, Osbert petitioned for Edward's canonization at the papal curia in autumn 1139.[14] Lukewarm support for this canonization bid came from Henry, bishop of Winchester, and the chapter of St Paul's. King Stephen's letter, which was apparently drafted by Osbert himself, is the only enthusiastic one.[15] In this, the incorruption of Edward's corpse – linked with his virginity – is stressed, and he is placed in the context of English kings who were holy by virtue of virginity, as opposed to martyrdom.[16] Osbert seems to have impressed Innocent II, but the petition was refused on the grounds that it was insufficiently supported by the testimony of bishops and abbots: it was felt that a saint for the whole realm should have more supporters throughout the realm.[17]

A second canonization bid, coordinated by Laurence, abbot of Westminster (*c.*1158–73) was successful. Presumably in response to Innocent II's objection, Laurence provided letters showing more widespread support for Edward's cause than in 1139.[18] A party was dispatched to the papal curia, bearing, in addition to the letters, a book of miracles, probably Osbert's *Vita beati Ead.*, and Edward was duly canonized by Alexander III in February 1161.[19]

Aelred of Rievaulx was commissioned by his kinsman Abbot Laurence to write a further *vita*, which was presented on 13 October 1163 at the translation of Edward's corpse.[20] Aelred's *vita* is based on that of Osbert, with additional elements including those from chronicles.[21] It was Aelred's *vita*, rather than either of the earlier texts, which was to enjoy medieval circulation in its own right and to be adapted for both subsequent texts and other media.[22] These, then, are the texts with which we are concerned. How do they portray Edward's virginity?

The Anonymous's account of Brihtwald's vision seems to set the scene for Edward's celibacy. Brihtwald, bishop of Wiltshire, having bewailed the desolation of the realm, falls asleep and in a vision sees St Peter consecrate a seemly man as king, and 'assign him a celibate life [*celibem ei uitam designare*]' (1992, p. 14).[23] When the king asks the apostle how the realm will fare, he is reassured: 'the kingdom of the English belongs to God; and after you He has provided for Himself a king according to His will' (1992, pp. 14–15). The phrase *celebs uita* is problematic. *Celebs* can imply celibate – either as a virgin or having abandoned sexual activity – or chastely monogamous.[24] Indeed, the Anonymous himself uses the term of Edith's brother Tostig's marriage:

> He renounced desire for all women except his wife of royal stock, and he governed the use of his body and tongue chastely, with more restraint, and wisely.

> *preter eandem regie stirpis uxorem suam omnium abdicans uoluptatem, celebs moderatius corporis et oris sui prudenter regere consuetudinem.* (1992, pp. 50–1)

Brihtwald's vision, then, is ambiguous with regard to Edward's purported virginity, and *celebs uita* might suggest bachelorhood, sexually active and monogamous marriage, or celibacy, either consciously spiritually motivated or not. In the second part of the *Vita Æd.*, Edward is described as having been 'consecrated to the kingdom less by men than . . . by Heaven. He preserved with holy chasteness [*sancta castimonia*] the dignity of his consecration, and lived his whole life dedicated to God in true innocence' (1992, pp. 90–3), which seems to reinforce the notion of sexual purity. Pierre J. Payer argues that, for moral philosophers and theologians, *castitas* 'is invariably associated with the rational control of lust'.[25] However he also points to a continued ambiguity about the exact definition and usage of terms such as *castitas*, *continentia* and *pudicitia* in the thirteenth century.[26]

Unfortunately, the single extant manuscript of the *Vita Æd.* is damaged at the point where a description of Edith and, presumably, of Edward's marriage and married life might be. Barlow makes a convincing case for his interpolation of Richard of Cirencester's account of Edith and her marriage to Edward into the Anonymous's *vita*.[27] Although his main source was Aelred's *vita*, Richard 'lifted' three passages from a manuscript similar to that which contains the extant *Vita Æd.*[28] Additionally, a passage of some 500 words, as yet untraced to any extant manuscript, treats of Edith and her marriage.[29] In this, the chastity is essentially Edith's, inculcated by her education at Wilton, and rendering her the perfect match for Edward:

> Christ had indeed prepared her for His beloved Edward, kindling in her from very childhood the love of chastity [*castitatis*], the hatred of vice, and the desire for virtue. Such a bride – whose every virtue it is completely beyond our ability to describe – was therefore entirely suitable for this great king.[30]

Edward is depicted as enthusiastically embracing the match: 'Edward agreed all the more readily to contract this marriage because he knew that with the advice and help of . . . Godwin he would have a firmer hold on his hereditary rights in England.'[31] In the light of the celibacy and/or chastity alluded to in the account of Brihtwald's vision, this passage may be suggesting that Edith and Edward are celibate by mutual choice and inclination. Although Edith is described as returning to the king's bedchamber after her repudiation (1992, pp. 44–5), for the most part she is described as Edward's daughter or mother.[32]

Monika Otter's recent work corroborates the notion that, in the *Vita Æd.*, such virginity as there is, is Edith's. She draws attention to the epithalamium which ostensibly celebrates Wilton, and convincingly argues that it is a thinly veiled epithalamium to Edith as a spiritual mother, whose power is intrinsically linked with the prosperity of the realm.[33] Thus Edith's barrenness is presented as spiritually motivated chastity which produces spiritual fecundity. To this end, the Anonymous hints that the marriage was chaste by mutual agreement. We see, then, that while the *Vita Æd.* does not overtly articulate the story of a mutually chosen and spiritually motivated celibate marriage, it nonetheless can be seen as suggesting one.

Barlow states that 'Osbert of Clare . . . produced the first full-blown account of the chaste marriage.'[34] As we will see, Osbert certainly is wresting chastity from Edith and situating it – and its concomitant spiritual value – with Edward. Nonetheless, his is in fact still not a 'full-blown account of the chaste marriage'. On the contrary, in the *Vita beati Ead.*, Edward's virginity in marriage is little dwelt upon compared to his virginity in death.

In his introductory letter to Alberic of Ostia, Osbert points to four attributes of Edward. First, he was a distinguished and great king; second, his holiness is proven by miracles: 'as has been so often shown to the world by heavenly miracles, [he] deserves, as confirmed by signs, to be celebrated with a feast among men on earth' (p. 65). Third, he was a virgin, which has rendered his corpse incorruptible: '[his] form of integrity . . . still today shows in the flesh with how much purity of mind he cultivated the title of virginity [*titulos virginitatis*]' (p. 66). The incorruption of Edward's corpse had been discovered in 1102, as recounted by Osbert (pp. 121–3), and is associated in his text with Edward's virginity. Finally, Edward was a patron of justice (p. 66).

Osbert's account of Brihtwald's vision (p. 72) is essentially the same as the Anonymous's.[35] His account of Edward's marriage, however, differs.[36] Having described the king's appearance and character, Osbert tells us that 'the virgin mother of God dwelt always in [Edward's] heart, always on his lips. Having become an abode of virginity [*virginitatis factus domicilium*], he held up the virginal way of life as a model for himself' (p. 74). Edward, however, is urged to marry. Osbert briefly portrays the marriage as an assault on Edward's chastity perpetrated by others: 'some men . . . strove that his modesty should be shipwrecked [*ut naufragium incideret eius pudicitia*]' (p. 74). Both Osbert and his Edward, however, quickly seem reconciled to the choice of Edith, as Osbert immediately goes on to extol her virtues (although not as much as in Richard of Cirencester's account), and we are told that 'merciful God, who preserved his blessed confessor Alexius a virgin, kept . . . St Edward the king all the days of his life in the purity of the flesh [*in carnis puritate*]'.[37] As in the Anonymous's *Vita Æd.*, Edith is described as Edward's daughter – 'the excellent queen served him as a daughter, and from the beginning of their marriage arrayed him in many kinds of embroidered robes'[38] – and safeguards the secrecy of their chaste marriage: 'she preserved the secret of the king's chasteness [*castimoniam*] of which she had learned, and kept those counsels that she knew'.[39] Osbert concludes this passage with a reminder that 'even today [Edward's] flesh remains in an urn entirely incorrupt' (p. 75), before turning to Edward's first vision within the narrative.

After this passage, Edward's chastity is barely touched upon until those passages which deal with his death and post-mortem career. Immediately before the account of Edward's miraculous cure of a young woman, also recounted in the *Vita Æd.*, Osbert, like the Anonymous and with very similar wording, recalls Brihtwald's vision and Edward's subsequent chastity: '[Edward was] consecrated by the adminstration of divine grace. Indeed the dignity of this great consecration always increased day by day, which perpetual chasteness [*castimonia*] accompanied, leading him to glory, lest through legitimate joining of the flesh he should veer towards ruin' (pp. 92–3). Osbert renders Edward's *castimonia* more explicitly non-sexual than does the Anonymous, by emphasizing that sexual relations with Edith would have been licit. Osbert places two further references to a chaste marriage with Edith rather than Edward. As Edward sickens, his patronage of Westminster is taken over on his behalf by Edith, 'whom he had possessed only in appearance and whose secrets this man of God did not know in the flesh'.[40] Similarly, during the account of Edward's death, Edith is described as 'she in whom no corruption of the flesh inhered, even though it would have been permitted by law' (p. 110). These last two examples, however, are at the point of Edward's death and thus, arguably, associated more with Edward's corpse than his living body.

What, then, can we say about the portrayal of Edward's virginity in Osbert's *Vita beati Ead.*? Osbert has developed the notion of mutually chosen celibacy suggested by the Anonymous, and has expanded on the frequently ambiguous comments of the earlier work. However, there is an important qualification: Edward's virginity is for the most part important to Osbert only in relation to the incorrupt corpse, revealed in 1102. His account of this provides the denouement of Osbert's *vita*, and is flagged at several points throughout the text. With but a few exceptions, wherever Edward's chastity is mentioned or alluded to, it is in connection to his dying, death and/or the incorruption of his corpse. Even the account of his marriage is concluded with a reference to his corpse. At one point Osbert misses what would seem to be an ideal opportunity to underline Edward's lived virginity, as he describes the horror of Edward's subjects at his proposed pilgrimage to Rome: they feared that the king might die or meet some injury en route, depriving the realm of royal heirs (p. 78). Although Osbert has previously mentioned the secrecy of the king and queen's chastity, it is surprising that he does not take this opportunity to comment again on the spiritual value of Edward's chastity. It is less surprising, however, if we see that Osbert is quite simply not interested in Edward the man as virgin. Instead, his interest is in Edward the virgin corpse.

This corroborates Barlow's model of the impetus behind the development of Edward's cult in the 1130s, culminating in Osbert's *vita* and the first canonization bid. Barlow sees this as a fundamentally Westminster-based process, and specifically Osbert-driven.[41] During a period of exile from Westminster, Osbert wrote a letter of self-justification to Abbot Herbert, in which he bewails the material state of Westminster Abbey, referring to

> the dilapidation of the church, the starving of the servants, the ruin of the monastic buildings, roofs out of repair, meals of the seniors cut down, the resources of the treasury diminished, walls and battlements broken and ruined, all that the brethren needed indiscreetly wasted by alien hands without your knowledge.[42]

This was not, it seems, mere hyperbole on Osbert's part; indeed, all was not well with the material fabric and financial position of the abbey.[43] Osbert's inventiveness in his determination to secure the rights and prestige of Westminster is seen in his part in the forgery of charters identified as the 'Westminster forgeries'.[44] Similarly, the material advantages of Edward's virginity and saintly corpse would have been desirable, to say nothing of the added prestige they guaranteed, and perhaps even more welcome in the light of the hostility existing at this time between Westminster Abbey and St Paul's in London.[45]

Having seen, then, the possible advantages of Osbert's highlighting Edward as a saintly corpse, let us return to one other aspect of Edward's virginity: it is static. Neither tested nor actively maintained, it just *is*. This must be placed in the context of medieval perceptions of virginity. Much work is still to be done on medieval representations of virginity, especially of male virginity. One needs to be aware of the danger of analysing different genres or genders according to a uniform template. However, two models of virginity recently proposed are apposite here. Kathleen Coyne Kelly has shown that, whereas female virginity is assaulted by violence or the threat thereof, male virginity is assayed, often by seduction.[46] Further, Sarah Salih has shown that virginity 'cannot be self-evident, but must be constituted perform-atively'.[47]

Osbert's Edward does not conform to either of these models. The only suggestion of struggle in the chastity of Osbert's Edward occurs in a description of Edward in an account of a miraculous cure: 'the king, offering a daily sacrifice to God in the dove and the turtle-dove, furnishing an example of chastity and of innocence to those who imitated him' (p. 95).[48] Admittedly, we do have here a suggestion of personal sacrifice, but it is as nothing compared to the struggles of another saintly noble layman, Gerald of Aurillac (CE 855–909). Gerald's virginity is constructed as being achieved through a mixture of divine assistance and personal determination, in spite of the devil's anger that Gerald had avoided the shipwreck of his modesty (*naufragium pudoris*): 'he constantly suggested lustful thoughts to him'.[49] Gerald almost succumbs, after a lengthy struggle, to the charms of a girl brought before him by the devil. Fortunately, God intervenes and renders the girl hideously deformed to Gerald's eyes just as he is about to take her.[50] Later, the 'horror he felt for carnal obscenity may be judged from the fact that he never incurred a nocturnal illusion without grief'.[51] That nocturnal illusions were incurred at all imbues Gerald's chastity with a sense of struggle: it is not presented as a fait accompli, but is performative and actively maintained.

William of Malmesbury's *Vita Wulfstani*, written in the second quarter of the twelfth century, also depicts struggle and danger in the attempted shipwreck of a saint's modesty (*naufragium pudoris*).[52] A local girl sets out to tempt Wulfstan, with dancing, lewd gestures and come-hither looks. Eventually she is almost successful: 'he . . . panted with desire, completely reduced by her disarming gestures', but he comes to his senses and flees into some prickly bushes. A miraculous cloud descends upon him and cools his ardour, after which he is so free from lustful thoughts that he is not even troubled by nocturnal emissions.[53] Even so, Wulfstan's chastity is still explicity maintained: his chasteness (*castimoniam*) is 'an integrity as briskly maintained by him as its loss was keenly pursued by others'.[54]

By contrast, in the *Vita beati Ead.*, Edward's celibacy is neither explicitly threatened nor maintained by struggle. Instead it is simply presented as a fait accompli: 'having become an abode of virginity' (p. 74). Whilst the phrase suggests that Edward was not always virginal, the *vita* gives no account of his achieving that state. Osbert makes a brief gesture towards presenting Edward's celibacy as assayed, as he describes Edward's subjects intending the shipwreck of his chastity, but from the very next sentence, we see that the plan was not dastardly:

> there was a discussion about the consort who should cleave to the royal side, and it was decided to seek a wife worthy of such a husband from among the daughters of the princes. One alone was found in that people, inferior to none, superior to all.[55]

This is not to say, though, that virginity was not important to Osbert. On the contrary, it was a concept dear to his heart.[56] The swift move in *Vita beati Ead.*, from potentially shipwrecked chastity to reconciliation to a suitable marriage, contrasts with an analogous situation in Osbert's *vita* of Ethelbert, eighth-century king of East Anglia.[57] As Ethelbert's magnates urge him to marry, Osbert dwells in far more detail on Ethelbert's internal dilemma and reluctance to forsake virginity, before his eventual acceptance of the match.[58] For Edward, however, no such internal dilemma is depicted. Virginity simply defines Edward's body as a site of saintly power. Westminster Abbey, in turn, becomes a locus of saintly power. Osbert's *vita*, then, seems to be part of the trend outlined by Susan J. Ridyard, by which post-conquest authors adopted pre-conquest Anglo-Saxon saints to further the interests of specific religious communities.[59] Osbert in particular seems to have written *vitae* to this end, perhaps expressing gratitude to those houses with which he had 'a significant personal connection'.[60] The virginity of Osbert's Edward is situated in his corpse, and nuanced to further Westminster's interests. The virginity of a dead virgin is stable. To find an Edward whose virginity is lived and performative, we need to turn to Aelred.

In the prologue, Aelred places Edward in the company of kings who 'reigned with justice and holiness and sought to be of use to the people rather than to rule over them'. This *rex iustus* exercised 'self-restraint in the midst of so much wealth and luxury'.[61] In his preface, Aelred's first comment on Edward after the modesty topos is: 'I found here someone more than man: someone who "in his days pleased God and was found righteous", who, after the salvific seed had been conceived, not satisfied with the thirty- or sixtyfold return, ambitiously rose to the hundredfold harvest of virginity.'[62] Aelred elaborates on Osbert's account of Edward's exile in Normandy, stating that he 'was immune from the vices with which that age or that kind of man are wont to be entangled . . . He kept his body chaste [*castus*]' (col. 742). This is followed by the chapter dealing with Brihtwald's vision. The vision itself is recounted in much the same way as by the Anonymous and Osbert: '[the apostle] gave [Edward] counsels of salvation, particularly commending the celibate life [*caelibem vitam*]' (col. 743). Although there is the same potential ambiguity about the exact meaning of *celebs* as outlined above, the intensifier *praecipue* draws attention to the value of a celibate life.

Aelred's treatment of Edward's vow to make a pilgrimage to Rome eliminates the ambiguity of Osbert's account noted above. Not only does Aelred insert the vow itself, during the period within his narrative of Edward's exile,[63] he also removes the suggestion that the king's subjects anticipated heirs to the kingdom, which Osbert included in *Vita beati Ead*. It is Aelred's treatment of Edward's marriage, however, that shows the most marked change in the representation of his chastity. Here, for the first time, we get a sense of Edward's chastity being fragile when his nobles suggest he should marry: 'the king was aghast, frightened about the treasure which he kept in an earthen vessel, fearing that it could easily be destroyed by heat' (col. 747). This motif of fragile virginity was to be applied in stronger terms in treatises addressed to women. Aelred himself expands upon a similar reference to 2 Corinthians 4:7 in *De Institutis Inclusarum* by explicating Ecclesiasticus 34:9, introducing the notion that heat might threaten the 'treasure', but is necessary to prove its worth:

> Bear in mind always what a precious treasure you bear in how fragile a vessel . . . 'The man who has not been tested is not accepted.' Virginity is the gold, the cell is the crucible, the devil is the assayer, temptation is the fire. The virgin's flesh is the earthenware vessel in which the gold is put to be tested. If it is broken by the intensity of the heat the gold is spilt and no craftsman can put the vessel together again.[64]

Here the notions discussed above – that virginity is both fragile and performative, proven through being tested – are encapsulated. Aelred stops short of making Edward's virginity as persistently vulnerable as virginity is in texts addressed to women, but it is still notably more fragile than that presented by Osbert. Unlike Osbert, Aelred dwells on Edward's dilemma: 'but what to do? If he refused more stubbornly, he was afraid lest the sweet secret of his resolve might be betrayed: if he agreed to their pressure, he dreaded the shipwreck of his modesty [*naufragium pudicitiae*].' Aelred's courtiers are correspondingly more insistent than Osbert's: 'they insisted, in season and out of season'. The threatened 'shipwreck' seems far more alarming to Aelred's Edward than to Osbert's, and closer to those of Gerald and Wulfstan. This is reinforced by the impassioned prayer Aelred puts into Edward's mouth:

> O Good Jesu, your mercy once preserved three boys unscathed in the Babylonian furnace. By your aid Joseph kept his chastity . . . The noble Susannah, supported by your aid, vindicated her virtue against the libidinous priests. Holy Judith preserved the city from siege through her singular chastity, which was neither shaken nor even tempted among the royal banquets and brimming cups of Holophernes . . . And far above all these, you willed . . . your Mother, to be both spouse and virgin, nor did the sacrament of matrimony bring an end to her virginity . . . Come to my aid, therefore . . . help me to undertake the sacrament of marriage in such a way as not to endanger my modesty [*pudicitiae*]. [65]

As in Richard of Cirencester's account, the childhood education of Aelred's Edith has rendered her a worthy helpmeet for Edward: 'she it was that Christ prepared for his beloved Edward, inspiring her from childhood with a desire for chastity [*castitatis*], hatred of vices and love of virtue'.[66] Here, for the first time in Edward's hagiography, we have the explicitly mutually chosen chaste marriage which was to feature in subsequent versions of his story:

> the king and queen, once united, agreed to preserve their chastity [*castitate*] . . . She became a wife in heart, but not in flesh: he a husband in name, not in deed. Their conjugal affection remained, without the conjugal act, as did the embraces of a chaste love without the defloration of her virginity. He loved, but was not corrupted; she was beloved but not touched, and like a second Abishag warmed the king with her love but did

not dissipate him with lust; she was a delight to his will, but he did not soften in his desires. (col. 748)[67]

Aelred further insists that their chastity was spiritually rather than politically motivated.[68] He makes the link between Edward's celibacy and his visionary powers more explicit than do the Anonymous and Osbert:

> sure witness to the king's chastity [*castitati*] is borne by his pure mind, for, drained of all the dregs of pulsating vice, and detached, it could regard present things and know future things, more or less as if they were placed before his eyes, as the following chapter will declare. (col. 748)[69]

Aelred's Edward, then, is a virgin in life, not just in death as in Osbert's *vita*. Aelred attributes not only Edward's visionary powers but also his miraculous healing powers partially to his chastity:

> 'happy the man who is found without stain, who goes not after gold nor places his trust in a well-filled treasury'. He was 'found without stain' because of the privilege of his chastity [*castitatis*]. He 'went not after gold' but rather gave it away. He 'put no trust in his treasury' since he did not so much diminish as extinguish it in God's cause . . . He has done wonderful things in his lifetime, restoring sight to the blind, steps to the lame; dispersing fevers, healing the paralytic and curing the different ills of mankind.[70]

Aelred also introduces the miracle of the ring, in which Edward gives his ring to a pilgrim, who transpires to be John the Evangelist, who holds Edward 'in great affection for the sake of his chastity (*castitatis*)', thus emphasizing both Edward's devotion to John and Edward's chastity.[71] The introduction of John as a spiritual patron and exemplar is, as pointed out by Marsha L. Dutton, in accordance with a devotion to the evangelist apparent elsewhere in Aelred's works,[72] but notwithstanding, it also serves to underline Edward's virginity more than Osbert had done.

Upon Edward's death, therefore, references to his virginity are an extension of those within the narrative of his lifetime. When we hear, for example, that 'the glory of the stripped body increased their amazement, for it shone so glitteringly with snowy whiteness that the splendour of his virginity [*virginitatis*] could not escape even the most incredulous' (col.

776), this is in the context of Edward's lived virginity. In Aelred's *vita*, Edward is a virgin king, whose virginity is assayed but maintained, and demonstrated to have conferred saintly powers in life, which sets the scene for his posthumous career as a virginal and saintly corpse.[73]

In all three *vitae*, Edward is a *rex iustus*:[74] virginity is not the only feature of his twelfth-century saintly character. In this respect he corroborates Salih's contention that while 'several male saints are approvingly referred to as chaste or virginal . . . their sexual status is rarely the locus of their sanctity, as is often the case for women'.[75] However, there is a marked difference in the presentation of his chastity. The Anonymous hints at a celibate marriage, with an emphasis on Edith's resulting spiritual fecundity. Osbert wrests the virginity from Edith and places it squarely with Edward, although it is not a lived virginity – it serves rather to manifest posthumous saintly virtue. Aelred is the first to develop the notion of a lived, performative virginity for Edward. To the Anonymous, Edward is Edith's husband; to Osbert, he is a virginal saintly corpse; to Aelred, he is virgin king in life, then saintly virgin corpse.

The shift in Edward's virginity proposed here continues in texts beyond the remit of the current chapter. Thus, for example, the *Estoire de Seint Aedward* of the mid-thirteenth century expands on Aelred's version of both Edward's dilemma at the proposed marriage's threat to his virginity and the mutual choice of celibacy of Edward and Edith.[76] Edward is described as saintly by virtue of his having conquered '[his] flesh, the devil and the world'.[77] Edward's virginity, finally, is a martyrdom: 'By the conquest over fleshly lust / Well ought he to be called a martyr.'[78] It was this aspect of Edward's sanctity which was to prove particularly appealing to Richard II.[79]

We have seen that, for Osbert, Edward's virginity is situated in his corpse, presumably to further Westminster Abbey's interests, and that the localized nature of the first canonization bid was cited as the reason for its rejection. The second bid addressed this objection with letters from throughout the realm. In their current form, seven out of the thirteen extant letters supporting this bid draw attention to Edward's virginity – in the context of his incorrupt corpse.[80] Presumably the geographical spread of the supporting letters helped to mitigate the Westminster bias of Osbert's *vita*. The extant letter from Alexander III conferring saintly status on Edward, however, does not mention his virginity, commending instead miracles which Edward had performed in life and death.[81]

Aelred's *vita*, perhaps in response to the papal letters of 1139 and 1161, offers a new version of Edward's virginity, and hence of his sanctity. Explicitly linked to prophetic and healing powers, it renders Edward like other models of saintly virginity, and hence more widely appealing beyond the immediate confines of Westminster. It was indeed this text which proved more to the tastes of subsequent patrons, translators, artists and audiences beyond Westminster. A marked change in monastic literary tastes in the mid-twelfth century has been identified, in which writers such as Osbert were supplanted by a new style, less ornate and wordy.[82] This may account for the popularity of Aelred's *vita* over its predecessors. However, the shift in the depiction of Edward's virginity itself might have contributed to the eventual triumph of Aelred's Edward.

This interpretation, then, does not challenge Barlow's overall model of Osbert's *vita* being driven by Westminster Abbey's concerns and by Osbert specifically. The identification of changing nuances in Edward's successive constructed virginities, however, does add to our understanding of the concerns which drove the development of his cult, providing a register of attitudes to both Edward and saintly virginities in the twelfth century on which to build.

Notes

I would like to thank Katherine J. Lewis, Victoria Thompson, Sarah Salih, Anke Bernau, Peter Biller and Felicity Riddy for their advice and encouragement for this chapter.

[1] Frank Barlow, *Edward the Confessor*, 2nd edn (New Haven: Yale University Press, 1997), p. 82.

[2] Ibid., p. 84.

[3] Thus Paul Binski, 'Reflections on *La estoire de Seint Aedward le rei*: hagiography and kingship in thirteenth-century England', *Journal of Medieval History*, 16 (1990), 333–50, for example, on the mid-thirteenth-century *La estoire de Seint Aedward le rei*.

[4] On the multiplicity of masculinities, see, for instance, Jacqueline Murray (ed.), *Conflicted Identities and Multiple Masculinities: Men in the Medieval West* (New York: Garland, 1999). On virginities, see, for example, Sarah Salih, *Versions of Virginity in Late Medieval England* (Cambridge: Brewer, 2001).

[5] 'La vie de S. Édouard le Confesseur par Osbert de Clare', ed. Marc Bloch, *Analecta Bollandiana*, 41 (1923), 5–131; hereafter Osbert, *Vita beati Ead.* References to Bloch's introduction will be cited as Bloch, 'La vie'.

Translations of the Latin text are mine (unless otherwise stated), with the unfailingly patient guidance of Jim Binns, for which I would like to note immense gratitude. I am also indebted to Jill Yeomans for her assistance with Bloch's introduction. Throughout this chapter, published translations are used where possible, but on occasion, where the published translation has preferred a flowing modern translation to literal translation, I have altered the translation slightly. Where the translation cited here differs greatly from a published translation, the Latin edition only will be referenced. Elsewhere, the relevant passage in the published translation will be referenced in brackets, even if the translation here differs slightly, so that the reader is able to refer easily to the sources.

[6] *The Life of King Edward Who Rests at Westminster: Attributed to a Monk of Saint-Bertin*, trans. Frank Barlow (1st edn, London: Thomas Nelson & Sons, 1962; 2nd edn, Oxford: Clarendon Press, 1992); hereafter Anon., *Vita Æd.* For the most part, the 2nd edn is cited here, but I have also occasionally cited the 1st edn, therefore (1962) or (1992) will denote the 1st or 2nd edns respectively. References to Barlow's introduction will be cited as Barlow, *Vita Æd.* (1962) or (1992).

[7] *PL*, 195, cols 737–90; hereafter Aelred, *Vita S. Ed. Life of St. Edward the Confessor*, trans. Jerome Bertram, 2nd edn (Southampton: St Austin Press, 1997); hereafter (Aelred, *Life*), where my own translations are not used.

[8] Barlow, *Edward the Confessor*, p. 82.

[9] An exhaustive list is neither practical nor necessary here, but in addition to Barlow, *Vita Æd.* and *Edward the Confessor*, see, for example, Pauline Stafford, *Queen Emma and Queen Edith: Queenship and Women's Power in Eleventh-Century England* (Oxford: Blackwell, 1997); Monika Otter, 'Closed doors: an epithalamium for Queen Edith, widow and virgin', in Cindy L. Carlson and Angela Jane Weisl (eds), *Constructions of Widowhood and Virginity in the Middle Ages* (New York: St Martin's Press, 1999), pp. 63–92.

[10] Barlow, *Vita Æd.* (1992), pp. xxix–xxxiii.

[11] Eleanor K. Heningham, 'The literary unity, the date and the purpose of the Lady Edith's book, "The life of King Edward who rests at Westminster"', *Albion*, 7 (1975), 24–40.

[12] Stafford, *Queen Emma and Queen Edith*, pp. 40–1.

[13] On Osbert's eventful and troubled career, see J. Armitage Robinson, 'Westminster in the twelfth century: Osbert of Clare', *Church Quarterly Review*, 68 (1909), 336–56; repr. as 'A sketch of Osbert's career', in *The Letters of Osbert of Clare, Prior of Westminster*, ed. E. W. Williamson (1929; repr. Oxford: Oxford University Press, 1998), pp. 1–20; Susan J. Ridyard, *The Royal Saints of Anglo-Saxon England: A Study of West Saxon and East Anglian Cults* (Cambridge: Cambridge University Press, 1988), pp. 16–37; Emma Mason, *Westminster Abbey and its People, c.1050–c .1216* (Woodbridge: Boydell, 1996), pp. 89–91. Brian Briggs's current doctoral work on Osbert is eagerly awaited.

[14] Barlow, *Edward the Confessor*, pp. 274–7; Mason, *Westminster Abbey*, p. 39; Bernhard W. Scholz, 'The canonization of Edward the Confessor', *Speculum*, 36 (1961), 38–60 (39–40).

[15] *Letters of Osbert*, ep. 16–18, pp. 85–7; Robinson, 'Westminster in the twelfth century', p.18.

[16] *Letters of Osbert*, ep. 17, pp. 85–6.

[17] Ibid., ep. 19, pp. 87–8. On the political factors which may also have influenced Innocent's decision, see Mason, *Westminster Abbey*, p. 302; Barlow, *Edward the Confessor*, p. 276; Scholz, 'Canonization of Edward the Confessor', 47–8.

[18] Barlow, *Edward the Confessor*, pp. 278–9. Thirteen of the letters are extant (reproduced in ibid., appendix D, pp. 309–24). On these letters, see below. The extent of Osbert's involvement in this second bid is uncertain; ibid., p. 280, n. 6; Robinson, 'Westminster in the twelfth century', p. 19.

[19] Scholz, 'Canonization of Edward the Confessor', 50; Barlow, *Edward the Confessor*, p. 280. Alexander's letter is reproduced in ibid., pp. 323–4.

[20] Aelred, *Vita S. Ed.*, cols 739–40 (Aelred, *Life*, pp. 17–18); cf. *The Life of Aelred of Rievaulx by Walter Daniel*, trans. F. M. Powicke (London: Nelson & Sons, 1950), pp. 41–2. The translation was delayed until the king was able to attend; Barlow, *Edward the Confessor*, pp. 281–3; Mason, *Westminster Abbey*, p. 53.

[21] Aelred, *Vita S. Ed.*, col. 740 (Aelred, *Life*, p. 18).

[22] Grace E. Moore, *The Middle English Verse Life of Edward the Confessor* (Philadelphia: University of Pennsylvania, 1942), pp. xli–xlii; Paul Binski, *Westminster Abbey and the Plantagenets: Kingship and the Representation of Power 1200–1400* (New Haven: Yale University Press, 1995), pp. 56–8. On the nun of Barking's Anglo-Norman verse life of the late twelfth century, for example, see Jocelyn Wogan-Browne, *Saints' Lives and Women's Literary Culture, 1150–1300* (Oxford: Oxford University Press, 2001), pp. 249–56. On the mid-thirteenth-century *La estoire de Seint Aedward le rei* (generally attributed to Matthew Paris and now Cambridge University Library MS Ee.3.59, printed in *Lives of Edward the Confessor*, ed. Henry R. Luard, Rolls Series, 3 (London: Longman, Brown, Green, Longmans & Roberts, 1858), pp. 25–157, with translation at pp. 161–311; hereafter cited as Luard, *Estoire*), see Binski, 'Reflections on *La estoire*', pp. 333–50.

[23] My translation. Barlow renders this 'assign him the life of a bachelor'; Barlow, *Vita Æd.* (1992), p. 15.

[24] The primary definition is 'unmarried, single'; Charlton T. Lewis and Charles Short (eds), *A Latin Dictionary* (Oxford: Oxford University Press, 1879), p. 262; see Barlow, *Edward the Confessor*, p. 218, n. 8. However, Latham defines it as 'celibate'; Ronald E. Latham (ed.), *Dictionary of Medieval Latin from British Sources* (London: Oxford University Press for the British Academy, 1975–97), fasc. II/C (1981), p. 237. Aldhelm, for example, used words associated with *virginitas* or *castitas* more frequently than those with *celebs*. The latter appears in the prose *De virginitate* just five

times, according to the index of *Aldhelmi Opera*, ed. Rudolfus Ehwald, Auctores Antiquissimi, 15 (Munich: Monumenta Germaniae Historica, 1984). On two instances it could refer to virgins and/or chaste individuals (XXV, p. 260; XLV, p. 298); on the remaining three, he appears to use it synonymously with *virgines* (X, p. 239, XVIII, p. 247; XXI, p. 252). I am indebted to Emma Pettit for drawing my attention to this text and for her assistance with it. *Castitas* and *virginitas* (and associated vernacular terms) are similarly ambiguous; see Dyan Elliott, *Spiritual Marriage: Sexual Abstinence in Medieval Wedlock* (Princeton: Princeton University Press, 1993), pp. 5–6; Kathleen Coyne Kelly and Marina Leslie, 'Introduction: the epistemology of virginity', in Kelly and Leslie (eds), *Menacing Virgins: Representing Virginity in the Middle Ages and Renaissance* (London: Associated University Presses, 1999), pp. 15–25 (pp. 16–17); Kathleen Coyne Kelly, *Performing Virginity and Testing Chastity in the Middle Ages* (London: Routledge, 2000), pp. 3–7.

[25] Pierre J. Payer, *The Bridling of Desire: Views of Sex in the Later Middle Ages* (Toronto: University of Toronto Press, 1993), p. 138.

[26] Ibid., pp. 154–5. He suggests that '"continence" [eventually] lost out to "chastity" as the preferred term for the virtue covering sexual matters', partially because of the notion of restraint usually associated with the term.

[27] Barlow, *Vita Æd.* (1992), pp. xxxix–xl. This Westminster monk, writing in the second half of the fourteenth century, wrote a 'completely derivative' work (the phrase is Barlow's, *Vita Æd.* (1992), p. xxxix); Richard of Cirencester, *Speculum historiale de gestis regum Angliae*, ed. John E. B. Mayor, Rolls Series, 30, 2 vols (London: Longmans, Green & Co., 1863–9).

[28] Barlow, *Vita Æd.* (1992), p. xxxix, highlights pp. 14–18, 18–20 and 122–4 of Anon., *Vita Æd.* These passages are indeed remarkably close to Richard's text: *Speculum historiale*, vol. 2, pp. 210–11, 212 and 291–2 respectively.

[29] Barlow, *Vita Æd.* (1992), pp. xxxix–xl, with regard to Richard of Cirencester, *Speculum historiale*, vol. 2, bk 4, ch. 11, pp. 221–3. Barlow deduces that this represents just under half of the lacuna, and includes it in Anon., *Vita Æd.* (1992), pp. 22–5.

[30] Richard of Cirencester, *Speculum historiale*, vol. 2, p. 221 (Barlow's translation in Anon., *Vita Æd.* (1992), pp. 22–3).

[31] Richard of Cirencester, *Speculum historiale*, vol. 2, p. 223 (Barlow's translation in Anon., *Vita Æd.* (1992), pp. 24–5).

[32] Anon., *Vita Æd.* (1992), pp. 24–5, 90–1, 122–3. On the implications of this, see Barlow, *Edward the Confessor*, pp. 299–300; Stafford, *Queen Emma and Queen Edith*, p. 47.

[33] Otter, 'Closed doors', pp. 63–92, discussing Anon., *Vita Æd.*, pp. 72–5.

[34] Barlow, *Vita Æd.* (1992), p. lxxiv.

[35] Ibid., appendix A, pp. 128–9.

[36] With, that is, the important caveat that we only have the Anonymous's account in a fourteenth-century copy, if we accept Barlow's argument, see n. 28 above.

[37] Osbert, *Vita beati Ead.*, 75 (Barlow's translation in Anon., *Vita Æd.* (1962), p. 15).

[38] Osbert, *Vita beati Ead.*, 75 (Barlow's translation in Anon., *Vita Æd.* (1962), p. 15); she is also 'sister' at Osbert, *Vita beati Ead.*, 110–11.

[39] Osbert, *Vita beati Ead.*, 75 (Barlow's translation in Anon., *Vita Æd.* (1962), p. 15).

[40] Osbert, *Vita beati Ead.*, 105 (Barlow's translation in Anon., *Vita Æd.* (1992), pp. 112–13). Osbert's likening Edward to David in connection with his chaste relationship with Abishag in the prologue might conceivably be interpreted as a reference to Edward's celibacy (cf. 1 Kings 1:1–4, 15); Osbert, *Vita beati Ead.*, 67. However, it should also be noted that this biblical passage had been interpreted in terms of David embracing and being warmed and renewed by Wisdom; see, for example, *Select Letters of St Jerome*, trans. F. A. Wright (London: Heinemann, 1933), ep. 52, pp. 191–9. In the context of Osbert's prologue, which praises Edward as a king who is humble, lacks avarice, but exercises philosophical rule and fair-minded justice, it seems that the latter model is more appropriate here, thus reinforcing the notion of Edward as *rex philosophicus*.

[41] Barlow, *Edward the Confessor*, pp. 272–6.

[42] *Letters of Osbert*, ep. 2, p. 51; trans. Robinson, p. 5. Robinson places this letter before 1123, p. 9; cf. Osbert's complaint about violent despoilers of the abbey's property: *Vita beati Ead.*, p. 105.

[43] Mason, *Westminster Abbey*, pp. 33–6.

[44] Pierre Chaplais, 'The original charters of Herbert and Gervase, abbots of Westminster (1121–1157)', in Patricia M. Barnes and C. F. Slade (eds), *A Medieval Miscellany for Doris Mary Stenton*, Pipe Roll Society, NS, 36 (London: Pipe Roll Society, 1962), pp. 89–110.

[45] Scholz, 'Canonization of Edward the Confessor', 40–1.

[46] Kelly, *Performing Virginity*, especially pp. 91–118; see also Kelly, 'Menaced masculinity and imperiled virginity in the *Morte Darthur*', in Kelly and Leslie (eds), *Menacing Virgins*, pp. 97–114 (pp. 99–100), and Maud Burnett McInerney, 'Rhetoric, power and integrity in the passion of the virgin martyr', ibid., pp. 50–70.

[47] Sarah Salih, 'Performing virginity: sex and violence in the *Katherine group*', in Carlson and Weisl (eds), *Constructions of Widowhood and Virginity*, pp. 95–112 (p. 100).

[48] This renders more explicit the Anonymous's simpler 'the king, of dove-like purity'; Anon., *Vita Æd.* (1992), p. 94.

[49] Odo of Cluny, *De Vita Sancti Geraldi Auriliacensis Comitis*, PL, 133, cols 639–703 (col. 648) ('The *Life* of Saint Gerald of Aurillac', trans. Gerard Sitwell, in *Soldiers of Christ: Saints and Saints' Lives from Late Antiquity and the Early Middle Ages*, ed. Thomas F. X. Noble and Thomas Head (London: Sheed & Ward, 1995), pp. 295–362 (p. 304)).

[50] *Vita Geraldi*, col. 648 ('*Life* of Gerald', p. 304).

[51] *Vita Geraldi*, col. 662 ('*Life* of Gerald', p. 319).

52 *The Vita Wulfstani of William of Malmesbury*, ed. Reginald R. Darlington, Camden Society, 3rd ser., 40 (London: Royal Historical Society, 1928), p. 6 ('The *Life* of Bishop Wulfstan of Worcester', trans. Michael Swanton, in *Three Lives of the Last Englishmen* (New York: Garland, 1984), pp. 89–148 (p. 94)).

53 *Vita Wulfstani*, pp. 6–7 ('*Life* of Wulfstan', pp. 94–5).

54 *Vita Wulfstani*, p. 11 ('*Life* of Wulfstan', p. 99).

55 Osbert, *Vita beati Ead.*, 74–5 (Barlow's translation in Anon., *Vita Æd.* (1962), p. 14).

56 See, for example, his letter to Adelidis, abbess of Barking, on the armour of chastity and the virtues of the saintly virgins; *Letters of Osbert*, ep. 42, pp. 153–79. See also the prologue on virginity in his *Vita Edburge* in Ridyard, *Royal Saints*, pp. 259–308 (p. 263). On his devotion to the Blessed Virgin and St Anne, and his role in the revival of the Feast of the Conception of the Blessed Virgin, see Robinson, 'Westminster in the twelfth century', pp. 11–14.

57 The *vita* is partially incorporated into Richard of Cirencester, *Speculum historiale*, vol. 1, pp. 262–94. I am grateful to Brian Briggs for pointing out this reference to me. On Richard's treatment of the text, see Robert Bartlett, 'Rewriting saints' lives: the case of Gerald of Wales', *Speculum*, 58 (1983), 598–613 (601, n. 14).

58 Richard of Cirencester, *Speculum historiale*, vol. 1, pp. 266–7, 270–5; discussed by Bartlett, 'Rewriting saints' lives', 602–3, 607. I was gratified to see that Bartlett highlights an increased focus on the dangers and trials of marriage in Gerald of Wales's rewriting of Osbert's *vita* of Ethelbert, similar to that about to be proposed for Aelred's *vita* here. I hope to be able to develop elsewhere the rewriting of virginity in *vitae* other than Edward's.

59 Susan J. Ridyard, '*Condigna veneratio*: post-conquest attitudes to the saints of the Anglo-Saxons', *Anglo-Norman Studies*, 9 (1987), 179–206.

60 Ridyard, *Royal Saints*, p. 21.

61 Aelred, *Vita S. Ed.*, col. 738 (Aelred, *Life*, p. 16).

62 Aelred, *Vita S. Ed.*, cols 739–40 (Aelred, *Life*, p. 17); cf. Matt. 13:8, 23. This formula was popular in medieval treatments of virginity; see Payer, *Bridling of Desire*, pp. 175–7.

63 Aelred, *Vita S. Ed.*, col. 744 (Aelred, *Life*, p. 28).

64 'The "De Institutis Inclusarum" of Aelred of Rievaulx', ed. C. H. Talbot, *Analecta sacri ordinis Cisterciensis*, 7 (1951), 167–217 (189) ('A rule of life for a recluse', trans. M. P. Macpherson, in *Aelred of Rievaulx: Treatises and Pastoral Prayer*, ed. M. Basil Pennington (Kalamazoo: Cistercian Publications, 1971), pp. 41–102 (p. 63)). Other examples are discussed by Barbara Newman, 'Flaws in the golden bowl: gender and spiritual formation in the twelfth century', *Traditio*, 45 (1990), 111–46 (123–5).

65 Aelred, *Vita S. Ed.*, col. 747 (Aelred, *Life*, p. 34).

66 Aelred, *Vita S. Ed.*, col. 747 (Aelred, *Life*, p. 35).

67 Edith is not daughter, sister or mother at this point, as in the earlier *vitae*, but she is 'sister or daughter' at Edward's deathbed; Aelred, *Vita S. Ed.*, cols 774–5 (Aelred, *Life*, pp. 93–4).

68 Aelred, *Vita S. Ed.*, col. 748 (Aelred, *Life*, p. 36), presumably rebutting suggestions such as that made by William of Malmesbury: 'The king's policy with her was neither to keep her at a distance from his bed nor to know her as a man would; whether he did this out of hatred for her family, which he prudently concealed to suit the time, or whether from a love of chastity, I have not discovered for certain': *Gesta regum Anglorum: The History of the English Kings*, trans. Roger A. B. Mynors, completed by Rodney M. Thomson and Michael Winterbottom, 2 vols (Oxford: Clarendon Press, 1998), vol. 1, bk 2, ch. 197, pp. 353–5.

69 The notion that detachment from worldly things conferred visions is reiterated, without an explicit reference to chastity, at Aelred, *Vita S. Ed.*, col. 760 (Aelred, *Life*, p. 59).

70 Aelred, *Vita S. Ed.*, col. 754 (Aelred, *Life*, p. 47). This connection is made again: 'he was particularly distinguished by the special grace of giving sight to the blind, because, as it was believed, of his inner purity. As his unusual chastity (*munditia*) kept the gaze of his heart clear, just so did he dispel darkness from the outward eyes of others'; Aelred, *Vita S. Ed.*, col. 762 (Aelred, *Life*, p. 64).

71 Aelred, *Vita St Ed.*, cols 769–70, col. 770 (Aelred, *Life*, pp. 81–4, p. 84). Although this episode is included in the abbreviated Cambridge manuscript of Osbert's *Vita beati Ead.*, it is generally held to be an addition of Aelred's; see Bloch, 'La vie', 58–60; Barlow, *Vita Æd.* (1992), p. xxxviii, n. 107; Binski, *Westminster Abbey,* p. 55; Lan Lipscomb, 'A distinct legend of the ring in the *Life of Edward the Confessor*', *Medieval Perspectives*, 6 (1992), 45–57 (46–8); Marsha L. Dutton, 'Aelred, historian: two portraits in Plantagenet myth', *Cistercian Studies Quarterly*, 28 (1993), 113–44 (125, 133–5).

72 Dutton, 'Aelred, historian', 135; cf. *De Institutis*, pp. 196–7, 205 ('A rule of life', pp. 73–4, 86–7).

73 See the emphasis on the connection of his virginity with his saintly posthumous power at Aelred, *Vita St Ed.*, col. 775 (Aelred, *Life*, p. 96); col. 780 (Aelred, *Life*, p. 105); col. 782 (Aelred, *Life*, p. 108).

74 See, for example, Anon., *Vita Æd.* (1992), pp. 18–21; Osbert, *Vita beati Ead.*, 66; Aelred, *Vita S. Ed.*, col. 738 (Aelred, *Life*, p. 16). I hope to return to the portrayals of Edward's kingship elsewhere.

75 Salih, *Versions of Virginity*, p. 17.

76 Luard, *Estoire*, ll. 1093–1124, 1224–78. Edward's devotion to St John the Evangelist is also further emphasized, in the context of Edward's virginity, at ll. 668–73, 1097–8 and 1111–14. See also the Anglo-Norman verse life written by the nun of Barking, which, according to Wogan-Browne, presents 'a saint-king who is a virgin visionary'; Wogan-Browne, *Saints' Lives*, pp. 249–56 (p. 249).

77 Luard, *Estoire*, l. 21; cf. ll. 23–31 and 1255–60.

78 Ibid., l. 1255–6.

79 Katherine J. Lewis, 'Becoming a virgin king: Richard II and Edward the

Confessor', in Samantha J. E. Riches and Sarah Salih (eds), *Gender and Holiness: Men, Women and Saints in Late Medieval Europe* (London: Routledge, 2002), pp. 86–100.

80 Barlow, *Edward the Confessor*, appendix D, pp. 310–24. One further letter refers more generally to 'pleasures of the flesh' (*carnis . . . voluptates*), p. 313.

81 Ibid., appendix D, pp. 323–4.

82 Rodney M. Thomson, 'Two versions of a saint's life from St Edmund's Abbey: changing currents in twelfth century monastic style', *Revue Bénédictine*, 84 (1974), 383–408; cf. Bartlett, 'Rewriting saints' lives', 598–613.

8

Alchemy and the Exploration of Late Medieval Sexuality

JONATHAN HUGHES

The late Middle Ages and early Renaissance saw the flowering of an alchemical medicine centred on female sexual and reproductive functions in a specific, medical, biological way that had profound intellectual, philosophical, political and scientific ramifications. This chapter is an attempt to trace the often convoluted and contradictory interrelationships between reproductive heterosexuality and virginity in alchemical writings of the later Middle Ages and the Renaissance. Sometimes these contradictions offer an unfamiliar perspective on both heterosexual sex and virginity. Alchemical and medical concepts of sexuality and virginity were distinct from, and sometimes sharply at odds with, the clerical view that virginity was always the highest state. Alchemy was predicated on sexual symbolism, and alchemically informed sexual imagery permeated late medieval culture. Both the individual body and the body politic required sexual regulation, enabling alchemical thought to influence matters as diverse as witchcraft accusations and the imagery of kingship. Alchemical and medical conceptions of sexuality were largely heteronormative, assuming reproduction to be the inevitable goal of sexual activity. The female principle was valued for its generative power, which could then be appropriated by the male alchemist. The alchemist, usurping the role of maternity, harnesses woman's creative erotic energy. The triumph of art over nature becomes a triumph of man over woman.[1] There is no room for the virgin in this paradigm, and women perceived as post-sexual could be regarded with suspicion. And yet, on the level of treatment of the individual body, alchemical thought could also be aligned with the broader and more diffuse understanding of sexuality found in mystical writing, in which virginity may coexist with sexual pleasures. This had repercussions in the wider spheres of science and politics, encouraging an understanding that the fulfilment and expression of self, whether within the individual or the wider body politic, depended on an acceptance and expression of sexuality that might have little to do with the act of sexual intercourse itself. From an alchemical perspective chastity or virginity could be extolled if allowance was made for the expression of sexual identity and the achievement of sexual relief in the interests of the health of body and soul or the political equivalent.

Sexual chemistry

Myths explain the origins of alchemy in terms of female sexuality. Metals were believed to grow organically within the earth, like an embryo developing within its mother's womb. *The Mirror of Alchimy*, widely circulated in the fifteenth century and attributed to Roger Bacon, maintained that the natural force of fires within the mines of the earth dried out and coagulated the thicker or grosser water into quicksilver (female) in the belly and veins of the earth and into sulphur (male) in the mountains.[2] Lying within the womb of the earth some metals, such as gold, reached maturity while others did not. From this belief arose the alchemical myth that the womb of the earth could be created artificially within the laboratory. The model was the female body, the earth that provided the warmth and nutrition necessary for the birth of the stone. Alchemy also shows a desire to have its own mythical maternal origins. Zosimos of Panoplis, who lived in Alexandria in *c.*300 CE, preserved the myths of the female origins of alchemy in Egypt, referring to one text containing the account of Isis the prophetess explaining the mysteries of alchemy to her son.[3] Zosimos also alluded to female experts in the art who may have existed. One was a Jewess, Maria Prophetissa, legendarily identified with Miriam, the sister of Moses.[4] By the sixteenth century practical instructions on distillation attributed to Maria the Prophetess were included in manuscripts containing the alchemical works of Roger Bacon and George Ripley.[5]

Despite such validations of imaginary mothers, medieval medicine was dominated by notions of male superiority, illustrated by the alchemical evolution of base matter to gold. Fourteenth- and fifteenth-century alchemy reinforced this view with the idea that the application of heat could accelerate the evolution of heavy gold from dull, wet earth. The process was represented in an emblematic alchemical scroll known as the *Ripley Scroll*. Some twenty-two copies of this 8-foot long scroll survive, most from the sixteenth century; the earliest, based on the vivid sexual allegories of Sir George Ripley, an alchemist prominent at the courts of Henry VI and Edward IV, was made around 1460.[6] The scroll shows the scattering of male seed or sperm in moist elemental water. The stone, symbolized by the bird of Hermes perched on a globe, has evolved from the primitive, primeval female elements of water and mercury, symbolized by the moon (*Luna*), out of the depths of a primeval state of existence (what we might term the unconscious) represented by a putrefied toad, a serpent woman and a dragon. Essential to this process is the fire of choler, the ripening and drying masculine energy represented by the sun. Philosophic water or mercury could, if joined with the male sulphur, evolve with the application of drying heat into gold. Ripley advised his followers to be patient until the water be dried to powder with nourishing heat 'for sperme and heate are as sister and brother'.

Medieval alchemy is a celebration of male perceptions of the feminine. The opposite of *Sol*, the highly evolved masculine sun, is the maternal earth, the receptacle and nourisher of sperm. Water is seen as the primeval sea, the source of life, and yet also has potentially devastating destructive power, like Noah's flood. The female is the elemental principle: her menstrue, like lead, was seen to be essential to the commencement of the work, and the alchemist saw himself as Noah cautiously navigating leaden waters, those unpredictable primitive forces governed by the inconstant moon, the conjugal partner of the sun. Understanding mercury, unstable, volatile and unpredictable, governed by the moon, is the key to the mastery of alchemy. In a mid-fifteenth-century alchemical treatise quicksilver is described as wild water in the earth, a subtle, white substance evenly joined by art's heat which always flees from a plain place and cannot be fixed; and yet from this cold, moist substance all metals are engendered.[7] Elusive in its virgin state, it could be controlled only by making it breed. Woman, like mercury, was viewed with a mixture of fear, awe and incomprehension. From the male perspective *Luna* rather than *Sol* represented the unconscious, and one of the spiritual functions of alchemy was to apply choler, fire and light (or reason) to chthonic, maternal forces to facilitate the development of self. The first step in the great work therefore was to fix unstable mercury.

The medieval alchemist created in his laboratory a feminine world of vessels and water. He entered the body of mother earth, the monster or dragon, and extracted from the womb of the earth precious metals. Like the Siberian shaman who assumed the role of mother, he attempted to acquire the secrets of maternity to extract from nature her creative powers.[8] Alchemists therefore continued to explain their work of heating combinations of metals in the quest to conceive and grow gold in terms of sexual metaphor. The furnace, warmed with a carefully regulated heat, was like the trunk of the human body heated by the liver. Within this heated furnace the alchemist placed a glass vessel or alembic, which he described as a matrix or womb. Within this vessel various forms of sexual conjunction took place. The fourteenth-century alchemist John Dastin declared: 'let male and female together ever meet'.[9] In the *Testamentum* ascribed to Ramon Lull, which was translated from Catalan into Latin in England in 1456, magnesia is called a white earth in which 'our gold', the masculine, fiery principle, is planted and from whose whiteness, with time and patience, the stone grows.[10] This assumes that the process of gestation of base metal into gold should be stimulated by the introduction of the seed of gold, described as semen, and symbolized by *Sol*. In *The Mirror of Alchimy* gold is proclaimed 'a perfect masculine body, without any superfluity of diminution' which could perfect imperfect bodies mingled with it by melting.[11] The alchemical conjunction most frequently took the form of a fusion of the male semen or red sulphur, symbolized by the sun (*Sol*), with the female mercury, symbolized by the moon (*Luna*). In the *Ripley Scrolls*, this marriage was represented in colourful emblematic images of a red king (*Sol*) and a white queen (*Luna*). Richard Carpenter (d. 1503), the probable author of verses subsequently attached to the scrolls, wrote of the alchemical marriage as a planetary conjunction of sun and moon. Explicit sexual imagery occurs in these scrolls and other related illustrations of Ripley's works, including the copulating king and queen and showers of semen from the sun. In *The Compound of Alchemy*, written for Edward IV in 1471, Ripley explained the beginning of his alchemical work in the alembic in terms of the sexual restlessness and fulfilment of the womb. Prostitutes, he claimed, do not bear children because their wombs never close after copulation, and he gave instructions to close up the matrix after conception and to nourish the seed with temperate heat.[12]

Conception was followed in alchemy by gestation and alchemists were therefore interested in menstruation. Thomas Norton celebrated a successful alchemical conjunction by exclaiming

> How the semynale sede and masculine
> Hath wrought and wonn the victorie
> Upon the menstruallis worthely.[13]

As the alchemist tended his fire and fed the conjoined mercury and sulphur with base matter, including 'menstrue', he meditated on the process of conception and gestation within the womb leading to the birth of the stone, equated with the child or *homunculus* (the artificially created child). In a tract attributed to Roger Bacon on 'the withdrawing of the accidents of age', occurring in a mid-fifteenth-century alchemical collection made by John Vale, secretary to Thomas Cook, Lord Mayor of London, there is a meditation on the way the conjoined sperm of the man and woman is nourished in the matrix by menstrual blood which with natural heat fosters 'the growth of an embryo that takes the shape of a man after thirty days'.[14] A close description of the gradual formation of the hair, cheeks and mouth of the foetus follows. After four months in the case of a female, and five months for a male, the child develops nails and begins to move in the womb. The writer asserts that the nourishing of the child with menstrual blood from the walls of the womb is vital to this process. Such a description leads one to assume that the author had seen or heard of autopsy reports of foetuses in various stages of development, and that for him the glass alembic served as a source of empathetic meditation on the process of gestation within a pregnant woman's womb.

One of the persistent sexual myths of alchemy is that of the symbolic alchemical couple, implying that heterosexual activity is fundamental to alchemical process. The most famous pairing in the late Middle Ages is that of Nicholas Flamel (d. 1418) and his wife Peronelle ('flame perennially'). Flamel, a wealthy scrivener, was supposed to have come across alchemical secrets in a cabbalistic book, *The Book of Abraham*, and he and his wife performed the lesser work of converting mercury to silver on 17 January 1383. On 25 April of that year they were alleged to have transmuted mercury into pure gold. However, although the couple did exist and were buried in the church of the Holy Innocents in Paris, their involvement and enrichment through alchemy is a myth. The *Exposition of the Hieroglyphicall Figures*, recounting this story, is a forgery foisted on the pious Parisian bookseller by French publishers in 1624.[15] The combining of opposites (male and female) in alchemical experimentation must have inspired alchemists to meditate on sexual chemistry, and spilled over into an actual sexual experiment in the cross-matching of the wives of John Dee and Edmund Kelly following the instructions given by the spirit medium, Madini, to Kelly in Dee's scrying glass. Ostensibly the two alchemists were trying to prove their faith in and obedience to the guidance of their guardian spirits, but the two wives, especially Joan Dee (who hated Kelly) were passive and reluctant participants in this wife-sharing experiment. The women's participation thus reinforced a familiar binary division between male agents and female material.

In terms of alchemical, sexual metaphor women played an equal share in the conjunction of mercury and sulphur, and in the ensuing gestation of the homunculus or philosopher's stone the emphasis was entirely on the workings of the woman's womb. But as actual women played so little part in the theory or practice of alchemy these explicit allegories and meditations on the female body must be seen as largely a projection of male practitioners and theorists. Their assumptions were based on the medical philosophy of the romanized Greek physician Galen of Pergamum (129–c.200/216 CE). According to Galen males reached their full potential by amassing a decisive surplus of heat, a fervent vital spirit, in the early stages of coagulation in the womb. The hot ejaculation of male seed proved this. Women were failed males, lacking the necessary vital heat. Their lack of heat gave them greater liquidity, which made them clammy, softer, colder and more formless than men. They were identified with the element from which the alchemical work began, formless water,[16] the *prima materia*, symbolized by the toad which, when it puffed and expanded itself, represented the womb. Ripley informed his followers

> water is the secret and life of everything,
> For of water each thing hath his beginning
> As showeth in women.[17]

Periodic menstruation, necessary for the maintenance of a woman's humoral balance and health, proved that their bodies, defective in heat (the principle of life) were unable to burn up the nutriments and the heavy surpluses that coagulated within them. This build-up of poisonous humours was believed to be so great that it was maintained in a popular work on human reproduction, *The Secrets of Women*, that during menstruation a woman could sully and stain mirrors with her glance.[18] Such fears were also expressed in standard alchemical texts. *The Mirror of Alchimy* claimed: 'Aristotle saith in his booke of sleep and watching that if a menstruous woman behold her selfe in a looking glasse, she will infect it, so there will appearee a cloude of bloud.'[19] The sexual biology of women who were not contained by pregnancy held manifold dangers. Yet such surpluses were needed to nurture and contain the hot seed that produced children. Galenic theory implied that creation purposely made one half of the human race imperfect. Ripley, aware of this paradox, wrote 'And were not heate and moysture continuall, sparme in the wombe might have no abiding.'[20] Woman and the alchemical ingredients associated with her were valued for their capacity to generate or become something else.

Alchemy and the individual body

Medical assumptions about the importance of a clear sense of sexual identity and sexual release for the maintenance of humoral balance and health within both the individual body and the body politic ran counter to the Church's privileging of virginity throughout the Middle Ages. According to the chroniclers William of Newburgh and Roger of Howden, writing eight decades after the event, when Archbishop Thomas of York lay dying in 1114, he was told by his doctor that intercourse with a woman was the only remedy for his illness. Some advisers urged him to accept this guidance, claiming that God would not be offended by an act done only for medicinal reasons and not carnal lust. The prelate agreed and a beautiful woman was brought into his room. Later, however, when the doctor inspected the archbishop's urine it was revealed that Thomas had only feigned acceptance in order to placate his friends. When they rebuked him he replied 'shame upon a malady that requires sensuality for its cure'.[21] The tale is an exemplum of Thomas's holiness: it is assumed that most men would have chosen sin and health rather than virginal death. Edward IV possessed a copy of the *Secreta secretorum* with the alchemical additions of Roger Bacon in which the prince is advised to engage in regular sexual activity with young girls to maintain humoral balance.[22] A life of joy and health was to be found in the pleasures of music, eating and sex.

The key to maintaining health through sexual activity was moderation. Just as women were aged by frequent childbirth, it was believed men were aged by the expenditure of vital heat with frequent sexual intercourse.[23] Gilbert Kymer, physician and alchemist, composed a *Dietariam de Sanitatis Custodie* for Henry VI's uncle, Humphrey, duke of Gloucester, warning the promiscuous duke that too much sex and expenditure of semen dried and cooled the body, reducing its essential heat.[24] This is why excessively promiscuous men such as Edward IV were termed effeminate.[25] Sexual restraint could ensure the retention of masculine heat and energy. Lancelot, in Sir Thomas Malory's Arthuriad, combines Christian morality with a sense that sexual activity saps male energy. Answering a maid who asks him why he is wifeless, Lancelot explains:

> But for to be a weddyd man, I thynke hit nat, for then I muste couche with her, and leve armys and turnamentis, batellys and adventures. And as for to sey to take my pleasaunce with peramours, that woll I will refuse: in prenciple for drede of God, for knyghtes that bene adventures sholde nat be advoutres northir lecherous, for than they be nat happy nother fortunate unto the werrys; for other they shall be overcom with a sympler knyght than they be themselves, or else they shall sle by unhappe and hir cursednesse bettir men than they be hemself. And so who that usyth peramours shall be unhappy, and al thynge unhappy that is aboute them.[26]

There is a concern with the correct harnessing of sexual energy in Malory that has much in common with alchemists' views on the balancing of humours. Moderation rather than absolute virginity is the ideal.

For women the medical implications of the sexual urge were more specific as all their ailments and suspicions about their perceived fluidity and instability were related to the notion of the wandering womb, a concept endorsed by alchemists.[27] The reproductive telos of the medical view of sexuality meant that virginity could be a dangerous and unnatural state. The traditional Hippocratic view was that the womb, or matrix, the uterus and vagina, was one organ, like an upturned (weaker) vessel. In *The Sekenesse of Wymmen*, derived from the Trotula treatises and copied widely in the fourteenth and fifteenth centuries, the vagina is described as the 'mowthe of the moder, þat is to say hire priuy membre'.[28] The womb, if denied the moisture that came from sexual activity, wandered restlessly through the body in a search for moisture that was fundamentally a search for a child. In the course of its meandering it exerted pressure on organs including the heart, lungs and liver, causing various illnesses. Hysteria, mood swings, tender breasts, faintness, breathlessness and abdominal pains were all believed to be of uterine origin. Medical treatment was based on the assumption that the womb, blind to reason, could like a wild animal either be driven or lured back to its proper place in the woman's body with repulsive or pleasant odours. Fetid odours such as pitch or burnt hair were therefore applied to the nose and aromatic perfumes such as musk, rose water or opium were applied to the genitals.[29] The womb's hunger could only be appeased and its wandering stopped by sexual intercourse. Gynaecological tracts such as the *Treatise of Woman's Sicknesse* were explicit on the symptoms of sexual arousal in women and their medical implications: 'They fele mouche moystnesse and they haue much melancholy in womb and desire to be with man.'[30] The author maintained that a woman's moisture could dry up and cause illnesses if it were not refreshed with male sperm.

Alchemy was a science that embraced nature and saw heterosexual intercourse as essential to stabilizing both women and the body politic, which was conceived as female when unstabilized. Like much medical opinion on sex it ran counter to the Church's teaching on virginity while reinforcing some polarized views on the differences between men and women. However, in other respects physicians and alchemists encouraged frank investigation into the similarities between the sexuality of men and women and the possibility of a fulfilled healthy life, sometimes even outside conjugal relationships. A family of late medieval gynaecological treatises, some claiming the Salernitan female physician Trotula as their author, were all written by men but nevertheless drew sympathetically on the sexual experiences of women and their midwives.[31] Instructions were provided for wives to test for the fertility of their husbands by waiting for the appearance of an unpleasant smell and a worm, in a pot in which they had placed the man's urine on wheat bran. Women were even offered through medicine the choice of the sex of their child, and it was not necessarily assumed this would be male. If a woman desired a daughter she was advised to dry the testicles of a hare, powder them and place the powder in a potion. Then she should head towards the bed and 'go pley with her mate . . . and haue her desire'.[32]

Such autonomy was even extended to the maintenance of humoral balance outside the bonds of wedlock, and in ways which undermine the privileging of heterosexual penetration. The medical convention was that a woman's ovaries were testicles, which produced semen, though it was weaker than men's. The so-called Trotula treatises endorsed the medical tradition that a build-up of this corrupt seed, indicated by the appearance of moistness in the vagina, would cause illness in widows, virgins and nuns.[33] Galen and Avicenna specifically prescribed masturbation. The midwife was required to rub the genitals until the seed was ejected.[34] The Trotula treatises and other gynaecological tracts in circulation in the fifteenth century were less direct but ultimately just as explicit, prescribing peppers to encourage emission of humours through sneezing, good diet and hot baths to improve the balance of the humour of blood, make the woman leave her heaviness and become merry and glad. Such counsel is obviously opposed to the more ascetic teachings of the Church disseminated in sermons and during confession. Moreover, the same treatises recommended the midwife apply hot poultices, oils, baths and lotions and rub them around the genitals until there was a release of seed. Some of these potions, such as *aqua vitae*, were the product of alchemical distillation. Among the oils and herbs recommended in one treatise were known aphrodisiacs, such as comfrey, treacle or theriac, the miracle drug of the wealthy (like cocaine today) made from snakes' flesh which was regarded as hot, fiery and a potent restorer of vigour and which was to be rubbed around the mouth of the vagina.[35] Sexual activity between women in the form of simple rubbing or mutual masturbation was largely ignored in the Middle Ages and condemnation was reserved for the use of instruments.[36] Nevertheless, pessaries were also medically prescribed and inserted into the vagina until release was obtained. The erotically charged circumstances (some the length of a finger were made of silk, and soaked in oils and honey) imply that they served as penis substitutes. *The Sekenesse of Wymmen* suggests that linen cloth and honey be wrapped around the centre of a corn cob which is then placed in a woman's privy member and left in overnight. The object was always to 'delyuer hire of hire corrupt seed'.[37] The medical use of such pessaries as penis substitutes is confirmed by the recommendation in the same treatise that a linen clout moistened in hot oil be inserted in the vagina of those women who 'may not suffer a man's yerde [penis] for the greatnesse thereof' and who are constrained to suffer discomfort whether they wish to or not.[38] The author's sympathy was presumably aroused because these women were virgins being prepared for heterosexual penetration by rupturing the hymen. Specific

descriptions of the symptoms of female arousal at the point of release –
a build-up of heat about the mouth of the womb, an accumulation of
moisture, a pricking and hardness and a great desire for impregnation
– suggest a deliberate attempt to show the similarities between the
sexual organs of male and female at the point of excitement, which
includes female ejaculation: 'Women when they comen [copulate] with
men they be delivered of seed that passeth from the stones [testicles] of
the womb as men be delivered of seed that comes from the stones of the
yard.'[39] By obliterating difference between men and women in this area
of sexual desire and humoral release through the discharge of semen,
physicians were allowing women to exert some autonomous control
over their wandering wombs. Biblical proscriptions against masturbation applied only to men: women, if they practised masturbation, either
by themselves or with the help of midwives (or other women within the
context of a convent), could choose a life of relative good health and
sexual satisfaction outside the traditional role of wife and childbearer,
which, as recent cemetery excavations in Norwich and York reveal,
involved at least a 30 per cent chance of a childbirth-related death.[40]

A virginal life could be the site of further processes of interest to
alchemists. The fulfilment of the alchemist's work, the incarnation of
the son of man or *homunculus*, was in part a process of religious
meditation paralleled by the meditations of the late fourteenth-century
mystics, some of whom focused just as closely on sexual processes. The
anchorhold, like the alchemist's vessel, was an enclosed female space, a
womb and a refuge for Christ as Mary's womb once was.[41] The
addition of the alembic to the meanings of the already highly charged
space of contemplation further intensifies the processes and transformations which occur within it. The comparison in the *Ancrene
Wisse* of the anchorhold to a nest reads more like a description of the
vulva: 'hard on the outside, with thorns that prick, and on the inside
soft and yielding . . . Place [Christ] in your nest, that is, in your heart.'[42]
Holy women such as Hadewijch in the thirteenth century and
Catherine of Siena in the fourteenth wrote of the love of Christ in
sexual terms, dwelling on the wound on his side.[43] This wound appears
on prayer rolls, some juxtaposing images of the cross and the bleeding
wound with promises of protection for mother and child. These rolls
may have been used as birth girdles wrapped around the womb.[44] The
same image appears in books of hours in the shape of a mouth turned
vertically, bearing a close resemblance to gynaecological drawings of
the vulva and vagina so that it serves as a focus of meditation on the

mother's own 'wound'.[45] The Carthusian Margaret of Oignt (d. 1316), whose writings were well known in England, described Christ's incarnation and passion as one long powerful labour.[46] It is probable that some holy women identified Christ's wound with their own genitalia and in their intense identification with the suffering of Christ focused, like the alchemist, on the process of menstruation in which they shared their lord's bleeding and pain.

This preoccupation is most powerfully apparent in Julian of Norwich's *Revelation of Divine Love*. The wound of Christ, the subject of her meditations and source of the redemptive blood and water, resembles the maternal vagina:

> our lord . . . led forth the understondyng of his creture be the same wound into his side withinne. And then he shewid a faire delecytabil place, and large enow for al mankynd that shal be save to resten in pece and in love. And therwith he browte to mende his dereworthy blode and pretious water which he let poure al out for love.[47]

Julian, concentrating on the femininity of Jesus as the suffering mother of man, wrote in prose characterized by use of fluidity, liquidness and dominated by the theme of motherhood conveyed in terms of milk, tears and blood.[48] Her depiction of Christ as the lactating mother was influenced by the understanding that breast milk was transformed menstrual blood migrating upwards after the foetus had been formed and nourished.[49] In her intense identification with Christ's pain and his bleeding wounds she probably meditated on her monthly periods, her 'shewings' or manifestations (the word may then as today have had specific connotations of the manifestation of menstrual blood). Many married women, regularly either pregnant or breast-feeding, would have experienced relatively few periods before the onset of the menopause, but for a chaste anchoress in her sealed enclosure with only the cross, the mass and Christ's wound to think about, these shewings, with their associations with the monthly visitation of the host-like moon and their connotations of the death of the child, cleansing and rebirth, would have been experienced as powerful bodily manifestations of Christ's death and resurrection that only a woman could physically experience. Male contemplatives, on the other hand, could only strive for but rarely achieve the miraculous manifestation of stigmata. This may explain why Julian emphasized the bleeding of Christ as 'grete dropis of blode . . . like pellots . . . like to the dropys of water that fallen of the evys after a greate showre of reyne that fall so thick that no man may numbre them with bodily witte'.[50]According to Hildegard of Bingen the menstrual blood from a virgin is more sanguineous than a woman's because a virgin is still closed. When a girl is a pure virgin (like most anchoresses) her menstruation comes in drops from her blood vessels. After she has been deflowered the drops flow like a rivulet because they have been released through the act of a man.[51] Virgins' blood was sought after for use in alchemical distillations, most notoriously by the former companion-in-arms of Joan of Arc, Gilles de Rais, who was condemned in an ecclesiastical court in 1441 for using alchemical magic and murdering over one hundred children.[52]

Alchemy and the body politic

At the time of the original composition of the *Ripley Scroll*, alchemical meditations on the fusion of male and female opposites led to reflections on the role of men and women outside the laboratory in the wider sphere of the body politic. Men by definition had more precious heat than women and this, in the king, was seen as a vital source of energy for the well-being of the nation. Galen warned in his *Treatise on the Seed* that lack of heat from childhood could cause the male body to collapse back into a state of primary undifferentiation.[53] As Henry VI grew up to assume the mantle of heroic, masculine kingship bequeathed him by his formidable father, Henry V, he would have been closely watched by many hard clear eyes for any signs of a waning of this uncertain force of flickering heat, of any traces of softness that might betray his living in the half-formed state of a woman.[54] By the time he assumed full responsibility as king in the late 1430s he was giving indications of instability and suffered periods of depression and inertia. His physicians diagnosed his condition as premature senility and explained his suffering as the consequence of an excess of phlegm, derived from the element of water, the predominant humour of old men and women. There were frequent references to Henry VI's femininity as well as his simplicity and senility. Coppini, the bishop of Terni and agent of the duke of Milan, described Henry VI as 'a man more timorous than a woman, utterly devoid of spirit who left everything in his wife's hands'.[55] Henry's assertive queen, Margaret of Anjou, was probably behind the commissions of 1456/7, licensing physicians to find an alchemical cure for the ailing monarch. Margaret's physician, Master William Hattecliffe, was appointed to the March 1457 alchemy commission.[56] One of her servants, George Ashby, described the king in alchemical language as the 'water of life' and urged him not to drink too much (a cause of an excess of phlegm) and not to sleep too much (a sign of phlegmatic imbalance and one of the symptoms observed in the king).[57] It must have seemed in the 1450s that England was entering a barren and wintry old age under its phlegmatic king.

Attempts were made to rationalize the king's lack of masculine choleric vigour. The king's chancellor, Sir John Fortescue, adapted patristic teaching, equating virginity with a power that made humans equal to angels.[58] In *The Governance of England* he compared the king's power with that of an angel. But in the minds of many, the cause of the sickness of England's impotent Fisher King was virginity. In 1437 the papal tax-collector noted that the 16-year-old monarch avoided the sight and conversation of women, affirming these to be the work of the devil. Piero del Monte also claimed that those closest to the youth said that he preserved his virginity of mind and body for the present and firmly resolved to have no intercourse with any woman unless within the bonds of matrimony. This chastity was of course given a clerical ascetic gloss. John Capgrave compared the king to St Katherine, whose strength came from her virginity, and John Blacman stressed that Henry had relations only with his wife and then only to produce an heir. However, there was speculation that Henry was too chaste for the nation's good. A London draper was prosecuted in 1446 for attributing Henry's lack of an heir to pious scruples about sex. It took Henry and Margaret of Anjou eight years to produce a son, the only child they ever had, and there were rumours that the father was the duke of Somerset. This may explain the bypassing of Edward of Lancaster as heir of Henry VI in favour of Richard, duke of York, in the Act of Accord of 1459. It may be significant that Henry VI experienced a complete mental breakdown the year his child was born and on recovering his senses was reported to have remarked that the child must have been a gift from heaven.[59]

The alchemical medicine ministered to this sick king is vividly conveyed in the *Ripley Scrolls*, which show the application of masculine heat or choler to dry out moistness. Lions fighting around the fire of choler represent the struggle between the male and female poles. Masculinity is celebrated in the dominant image of the sun bursting through grey rain clouds. In some versions of the scrolls virility is even celebrated in images of sexually erect lions. However Henry, after suffering a wound in the neck at the First Battle of St Albans in 1456, was increasingly seen as incurable and attention was beginning to focus on his kinsman, Edward, earl of March, as a more complete, vigorous young man to redeem a sick land. The *Ripley Scrolls* all begin with the sun bursting through the clouds and the falling of a golden rain or sperm, an eloquent prelude to the emergence of the sun of March. Edward, the masculine opposite of his kinsman of the house of Lancaster, was born on 28 April, a child of the young and vigorous spring sun.[60] In the *Book of the York Barber Surgeons* it is demonstrated that this was when the moon was in the lusty sign of Aries, the time of year of blood, of the sanguine man, of the first element of air and the highest of the metals, gold.[61] Edward took the throne at the beginning of March and much was made in the poetry, genealogies and proclamations that accompanied his accession of his association with gold, the spring and the vigorous and new rekindling sun. In the spring of 1461, buoyed by an apparition of a parhelion, three suns in the sky before the Battle of Mortimer's Cross, the earl of March burst onto the political stage like the young ascendant sun he bore on his shield, adopting the alchemical cognomen of *Sol* to dispense the chilly mists of England's winter king. The *Ripley Scrolls* could now be interpreted as a celebration of the arrival of this masculine sun king. Because of his youth, beauty and charisma Edward of March attracted notions of virginity akin to that of Sir Galahad, which did not imply any diminution of masculine power. Poems celebrating Edward's role as the youthful redeemer such as *Edwardus Dei Gracia* addressed the young king as 'a Rose so white' and as 'Thou vergyne Knight of whom we synge, / Un-Deffiled sithe thy begynnyng.'[62] Henry VI was poignantly aware of this contrast between his own closeness to the feminine moon and that of his kinsman to the warm procreating sun. In 1471, while a prisoner in the Tower, he reflected that he had always, since he was a child, turned to the kingdom of heaven, and he told his chaplain Blacman 'of this earth I do not care . . . Our kinsman of March thrusts himself into it as is his pleasure.'[63]

Marriage and sexual union were as important to the health of the body politic as they were to the individual. Genealogical trees sometimes showed the evolution of the philosopher's stone from the four elements. One late fifteenth-century manuscript of alchemical recipes contains a genealogical tree branching from primordial chaos, through the various alliances of the four elements and seven metals created by

God, to the various combinations of the sanguine, melancholy and phlegmatic humours that comprise the different nations. England, in consideration of the long reign of Henry VI, was defined as a phlegmatic land governed by the moon.[64] If genealogical models were used to demonstrate alchemical processes, the reverse occurred and the genealogical evolution of families through British history culminating in the arrival of Edward IV was explained in terms of alchemical transmutation. History itself served as an alchemical furnace.[65] Women were a vital part of the process, but their role was perceived to be passive. But what happened when high-profile women did not behave in this predictably submissive way, when either their perceived sexuality or their exclusion from sexuality threatened the political schemes in which alchemists and physicians were so closely involved? There was a clear medical rationale for such behaviour. Mercury occupied the same essential female role in the alchemical work as the bride, the white lady, in politically arranged marriages. Both Elizabeth Woodville and her daughter Elizabeth of York were identified as the white lady on their marriages.[66] But mercury was a highly volatile, unpredictable substance that could drive an alchemist to despair as effectively as could any woman. When this was combined with medical notions of that roaming and irrational sexual animal, the womb, and women's susceptibility to lunar influences, then men, whether in the alchemist's cell or at councils deliberating policies for the common weal, believed they had cause to be fearful of prominent women, especially if they were post-menopausal widows in whom it was believed malignant humours accumulated.

These fears lay behind the increasingly frequent incidences of accusations and trials for witchcraft. The fire, water and vessels that represented the feminine *sanctum* entered by the alchemists could easily take on the sinister accoutrements of the witch. Disturbances in the body politic were linked to incidents of wet, cold weather, which indicated the rising of the negative female humour of phlegm associated with witchcraft, and with the occurrence of solar eclipses, when the choleric energy of the sun was believed to have been swallowed by the dark, chthonic, watery elements of the moon. When Henry VI's phlegmatic impotence became apparent, chroniclers, physicians and citizens began to look out for incidents of bad weather and eclipses and the witchcraft behind such phenomena. Chroniclers became preoccupied with water and its associations with disaster. The Brut chronicler recorded increasingly destructive wet summers that spoiled the harvests.[67] The *English Chronicle* recorded the appearance of a total eclipse of the sun in 1433, 'whereof peple was sore aferd'. Both the author of the *English Chronicle* and a Welsh chronicler in the household of Edward, earl of March, recorded a great frost on St Valentine's Day 1435 and crop failure, high wheat prices and famine (which are linked to the defection of Burgundy and the siege of Calais).[68] In 1441 occurred the very public trial for witchcraft of Eleanor Cobham, wife of Humphrey, duke of Gloucester, before the king and the lords spiritual. The duchess was accused of trying to bring about the death of Henry VI through necromancy and melting a waxen image of the king. She was also charged with casting medical horoscopes with her medical adviser, Thomas Southwell, with forecasting the young king's illness and death, and with trying to harness an unfavourable conjunction of watery planets to push the king over the brink. The duchess's penance was a very high-profile public humiliation, following which she was imprisoned for life. Eleanor confessed her witchcraft, and the possibility that there was some substance to the charges and that she was practising some form of alchemical magic (her husband Humphrey was a student of alchemy and employed an alchemist, Gilbert Kymer, as his physician) is suggested by the appearance of a vial of *aqua vitae* in her inventory.[69]

The main focus of fears about the effeminizing of the body politic was Queen Margaret of Anjou. She seemed to get stronger as her husband weakened and was blamed for effeminizing the king. Margaret's very arrival in England was presaged by storm. The Croyland Chronicle gives an account of the striking of St Paul's steeple by lightning followed by fire in 1444, and goes on to say that no man living 'had ever seen or even heard of the like'.[70] This account is succeeded by notice that in the following year the Lady Margaret landed in England. The *English Chronicle* combines an account of the parliament at Bury St Edmunds and the arrest of Humphrey, duke of Gloucester, with an observation that in 1446 'yn the monethis of Novembir and Decembir fille grete thundryng and lightnyng, with huge and grete wyndis'.[71] In February 1447, when Humphrey arrived at Bury St Edmunds to see the king, he was met by the treasurer of the household and told to go to his lodgings because it was so cold. He was then arrested during an extreme frost that killed some people.[72] This traumatic event and the subsequent loss of Normandy is followed by an account of an unnaturally blood-red sun appearing for several days, which made people think 'it sholde betoken sum harm sone afterward'.[73] Bale's Chronicle records for 1450, near the anniversary of Gloucester's death, a sudden fire (probably caused by lightning) at the royal palace at Eltham when Margaret of Anjou was in residence following a 'greet wedering of rayne and wynde'.[74] Margaret continued to be associated by chroniclers with malignant, phlegmatic forces of rain, lightning and mist. In 1459 the *English Chronicle* links a menstrual rainstorm in Bedfordshire, 'a blody rayne, whereof the rede dropys appered in shetes, the whiche a woman had hongen our for to drye', with the exile and attaining of the Yorkist lords.[75] Her invasion of England in 1471, it was noted, occurred during storms. The fact that many of the prominent political women of the fifteenth century, such as Eleanor Cobham, Elizabeth Woodville, Margaret of Anjou and Margaret Beaufort, were most powerful or disruptive when they were not sexually productive and probably post-menopausal may have encouraged men to draw the links between the practice of witchcraft and the menopause.

The unpredictability of the powerful woman was explained in alchemical terms by the ambiguous figure of the water witch, Melusine. Melusine was a metaphor for the feminine spirit of nature, the prim-eval mother of being that led to the production of the philosopher's stone. She stood for the perpetual cycle of generation and regeneration that eventually led to the balance between the four humours.[76] She was a manifestation of the earth mother that devours the dead and brings forth the newborn. From her body, which was like a sealed vessel, the waters of creation rose, and through her agency the sun and moon conjoined in marriage. Half-serpent, she is the naked figure winding her way down the tree of life in the *Ripley Scrolls*, presiding over the marriage of the sun and moon (Fig. 2). Identified with mercury, she was the source of life, the basis of the alchemical work, but also a potentially destructive power, at once medicine and poison. Though a loving wife and mother, a builder of castles and founder of a dynasty, Melusine remained, in her hybridity, mercurial and unfixable.[77] These paradoxes surfaced vividly into political life when Edward IV chose Elizabeth Woodville as his bride, against the wishes of his kinsman and mentor, the earl of Warwick. A key to Edward's motives, apart from Elizabeth's obvious physical qualities, may well have been alchemical symbolism. Her mother was Jacquetta of Luxembourg, the duchess of Bedford, and through her Elizabeth could claim descent from Melusine herself.[78] The court began to unravel as the powerful Neville family split into feuding factions. During the height of the king's troubles in

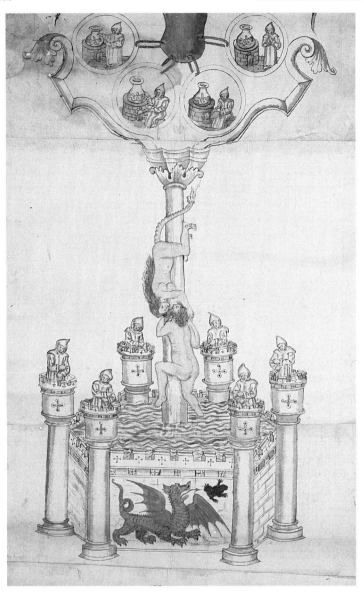

Figure 2 'Melusine', from the *Ripley Scroll*. Oxford, Bodleian Library, MS Ashmole 53.

1469, when Warwick was purging the court of Woodville influence, the mother of the queen was brought before him at Warwick Castle (where Edward was held captive) in August and accused by Thomas Wake and George, duke of Clarence, of sorcery. It was alleged that she had made a finger-length leaden image of a man-at-arms broken in the middle and made fast with line. Two other images were made to represent Edward and Elizabeth, and it was alleged that Jacquetta had used witchcraft and love potions (possibly menstrual fluid which would increase men's phlegmatic humours and make them weaker and more liable to do a woman's bidding) to cause the king to fall in love with her daughter.[79] As the disastrous political consequences of the marriage became apparent and Edward's reputation as a voluptuary grew, the demonic aspects of the king's falling into the clutches of these two descendants of Melusine would have preoccupied those prosecuting the charge of witchcraft.

This accusation demonstrates how both sexual and asexual women could be seen, in times of political upheaval, as serpents and witches undermining and disempowering the hero. The dragon vanquished by St George was often depicted as female with prominent pudenda, sometimes offering herself sexually in an effort to save her life.[80] As Edward's old friends and family drifted towards civil war, his court increasingly resembled Camelot, disintegrating around Guinevere and an enfeebled king, undone by the malign power of the mother and daughter who were the descendants of a serpent. This was a view that would have been endorsed in the Arthurian romances read at court and by the alchemists, who were keenly aware of the dual nature of Melusine as the agent of transformation and rebirth of the king and as the venomous serpent. Sir John Fortescue, a member of the 1456 alchemy commission, considered Yorkist England to be inflamed with a fever caused by the machinations of Melusine. He probably had the activities of Eleanor Cobham, Jacquetta of Luxembourg and Elizabeth Woodville in mind when he argued in *De Natura* against the female succession, the basis of Edward's occupation of the throne, and wrote:

> this was the crafty serpent nurtured on the poison of ambition which insinuating itself into the minds of princes, poisoned them so with malice of its virus that there was scarce no king who, inflamed by the angry venom growing therefrom, did not betake himself to the clash of arms by which he thought to appease the fire of that venom.[81]

The figure of Melusine, the half-woman, half-water witch using her sexuality to rob men of their power and further her own ambitions or those of her child, dominates Malory's depiction of a masculine court disintegrating around an unpopular queen. Viviane's messenger, the Lady of the Lake herself and Morgan le Fay all inhabit the realms of water.

Not surprisingly the second reign of England's King Arthur, Edward IV, was increasingly dominated by fears of witchcraft. On 12 April 1477 Clarence, delusional since his wife's childbirth-related death the preceding December, arrested his dead wife's attendant, Ankaretta Twynhot, without a warrant, on a charge of witchcraft, of killing her mistress with a venomous drink of ale laced with poison. She was executed at Warwick in Clarence's presence without a trial. In charging Twynhot with witchcraft, Clarence revived rumours of the queen's descent from Melusine. In the following year Dr Stacy, an Oxford astronomer and alchemist, and another astronomer, Thomas Blake, a chaplain of Merton College, established by art, magic and necromancy (according to their confessions) that the king would die in a short time and asserted this to a number of people in an attempt to 'shorten the king's life by sadness' (presumably by exacerbating his hypochondria). Blake was pardoned, but Stacy and Burdett were dragged to Tyburn on 19 May 1477 and hanged.[82]

This unprecedented infiltration of black magic into affairs of state and the increasing hostility towards powerful women at Edward's court were a direct response to the growing frustration with the way Edward, caught between his queen and his three regular mistresses, was becoming increasingly passive. By 1477 Edward's carnal past had come back to haunt him, and there was at this time a general perception that Edward had become disempowered by women. By this stage Edward may have come to believe, along with those pressing charges against his mother-in-law in 1469, that his profane marriage on the morning after Walpurgisnight had aroused in him a self-destructive and demonic sensuality. As his reputation for debauched satyrism increased, so too would have the belief that sexual excess had drained him of his vital heat and effeminized him. This may explain the extraordinary charge of witchcraft levelled at him by his brother Clarence, who encouraged rumours that 'the king our sovereign lord wrought him by nygromancy and used craft to poison his subjects such as he pleased'. Clarence also charged Edward with having designs on his life through witchcraft, and the imagery he used powerfully conveys that, in some minds at least, the sun had degenerated into a more occult consuming force: 'the king intended to consume him [Clarence] in likewise as a candle consumeth in burning.'[83]

Alchemy, with its imagery of scattering seed and its goal of creating life independent of women, was in some senses a masculine masturbatory fantasy. But there is in the heart of these sexual allegories a profoundly introspective dimension. The conjunction of *Sol* and *Luna*, the male and female poles, was envisaged within a single individual. The treatment of Henry VI expounded in Ripley's *Cantilena* and in the earliest version of the *Ripley Scrolls* depended on the integration of sexual opposites to make a whole personality. In his case this involved correcting an imbalance by encouraging the development of a more masculine sense of identity. The balancing of the sexual extremes (the *anima* and *animus*) to facilitate the individuation process was a more sophisticated aspect of the medical goal of humoral balance. The concept of the hermaphrodite was expounded by all alchemists. Mercury, while the female element of the alchemical marriage, could also be perceived as hermaphroditic in its volatility. The hermaphrodite features in the *Ripley Scrolls* in composite images of half-men, half-women, half-kings, half-queens, kings with breasts, representing the acceptance and acknowledgement of the male and female within the single personality that was necessary to achieve self- knowledge and growth. This was a Neoplatonic ideal in which the spirit, dulled by sexual and other forms of social intercourse, is burned, refined and distilled into pure gold. The various experiences of God among the late medieval mystics, passionate, associative, melancholy and erotic, similarly refer to a diffuse, introspective notion of sexuality.[84] The end-product of the process of perfection through alchemical masculinization is the hermaphrodite, a monster complete in itself and so removed from the heterosexual economy; that is, yet another figure of the virgin.

Notes

My thanks to Carole Rawcliffe and Frank Millard for their helpful suggestions and to Sarah Salih for her editing of this chapter.

[1] Sally G. Allen and Joanna Hubbs, 'Outrunning Atlanta: feminine destiny in alchemical transmutation', *Signs: Journal of Women in Culture and Society*, 6, 1 (1980), 210–19; Mircea Eliade, *The Forge and the Crucible: The Origins*

and Structures of Alchemy, trans. Stephen Corrin (New York: Harper & Row, 1971), pp. 43–52; Erich Neumann, *The Great Mother: An Analysis of the Archetype*, trans. Ralph Manheim (Princeton: Princeton University Press, 1963).

2   *The Mirror of Alchimy, Composed by the Thrice-Famous and Learned Fryer, Roger Bachon*, ed. Stanton J. Linden (New York: Garland, 1992), p. 10.

3   Marcellin Bertholot, *Collection des anciens alchimistes grecs* (Paris: Berthelot, 1888), p. 31.

4   Exodus 15:20–1.

5   Cambridge, Trinity College, MS R.14.45.

6   Oxford, Bodleian Library, MS Bodley Roll 1.

7   Cambridge, Trinity College, MS R.14.45, fol. 67.

8   Eliade, *The Forge and the Crucible*, pp. 43–52; Neumann, *Great Mother*.

9   John Dastin's Dream, in Elias Ashmole, *Theatrum Chemicum Britannicum* (London, 1652), pp. 258–9. The *Rosarius* is ascribed to Dastin in London, BL, MS Harley 3528, fols 171–5, and Oxford, Bodleian Library, MS Bodley Ashmole 1416, fols. 119–22. See also Lynn Thorndike, *A History of Magic and Experimental Science*, 8 vols (New York: Columbia University Press, 1923–58), vol. 3, pp. 92–4.

10 *Il Testamentum Alchemico Attributo a Raimundo Lullo: Edizione del testo latino e catelano del manuscritto Oxford, Corpus Christi College 244*, ed. Michaela Pereira and Barbara Spaggiari (Florence: Tavarnuzze, 1999), p. 15.

11 Bacon, *Mirror of Alchimy*, p. 6.

12 *George Ripley's Compound of Alchemy (1591)*, ed. Stanton J. Linden (Aldershot: Ashgate, 2001), p. 62.

13 *Thomas Norton's Ordinal of Alchemy*, ed. John Reidy, EETS, os, 272 (London: Oxford University Press, 1975), p. 83.

14 Cambridge, Trinity College, MS R.15.52, fol. 29; my translation.

15 Nigel Wilkins, *Nicolas Flamel: Des livres et de l'or* (Paris: Imago, 1993); *Nicolas Flamel, his Exposition of the Hieroglyphicall Figures*, ed. Laurinda Dixon (New York: Garland, 1994).

16 Bacon, *Mirror of Alchimy*, p. 11.

17 Ripley, *Compound of Alchemy*, p. 61.

18 Carole Rawcliffe, *Medicine and Society in Later Medieval England* (Stroud: Sutton, 1997), p. 175.

19 Bacon, *Mirror of Alchimy*, p. 53.

20 Ripley, *Compound of Alchemy*, p. 47.

21 Cited in Edward J. Kealey, *Medieval Medicus: A Social History of Anglo-Norman Medicine* (Baltimore: Johns Hopkins University Press, 1981), p. 41.

22 London, BL, MS Royal 12 Exv, fol. 22.

23 Cambridge, Trinity College, MS 0.2.5, fol. 131; Cambridge, Trinity College, MS R.14.45, fol. 2.

24 London, BL, MS Sloane 4, fols 127–209.

25 Philippe de Commynes, *Memoirs: The Reign of Louis XI, 1461–83*, trans. Michael Jones (Harmondsworth: Penguin, 1972), p. 181.

26 *Works of Sir Thomas Malory*, ed. Eugène Vinaver, 3 vols, 3rd edn (Oxford: Oxford University Press, 1947), vol. 2, pp. 270–1.

27 Laurinda S. Dixon, 'The curse of chastity: the marginalization of women in medieval art and medicine', in Robert R. Edwards and Vickie Ziegler (eds), *Matrons and Marginal Women in Medieval Society* (Woodbridge: Boydell, 1995), pp. 49–74; Barbara H. Traister, '"Matrix and the pain thereof": a sixteenth-century gynaecological essay', *Medical History*, 35 (1991), 436–51.

28 *The* Sekenesse *of* Wymmen: *A Middle English Treatise on Diseases of Women*, ed. M. R. Hallaert, Scripta, 8 (Brussels: Omirel, 1982), p. 33; London, BL, MS Sloane 2463, fol. 19.

29 *The Trotula: A Medieval Compendium of Women's Medicine*, ed. and trans. Monica H. Green (Philadelphia: University of Pennsylvania Press, 2001).

30 *Sekenesse of Wymmen*, pp. 31–2.

31 Three treatises traditionally attributed to Trotula were frequently copied and widely disseminated in nearly 100 manuscripts. John F. Benton, 'Trotula, women's problems and the professionalization of medicine in the Middle Ages', *Bulletin of the History of Medicine*, 59 (1985), 30–53. For Trotula texts see Oxford, Bodleian Library, MS Bodley 483, fols 82–117; Oxford, Bodleian Library, MS Douce 37, fols 1–42.

32 London, BL, MS Sloane 2463, fol. 230.

33 *Sekenesse of Wymmen*, p. 187.

34 Jacqueline Murray, 'Twice marginal and twice invisible: lesbians in the Middle Ages', in Vern L. Bullough and James A. Brundage (eds), *Handbook of Medieval Sexuality* (New York: Garland, 1996), pp. 191–222 (pp. 200–1).

35 London, BL, MS Sloane 2463, fol. 197v.

36 Murray, 'Twice marginal and twice invisible', pp. 200–1.

37 *Sekenesse of Wymmen*, p. 35; London, BL, MS Sloane 2463, fol. 197v.

38 London, BL, MS Sloane 2463, fol. 229v.

39 *Sekenesse of Wymmen*, p. 49.

40 Carole Rawcliffe, 'Women, childbirth and religion in later medieval England', in D. Wood (ed.), *Women and Religion in Medieval England* (Oxford: Oxford University Press, forthcoming); Brian Ayers, 'Excavations within the north-east bailey of Norwich castle', *East Anglian Archeology*, 28 (1985), 49–58; Jean D. Dawes and J. R. Magilton, *The Cemetery of St Helen-on-the-Walls*, *Aldwark* (London: Council for British Archaeology, 1980), p. 63.

41 See Anke Bernau, 'Virginal effects: text and identity in *Ancrene Wisse*', in Samantha J. E. Riches and Sarah Salih (eds), *Gender and Holiness: Men, Women and Saints in Late Medieval Europe* (London: Routledge, 2002), pp. 36–48, for further discussion of the boundaries of the anchoritic body and cell.

42 *Ancrene Riwle*, trans. M. B. Salu (Exeter: University of Exeter Press, 1990), pp. 59–60; see also Maud Burnett McInerney, '"In the meydens womb": Julian of Norwich and the poetics of enclosure', in John Carmi Parsons and Bonnie Wheeler (eds), *Medieval Mothering* (New York: Garland, 1996), pp. 157–83.

43 Caroline Walker Bynum, *Holy Feast and Holy Fast: The Religious Significance of Food to Medieval Women* (Berkeley: University of California Press, 1987), p. 173.

44 Rawcliffe, 'Women, childbirth and religion'; London, Wellcome Institute Library, MS Western 632; London, BL, Harley Charter 43.A.14; Curt F. Buhler, 'Prayers and charms in certain Middle English scrolls', *Speculum*, 39 (1964), 270–8 (274–5).

45 See book of hours in Cambridge, Trinity College, MS B.11.7, fol. 48v; Nigel Morgan, 'Longinus and the wounded heart', *Wiener Jahrbuch für Kunstgeschichte*, 46/7 (1993/4), 507–18; Madeline H. Caviness, *Visualizing Women in the Middle Ages* (Philadelphia: University of Pennsylvania Press, 2001), p. 120.

46 Rawcliffe, 'Women, childbirth and religion'; *The Writings of Margaret of Oignt, Medieval Prioress and Mystic*, ed. Renate Blumenfeld-Kosinski (Cambridge: Brewer, 1997), pp. 31–2.

47 Julian of Norwich, *A Revelation of Divine Love*, ed. Marion Glasscoe (Exeter: University of Exeter Press, 1986), p. 26 (Long Text, ch. 24).

48 For Christ as female see Caroline Walker Bynum, *Jesus as Mother: Studies in the Spirituality of the High Middle Ages* (Berkeley: University of California Press, 1982), pp. 110–69.

49 Bynum, *Holy Feast and Holy Fast*, pp. 270–2.

50 Julian, *Revelation of Divine Love*, p. 8 (Long Text, ch. 7).

51 Hildegard of Bingen, *On Natural Philosophy and Medicine*, ed. and trans. Margret Berger (Cambridge: Brewer, 1999), p. 80.

52 Jeffrey Burton Russell, *Witchcraft in the Middle Ages* (Ithaca, NY: Cornell University Press, 1972), pp. 262–3.

53 Galen, *De semine*, in *Galeni Opera*, 8 vols, ed. C. G. Kuhn (Leipzig: Knobloch, 1823), vol. 4, p. 586; Peter Brown, *The Body and Society: Men, Women and Sexual Renunciation in Early Christianity* (New York: Columbia University Press, 1988), p. 11.

54 Adapting Brown, *Body and Society*, p. 21.

55 *The Commentaries of Pius II Bks 97–99*, trans. Florence A. Cragg-Smith, Smith College Studies in History, 35 (Northampton, MA: Dept of History of Smith College, 1937–57), p. 579.

56 Ibid., p. 339.

57 'Dicta philosophorum et opiniones diversorum philosophorum', in *George Ashby's Poems*, ed. Mary Bateson, EETS, ES, 76 (London: Oxford University Press, 1899), p. 74; Anthony Gross, *The Dissolution of the Lancastrian Kingship: Sir John Fortescue and the Crisis of Monarchy in Fifteenth-Century England* (Stamford: Watkins, 1996), p. 42.

58 Joanna L. Chamberlayne, 'Crowns and virgins: queenmaking during the Wars of the Roses', in Katherine J. Lewis, Noël James Menuge and Kim M. Phillips (eds), *Young Medieval Women* (Stroud: Sutton, 1999), pp. 47–68 (p. 55).

59 R. A. Griffiths, *The Reign of King Henry VI: The Exercise of Royal Authority 1422–1461* (London: Benn, 1981), p. 255; Karen A. Winstead,

'Capgrave's St Katherine and the perils of gynecocracy', *Viator*, 25 (1994), 361–76 (368). Thanks to Katherine J. Lewis for discussion of this point.

[60] London, BL, MS Harley 543, fol. 130; London, BL, MS Cotton Domitian A.IX, fol. 83v; Cora L. Scofield, *The Life and Reign of Edward the Fourth, King of England and of France and Lord of Ireland*, 2 vols (London: Cass, 1967), vol. 1, p. 1.

[61] London, BL, MS Egerton 2572, fols 58–58v.

[62] *Political, Religious and Love Poems*, ed. Frederick J. Furnivall, EETS, os, 15 (London: Oxford University Press, 1866), p. 4.

[63] John Blacman, *Henry the Sixth: A Reprint of John Blacman's Memoir*, ed. M. R. James (Cambridge: Cambridge University Press, 1919), p. 16.

[64] London, BL, MS Harley 2407, fol. 10. See Jonathan Hughes, *Arthurian Myths and Alchemy: The Kingship of Edward IV* (Stroud: Sutton, 2002), pp. 77–115, for more detail.

[65] London, College of Arms, MS 20/25; Oxford, Bodleian Library, Bodley Ashmole Roll 26.

[66] Hughes, *Arthurian Myth and Alchemy*, pp. 301–5.

[67] *The Brut, or the Chronicles of England*, ed. Friedrich W. D. Brie, EETS, os, 131 (London: Oxford University Press, 1908), p. 512.

[68] *An English Chronicle of the Reigns of Richard II, Henry IV, Henry V and Henry VI*, ed. J. S. Davies, Camden Society, original ser., 64 (London: Camden Society, 1861), p. 55.

[69] A. R. Myers, *Crown, Household and Parliament in Fifteenth-Century England*, ed. Cecil H. Clough (London: Hambledon, 1985), p. 132.

[70] *Ingulph's Chronicle of the Abbey of Croyland with the First Continuations*, ed. Henry T. Riley (London: Bohn, 1854), p. 404.

[71] *English Chronicle*, p. 62.

[72] Ibid., pp. 62–3, 116; see also John Benet's Chronicle for 1400–62 in *Camden Miscellany*, 24, ed. G. L. Harriss and M. A. Harriss, Camden Society, 4th ser., 9 (London: Royal Historical Society, 1972), pp. 192–3.

[73] *English Chronicle*, p. 63.

[74] *Six Town Chronicles of England*, ed. Ralph Flenley (Oxford: Clarendon Press, 1911), pp. 140–1. My thanks to Frank Millard for showing me his work on prophecy and portent in relation to the fall of Humphrey, duke of Gloucester.

[75] Ibid., pp. 79–85.

[76] Paris, Bibliothèque Nationale, MS fr. 14765, fol. 135; Laurinda S. Dixon, *Alchemical Imagery in Bosch's Garden of Delights* (Ann Arbor: UMI Research, 1981), pp. 43–5.

[77] For a late medieval narrative of Melusine, see *Melusine, compiled by Jean D'Arras, Englisht about 1500*, ed. A. K. Donald, EETS, es, 68 (London: Kegan Paul, Trench, Trübner & Co., 1895).

[78] David MacGibbon, *Elizabeth Woodville, 1437–1492: Her Life and Times* (London: Arthur Barker, 1938); Anne F. Sutton and Livia Visser-Fuchs, ' "A most benevolent queen": Queen Elizabeth Woodville's reputation, her piety and her books', *The Ricardian*, 129 (1995), 214–45.

[79] G. L. Kittredge, *Witchcraft in Old and New England* (Cambridge, MA: Harvard University Press, 1928), p. 84; *Rotuli Parliamentorum*, vol. 6, pp. 232, 241; Henry A. Kelly, 'English kings and the fear of sorcery', *Medieval Studies*, 39 (1977), pp. 206–38.

[80] Samantha Riches, *St George: Hero, Martyr and Myth* (Stroud: Sutton, 2000), p. 141.

[81] *Works of Sir John Fortescue*, ed. Thomas Fortescue, Lord Clermont, 2 vols (London: privately printed, 1869), vol. 1, p. 331.

[82] Hughes, *Arthurian Myths and Alchemy*, pp. 288–90; Kelly, 'English kings and the fear of sorcery', 230–1.

[83] *Rot. Parl.*, vol. 6, p. 194.

[84] Jonathan Hughes, *Pastors and Visionaries: Religion and Secular Life in Late Medieval Yorkshire* (Woodbridge: Boydell, 1988), pp. 269–92.

9

The Jew, the Host and the Virgin Martyr: Fantasies of the Sentient Body

RUTH EVANS

In this same year [1290], in the kalends of July, there was a certain Jew in Paris, in the parish of Saint-Jean-en-Grève, who had done so much for a Christian woman that she brought him the body of Jesus Christ in a sacred host, which she had got during Holy Week, when she received the communion, and she handed it over to the Jew. When the Jew had got it as payment for his debt, he put the said host right in a cauldron of hot water, on Good Friday. And when the host was in the boiling water, he began to pierce it with his knife; and then the water became as if it were wholly red. And after that he took the said host out of the cauldron and began to strike it with a stick, which event was fully proved against the Jew by Bishop Simon Matifas. And it came about, according to the decision and assent of the experts who had been appointed to judge the case, who were Professors of the University of Paris in theology and canon law, that the said Jew was condemned to death and was burnt before all the people. And he was called the Good Jew, and his wife's name was Bellatine, and she had a daughter of twelve years old or thereabouts, whom the said Bishop Simon had baptized and lodged with the Filles-Dieu in Paris.[1]

This entry from the chronicle of St Denis is one of the earliest records of a fantasy about Jewish abuse of the eucharist that had wide currency throughout continental Europe well into the early modern period.[2] Other versions of the Paris case vary in length and detail, but the underlying *fabula* is clear enough: a Jew obtains from a woman the most precious symbol of Christian wholeness and community, the eucharist, and jealously tests its much-vaunted properties, boiling it and piercing it with various instruments until it bleeds, and (in some versions) injuring it with the instruments of the passion (hammer, nails, lance) or with judicial torture (lance, fire). Miraculously, the host transforms itself into another sign: a child or crucifix. As Miri Rubin observes of the various incarnations of this viciously anti-Semitic tale, '[t]he host's response was a truly eucharistic one, manifesting its real character: indestructible, changeable, full of mystery'.[3]

But the eucharistic *corpus Christi* (body of Christ) is not the only medieval body to be tested in this way. Numerous lives of female virgin martyrs (Katherine, Margaret, Juliana, Barbara, Agnes and so on), produced in England from the thirteenth to the sixteenth centuries, celebrate the triumph of a pure and inviolate Christian woman over the dark forces of pagan unbelief.[4] And the battleground is specifically that of the female body. *Seinte Margarete*, the well-known early Middle English version of the *vita* of one such exemplary Christian martyr, displays some striking similarities to the Paris accusation, even though it precedes it by almost ninety years.[5] Seized, humiliated and ritually tortured by the heathen governor Olibrius, the Christian virgin Margaret lives on through a variety of superhuman ordeals. First she is imprisoned, then stripped, hung up and flogged with rods. Then her flesh is ripped with awls and burnt with lighted tapers. Finally, she is thrown into a vessel of water. Margaret's body, like the abused eucharistic wafer, bleeds when pierced but remains intact – at least, until the final (phallic) sword severs (maiden)head from body.[6] As in the Paris host-desecration story, one of the effects of the miraculous indestructibility of the body in question is to bring about pious conversions.

I have deliberately brought these two narratives into proximity, but is there any reason to suppose that they might resonate with each other? *Seinte Margarete* was compiled in the early thirteenth century, and cannot claim the later host-desecration story as a contemporary intertext. Nor is it at all likely that the late thirteenth-century chroniclers of the so-called Paris story were consciously evoking early Middle English virgin martyr *passiones*. Each narrative belongs to a discrete locality (Paris; the south-west Midlands), circulates in very different milieux, and participates in different genres (historiography; hagiography). But there exist numerous later medieval English and early modern retellings of Margaret's legend and of those of the other virgin martyrs who undergo similar patterns of ritual abuse.[7] Each successive repetition of the same story or different version accrues new meanings as it is contextualized and recontextualized throughout the period, allowing for the possibility of it gaining associations with the anti-Semitic material. One such retelling is John Lydgate's *Legend of Seynt Margarete* (1415–26), which describes Margaret's body in terms that uncannily recall the eucharist: 'vertuous of kynde, rounde and small' (l. 34); 'white as melke' (l. 414).[8] Like the abused host she is first subjected to various injuries that make her bleed, and then cast in 'boylyng water' (l. 419). The narrative of Margaret's virginity, like the inviolacy of the eucharistic wafer in the host-torture legends, provides a fantasy of wholeness through which late medieval communities create their Christian identity by banishing the heathen or Jew to the outside. My focus in this chapter is on the English lives of the virgin martyrs. The case I want to make is that these narratives are shaped by the absent presence of the Jew, especially in his fantasized relation to the eucharist. If, as I will argue, the virgin's body is metonymically both Church and eucharist, then the narrative of what Jews do to the host is analogous to what pagans do to Christian virgins. Host and virgin are also related through a structure of parallel inversion: the host is an (apparently) insentient body that behaves as a sentient one when tested; the virgin is an (apparently) sentient body that is impervious to pain. But this does not mean that anti-Semitism and Christian evangelism are structurally equivalent. That would miss altogether not only their specific histories and constructions of the body, but also how each makes use of the other to articulate their different forms of power. Categories of sexuality and sexual identity, including virginity, also shape the bodies that matter (and do not matter) in anti-Semitic narratives, just as anti-Semitism shapes the cultural meanings of female bodies in English virgin martyr lives.[9]

This may seem a surprising claim, given that many of those English *vitae* were produced after 1290, the date when Jews were officially expelled from England (and, curiously enough, the date of the Paris accusation).[10] Furthermore, the host-desecration stories are confined to continental Europe, only appearing in England in the late fifteenth century, in the unique East Anglian *Croxton Play of the Sacrament* (*c*.1461).[11] And the opponents of female virgin martyrs are Romans or heathens, never Jews. I will deal in turn with these various objections, but I want to begin by looking at the category of medieval virginity itself. Because it eludes definition, virginity provides an apt example of the very signifying dynamic I aim to uncover, whereby the absent cultural narratives of anti-Semitism have the potential (in certain highly specified contexts) to transform the meanings of virginity, making the virgin and her *passio* the sites of Christian violence done to Jews. As several contributors to this volume acknowledge, virginity resists the question 'What is . . . ?' Neither a self-evident entity nor a fixed point of origin, it is not even necessarily dependent on the lack of previous sexual experience. As Margery Kempe recognizes in the early fifteenth century, virginity can be *willed*. Flickering between absence and presence, it is often most present when about to be lost. An effect of other discourses (legal, juridical, medical), it is nonetheless an effect that is not straightforwardly produced on or in the body. Its very confounding of categories may account for the repeated testing and anatomizing of the virgin's body in English virgin martyr hagiography, a testing that seeks confirmation of what cannot, finally, ever be confirmed. But how is this elusiveness relevant to anti-Semitism?

Since medieval English religious writings use the virgin's body to delimit the borders between the pure and the polluted, between Christianity and its others, the virgin and her tale necessarily carry within them the trace of what they have differed, and deferred, from in emerging as texts. As Jacques Derrida argues:

> [w]hether in the order of spoken or written discourse, no element can function as a sign without referring to another element which itself is not simply present . . . This interweaving, this textile, is the *text* produced only in the transformation of another text. Nothing, neither among the elements nor within the system, is anywhere ever simply present or absent. There are only, everywhere, differences and traces of traces.[12]

Derrida's description of how meaning is produced by *différance* (the differential spatio-temporal structure of language) implies that the *vitae* of the virgin martyrs are already sites of multiple meanings and intertextual crossings. But they also reverberate within the vast, open weave of 'language', transforming themselves in relation to a potentially inexhaustible range of other associations and contexts. The trace, as Kathleen Davis explains, 'carries within itself the mark of other elements that are, technically, absent'.[13] *Différance* accounts for how the Jew, host-desecration narrative and *corpus Christi* resonate within the textual weave. It is by no means coincidental that here Derrida might also be describing virginity. The hymen, paradoxical sign of both virginity and consummated marriage, is one of Derrida's names for *différance*: 'neither confusion nor distinction, neither identity nor difference, neither consummation nor virginity, neither the veil nor the unveiling, neither the inside nor the outside, etc.'[14]

The Book of Margery Kempe not only provides compelling historical evidence of just this paradoxical hymeneal logic but also links the virgin with the Jew. When the archbishop of York asks Margery Kempe why she goes about in white clothes and if she is a virgin, Kempe replies that she is a married woman. This puzzles her clerical interlocutors: 'Sum of þe pepil askyd whedyr [whether] sche wer a Cristen woman er [or] a Iewe.'[15] Christian or Jew, pure or impure: the white clothes of virginity are intended to draw a firm line between one physical state and another. But Kempe is married. Her white clothes – or, more accurately, the interplay between the outer signifiers of virginity and her married identity – signal the inherent paradox of virginity: neither the veil nor the unveiling. The contemptuous reference to Kempe's putative Jewish identity suggests that late medieval English vernacular culture links virginity's queerness to the dangerously ambiguous status of the Jew (and vice versa?): to what Louise Fradenburg calls 'the Jew's (non)occupation of interstices, of insides that are outsides'.[16]

Of course it is nothing new to claim that Jew and virgin meet at the borders of dirt and cleanness in the medieval English imaginary. As Jocelyn Wogan-Browne observes, 'Jewishness and virginity are intimately opposed in the construction of symbolic purity and filth.'[17] Early Middle English virgin martyr hagiography, as Robert Mills reminds us in this volume (referring to Wogan-Browne's pioneering work), invokes anti-Semitic discourse in the war against heresy.[18] This is unsurprising, given that the eleventh and twelfth centuries saw a great increase in anti-Jewish propaganda.[19] One of the ideological projects of the Fourth Lateran Council of 1215 was to draw boundaries around Christianity by violently excluding what it was not. Canon 68 of Lateran IV specified the wearing of distinguishing badges by Muslims and Jews; three years after its proclamation English Jews were made to wear the notorious badges of their difference.[20] The production of Christian identity through differentiation is seen in many texts about virginity and/or chastity that were produced in England while Jews still lived there (that is, before 1290). Rober le Chapelain's *Corset*, an Anglo-Norman exposition of the seven sacraments for his lay patron, Alain la Zouche (d. 1270), opposes

chastity and the Jew in its discussion of the sacrament of marriage.[21]
According to Rober, the roundness of the wedding ring (like that of the
eucharistic wafer?) symbolizes enduring love, and the whiteness of its
fine silver signifies that the woman is 'as white in chastity as a lily in
summer' (ll. 403–4). A *seigneur* who dishonours the proper form of
marriage is worse than a dog and behaves like the Jews.[22] If today we
believe, as Marjorie Garber puts it, that '[i]t is the dog that makes us
human', then, ironically enough, thirteenth-century English culture
believes that 'it is the Jew that makes us Christian'.[23] In *Seinte
Margarete* Olibrius's soldiers warn the governor that Margaret believes
'"o þe Lauered þe þe Gius fordemden ant drohen to deaðe, ant heðene
hongeden ant heuen on rode"' (in the Lord whom the Jews judged and
put to death, who was hanged by the heathen high on a cross) (p. 48,
ll. 16–17). This observation – which draws on the popular and enduring notion that the Jews were to blame for the death of Christ –
hints at the simultaneous identification of Margaret with Christ and of
Olibrius with the Jews. Not only is Olibrius identified in the text as
heathen but he also hangs Margaret up high, as the Jews did to Christ.
The injuries done to her body – beating, piercing – are reminiscent of
the buffeting and scourging of Christ by the Jews (and are the violent
inverse of what Christians later believe Jews do to the eucharist). The
other two Katherine group *vitae* also refer to Jews: in *Seinte Katerine*
Christ is the man whom 'þe Giws demden ant heaðene ahongeden'
(whom Jews condemned and heathens hanged), and *Seinte Iuliene*
refers to the 'giwes read' (Jews' advice).[24] The *Ancrene Wisse* (*Guide for
Anchoresses*), a virginity text closely associated with the Katherine
group, warns its audience of aristocratic women that the metaphorical
vinegar of envy will quench their love for Christ, making them like one
of the 'niðfule [envious] Giws'. Whoever carries sour thoughts in her
heart, the *Guide* declares, will be no better than a 'Giwes make'
(mate/equal).[25] Although it is true (and odd) that the persecutors of
virgins in twelfth- and thirteenth-century Britain are never represented
as Jews, the virginity texts themselves are sites where the chaste female
Christian is constructed through her opposition to the Jew.[26]

Jews may disappear from England after 1290, but they do not
disappear from English texts. For some time scholars have argued
that, despite the absence of Jews after the expulsion, a large number
of fourteenth- and fifteenth-century English texts (hagiographies,
romances, the mystery cycles, Chaucer's *Prioress's Tale*) are haunted
by the presence of what Sylvia Tomasch calls the 'virtual Jew'.[27] This

virtual Jew, Tomasch argues, is 'central not only to medieval Christian devotion but to the construction of Englishness itself'.[28] The early fifteenth-century Middle English Life of Edith of Wilton, an exemplary virgin, is a 'vengeance miracle' that explicitly deploys the opposition between the classical, intact virginal body and the grotesque, gaping body of the Jew to construct a fantasy of English Christian purity. According to Wogan-Browne, Edith's post-mortem assertion that her body is 'holle [whole] and sounde' differentiates her from the Jews, who 'euery gode-Friday at herre fundement [their anus] . . . done blede [bleed]', a reference not only to the widespread belief that Jewish men menstruated but, I would argue, to the Paris Jew's sacrilegious boiling of the host (which bleeds when pierced) on a Good Friday.[29] As Wogan-Browne brilliantly argues, 'in *Edith*, the long-expelled Jewish nation of England becomes an upturned and feminized anti-body to Edith's monastic and national purity'.[30] Edith's narrative is also haunted by the otherness of Paris (recalling the original site of the host-desecration story), since her devotion to St Denys 'promotes Wilton as a sacred site of national identity to rival St Denys in Paris'.[31]

Such violent production of Englishness also relies on an analogy between Christ and Edith. Her miracles are supposedly modelled on those of Christ, who allowed the Jews to slay him and only later took vengeance on them.[32] Margery Kempe's vivid 'eyewitness' account of Christ's passion shows how thoroughly an English born-again virgin has internalized the belief not only in the historical role of the Jews as Christ's tormentors but also in the right of devout Christians (and who better than virgins, who outrank all other categories of medieval women?) to put Jews on trial for their crimes. Kempe represents the Jews 'betyng hym & bofetyng hym in þe heued [head] & bobyng [striking] hym be-forn hys swete mowth', spitting in his face, and tearing the silk garment in which Christ is wrapped 'wyth gret violens' from his body so that it bleeds anew, nailing him to the cross and stretching the body to fit the boreholes. She imagines herself accusing them: 'ʒe cursyd Iewys, why sle ʒe my Lord Ihesu Crist?'[33] In this vision it is possible to see Kempe attempting to normalize the politically complex representation of torture in the York *Crucifixion* pageant (in which Christ's torturers are never identified as Jews) by rewriting Jews back into the scene in explicitly pernicious terms.[34]

But not all of Kempe's references to Jews are pernicious. When she is delayed in her journey north to see the abbess of Denny, she receives comfort from Christ, who tells her: 'I thanke þe for þe charite þat þu hast in þi preyer [prayer] whan þu preyist [pray] for alle Iewys & Saraʒenys [Saracens] & alle hethyn pepil þat þei xulde [should] comyn to Cristen feith.'[35] Here Jews are imagined as potential converts and recipients of Christian charity. The same formula reappears in the series of prayers with which her *Book* ends. Kempe prays 'for Iewys, & Saraʒinys, & alle hethen pepil', asking that the Lord remember 'þat þer is many a seynt in Heuyn whech sumtyme was hethen in erde [on earth]'.[36] Her imagined roll-call of 'heathen' saints must include several virgin martyrs born to heathen parents (Margaret, Katherine, Christine). But if we accept that Kempe may be including herself in the roll-call of converted saints, her idiosyncratic verbal formula hints at a more intriguing possibility. Just as Jews (and Saracens and heathens) can be 'remade' as Christians, so can married women remake themselves as 'intact' virgins through an act of will. This analogy relies on seeing Kempe's *Book* as her major submission in her bid for canonization, and on reading Kempe's self-representation as that of an allegorical 'heathen' who will be rewarded in the afterlife by canonization. If so, then the yoking together of Jews with heathen saints (because they both share in processes of conversion) suggests an analogy between Kempe's own 'willed' virginity (her perception, common enough in virginity literature of the time, that virginity is a state that can be willed and that can override sexual experience) and the processes of conversion. Jews may be linked with virgin saints because virginity itself, as Kempe understands it, represents a form of 'conversion': of remaking oneself according to the ideal of a truly devout Christian. This allows for a rather different alignment between virgins and Jews, one in which each shares in the same capacity for conversion.

But more usually what is at stake in English virgin martyr hagiography is the project of drawing a clear-cut boundary around Christianity. The Christian is defined by her difference from the heathen, whose difference allows her identity as a Christian to be properly recognized. Margaret's flesh may be lacerated, the white skin charred – 'te hude snawhwit swartede as hit snercte' (the snow-white skin blackened as it was scorched) (p. 74, l. 19) – but still her virgin body stands for the wholeness and unchangingness of the body of the Church, the *corpus verum* (true body). Lydgate's *Legend of Seynt Margarete* places great emphasis on Margaret's constancy: she is 'Ay vnmutable in hir stablenesse' (l. 19), 'hir herte roted on constaunce' (l. 21). When she later replies to Olibrius for the first time, 'Of chere nor colour ther was no variaunce; / Constaunt of herte, this holy blyssed mayde' (ll. 152–3). She symbolizes the faith that never changes. As Kathleen Coyne Kelly argues, 'the saint's virgin body . . . came to represent the "body" of the Church metonymically'.[37]

But her body is also a metonym for the *corpus mysticum* (mystic body): the eucharist.[38] As I have already argued in relation to Lydgate's Margaret, the virgin martyr's body is often described in eucharistic imagery: pure, white and round. Margaret is frequently compared to a pearl because of her Latin name, but such comparisons also evoke the virgin-as-host. In the prologue to his Life of Margaret in his *Legendys of Hooly Wummen* (1443–7) Osbern Bokenham remarks that the Latin etymology of her name (*margarita*, 'pearl') signifies that 'this uirgyne gloryous / May to a margaryte comparyd be', because she is 'whyht, lytyl, and eek verteuous'.[39] The lengthy elaboration of the etymology of Cecilia, in Chaucer's *Second Nun's Prologue and Tale* (*c.*1392–5), following a tradition established by Jacobus de Voragine, emphasizes her eucharistic aspects: her lily-like 'whitnesse' (VIII, l. 89), 'Cecilie the white' (VIII, l. 115), 'round and hool' (VIII, l. 117) – even her celestial likeness recalls the eucharist: 'swift and round and eek brennynge' (VIII, ll. 113–14), 'swift and bisy'. In a Vernon manuscript lyric, the *Six Miracles of God's Body* (*c.*1390), the host is also tireless in combating every sin, including that of sloth: 'Þis sacrament of þe Messe / Loueþ not such Idelnesse'.[40] A versified sermon in the Vernon manuscript known as *De festo corporis christi* (On the Feast of Corpus Christi) makes the virgin-as-host connection even more explicit. It singles out three famous virgin martyrs as having died for the 'bread of grace':

> Cecili, and Agnes, and Agace
> Diede for þis brede of grace
> Þerfore is riht heore [their] names to be
> Nempned [named] in þe Canone [canon (part of the
>   mass which includes the consecration)]
> ffor alle þeos [these] diȝede [died] in good entent
> ffor to Meyntyme [maintain] þe sacrament.[41]

This sermon boldly suggests that Cecilia, Agnes and Agatha were martyred not so much for Christ as for the body of Christ. Their deaths, it argues, keep alive the meaning of the host. These virgins are memorialized in the mass (as part of the litany of saints) because they (in their wholeness and purity) guarantee or underwrite the continued presence of the sacrament in the lives of Christian believers. In an extraordinary sleight of hand, the poem asserts that their absence maintains the sacrament as presence. This suggests that the body of the female virgin martyr is viewed, certainly in fourteenth-century England, as a metonym for the eucharist. But how do we read this metonymic status? As privilege or exploitation? Or as neither?

To some extent, a parallel can be drawn between the cultural status of the English virgin martyr's body and that of the bodies of fourteenth- and fifteenth-century continental women mystics. Kathleen Biddick argues that late medieval debates about transubstantiation engendered a crisis of signification over the meaning of 'Christ in a cake', a crisis that was linked to the phenomenal rise of female mystics. Their elaborate somatic performances, she contends, had little do with the appearance of a new, empowered female subjectivity. Rather, these pious women were the products of the clergy's desire to authenticate the troubled host. In Biddick's words, '[t]hey began to produce aura for the Corpus Christi'.[42] Their outré devotional practices are also defined by anti-Semitism, in particular by the blood-libel accusations sweeping across Europe: the tales that Jews abducted and ritually murdered little Christian boys. For Biddick, ' "Christendom" (*Christianitas*), Corpus Christi, and the Jew (as an anti-semitic category)' form part of a dense textual weave in which 'relations of the masculine and feminine' are also defined and redefined.[43] But Biddick's argument concerns female mystics, not virgin martyrs; she deals with historical, not virtual bodies; she is concerned with the polluting nature of blood rather than with eucharistic imagery, and she considers women and Jews more or less exclusively within a continental European context. Yet the emergence of huge numbers of *English* virgin martyr legends certainly coincides with the emergence of the Feast of Corpus Christi, around which coheres and condenses a mythology of wholeness and community, and which is concerned with the delineation of the borders of *Christianitas* through the violent expulsion of others, including Jews. The first appearance in England of the new feast is in 1318.[44] Between 1315 and 1325, England (along with much of Europe) was hit by severe famines and then in 1348 came the catastrophe of the plague, an event that was widely blamed on the Jews.[45] At the same time as the eucharist emerges as the most powerful signifier of late medieval European Christian wholeness, so also do narratives about its destruction at the hands of

Jews, narratives about the role of Jews in bringing disease and death, and narratives about the purity and fortitude of certain pious virginal women who profess the Christian faith even to their death.

Despite Biddick's warning that it is important not to judge the performances of continental female mystics, she tends to reduce them to passive ideological dupes, whose function is to cover over the gaps in the ideology of transubstantiation.[46] Of course, it is true that, like Kempe's white clothes, like the host, virginity seeks to cover the gap between inside and outside. But the lives of the English virgin martyrs do not merely serve to provide aura for the *corpus Christi* or to ward off the pollution of Jews. Although Kim Phillips in this volume makes the point that actual historical virgins were more often subjugated than empowered by their sexuality (because of the fears provoked by the preciousness of virginity), the virgins of medieval English hagiography cannot easily be read as victims.[47] But neither do they straight-forwardly enact a transgressive female *jouissance*. As Mills argues, their representations resist the binary opposition of oppressor and oppressed because their meanings are caught up within a proliferating range of historical contexts, including anti-Semitism.[48] William Paris's extraordinarily jaunty but pious life of *Christine* (*c.*1397–9) never mentions the Jews, but engages with the polarities of Jew/Christian, feminine/masculine, letter/spirit, blindness/insight that are present in the continental host-torture tales.[49] Many details in the poem confirm Christine as a version of the eucharist – for example, 'Hire flesche, þat was so white & shene [fair]' (l. 226) – and her martyrdom as host-torture: she is boiled in a cauldron of 'oile, pyche [pitch] & rosyne [resin]' (l. 309) where she imitates the host as Christ-child, 'al innocente / In credylle [cradle] rokkede' (ll. 317–18); she is put in a hot oven, where she remains miraculously unscathed.

But a reading of the text in these terms makes it clear that the moments where Christine seems to be most 'empowered' are also those in which her body functions as an agent of Christian imperialism. When her heathen father Urban orders that her flesh be scraped from her bones, Christine lobs a slice of that flesh back at her father's eye with the gleeful words: 'Haue here a morcelle, teraunte [tyrant]! take ite! / Of þe flesche was getyne of the' (that you produced) (ll. 239–40). Subversive as this appears (especially in its comic overturning of traditional medieval father–daughter relationships), it is also import-ant to recognize that it reworks the familiar polarity between Christian insight and Jewish blindness. Jews are often represented in medieval anti-Semitism as physically and spiritually blind (as in Christian representations of the allegorical figure of Synagoga), because of their Pauline association with the letter of the text.[50] The Christian virgin martyr opposes such blindness. In the prologue to Chaucer's *Second Nun's Tale*, the etymology of Cecilia's name includes the meanings 'the wey to blynde' (VIII, l. 92) and '[w]antynge of blyndnesse' (VIII, l. 100). This opposition is dynamically represented in *Christine* when Julian, the third tyrant, amazed at the maimed Christine's ability to keep talking, demands: 'Kytte [cut] oute hire tonge: it dos me woo' (it's hurting me) (l. 460). Repeating her previous *modus operandi*, Christine promptly throws her severed tongue at Julian's eye, as an ironic reminder of both his spiritual blindness and his insistence on the carnal letter: flesh hurts.

But in other details of the text the polarities start to undo themselves. In particular the extensive wordplay on Christine's name subverts and disperses apparently fixed gender and religious identities. For example, the narrator explains that Christine is able to resist her original heathen identity through the force of the Holy Ghost: 'Thus god cane of vncrystyne [unChristians/unChristines] make / Right holy martirs to be his' (ll. 55–6). Later we are told that 'Crist cristynde [christened/Christined] Cristyne' (l. 274). The onomastic word-play attempts to make Christine's name identical with the name of Christian, but the play on christening disseminates that secure identity by reminding Christians of their proximity to Jews. For Christine's very name bears witness to the sacrament of baptism through which, according to Augustinian theology, the exterior sign of Jewish circumcision is transformed into the interior identity of the Christian. Because Christine is female, the text invites us to see gender as structuring what it means to be a Christian. Sentience is crucial here. To what extent can the female body be generically Christian? Only to the extent that it is insentient, that it feels no pain? Repeatedly, the narrator tells us that Christine feels nothing: even in the boiling cauldron she 'felyde [felt] no wo' (l. 318). By contrast, her pagan opponents do suffer: Christine's tongue 'hurts' Julian. The Jew feels no pain when he stabs the bleeding host (nor does the host), but the violence he does to it (which is the violence that Christians do to Jews) comes back to haunt the virgin martyr *passio* with a difference. Is the eucharist also gendered? The virgin's extreme version of insentience, its displacement onto her torturers (which does not happen in the host-torture tales), reveals what has had to be repressed about the human body in order to make the virgin's body a coherent symbol of Christian wholeness. In both host-torture and virgin-torture the polarities between Jew and Christian are sustained by certain fantasies of the gendered body in which a Jew figures as carnal and a woman as spiritual. But Christine's insensitivity to pain also points to the limitations of these narratives as feminist fables, since real women do feel pain. Victim or victor? There is no way out of the aporia of reading: only further contexts (and readers) will suggest further meanings, will continue to make these narratives mean.

Because the vulnerable *female* body is so much on show in virgin martyr hagiography, critics readily acknowledge that gender and sexuality are at play in their legends. But they are also in play in the anti-Semitic host-desecration narratives. Rubin acknowledges the place of gender when she observes that the wife/mother in these tales is seen as 'misguided but pliant, impressionable, open to conversion'; a point of entry for the polluting forces of the Jew.[51] But this misses the ways in which gender and sexuality work at more fundamental levels in the host-desecration tales to sustain the differences between (impure) Jewish and (pure) Christian identities. When the Jew in the Paris case pierces the host with a knife, the reddening water evokes (blasphemously) not only Longinus' piercing of Christ but also the myth of Jewish men menstruating (referred to in the fifteenth-century Life of Edith), a myth that produces the incoherent gender and sexuality of the Jewish man. Other details sexualize the Jew, and – curiously – link his queerly feminized body with that of the virgin martyr and of the eucharist. The stabbing of the host also suggests, as in the narratives of the virgin martyrs, eroticized or sadistic meanings. I do not mean to suggest that the Jew obtains sexual satisfaction from the tortures. This is equally problematic in relation to the pagan torturers of female virgins. But the category of the Jew does not just serve to define and redefine relations with the Christian, and between masculine and feminine: it is itself already divided, already carries within itself the traces of these other sexualized meanings.

In mid-thirteenth-century Paris, one of the areas in which prostitutes plied their trade was La Grève, the parish in which the Paris host-desecration case is located.[52] There were also strict rules about the mingling of Jews and prostitutes: as Vern and Bonnie Bullough note, sexual intimacies between Jews and Christians were considered dangerous to Christianity.[53] The bishop's consigning of the Jew's daughter to the convent of the Filles-Dieu is rich with sexual connotations: this particular convent was originally founded to house penitent prostitutes.[54] As a polluting Jew, despite her baptism, she is still considered dangerously sexual. The conflation of penitent prostitutes with penitent former Jews suggests that Jewish female sexuality (like Jewish male sexuality) is viewed as deviant. As recently as 1969 a rumour was spread in Orléans 'that the Jewish proprietors of a new boutique were abducting younger female customers to sell into prostitution'.[55] This pernicious anti-Semitic 'rumour', a version of the medieval fantasy of Jews stealing and murdering young Christian boys, justifies the Jew's place 'outside' by producing him as a social deviant: a pimp. But in the medieval legend it is the Christian bishop who fulfils this role. Perhaps the medieval tale reveals what has had to be repressed about Gentile violence in the modern 'rumour'.

The Jew in the 1290 Paris case is the 'Good Jew': safely neutralized through being burnt like the host or the female virgin martyr. He does not speak. But the Jew answers back with a vengeance in a later English text. 'I am a Jew', declares Shylock famously in Shakespeare's *The Merchant of Venice*: 'Hath not a Jew eyes? Hath not a Jew hands, organs, dimensions, sense, affections, passions . . . ? If you prick us do we not bleed?'[56] Jonathan Dollimore reads this speech as an instance of what he calls 'the perverse dynamic', a dynamic that discloses 'not the reassuring static bedrock of common humanity but terrifyingly mobile proximities and connections between human diversity'.[57] Shylock's speech challenges its Christian auditors by drawing attention to Jewish proximity: to the figure of the Jew within Christendom as the outside insider and inside outsider. As Dollimore contends, Shylock's challenge lies in his interpretation of the law, a challenge that subverts notions of Christian mercy from within the law. But I also hear in this speech the echo of medieval Christian fantasies: of Jewish abuse of the host and pagan abuse of virgin martyrs. How can this be, in a post-Reformation text? Yet virgin martyrs live on. John Foxe's Protestant *Book of Martyrs* (1563) has no Margaret or Juliana, but it does include Katherine (albeit with large reservations).[58] Both host-torture and virgin-torture resonate in Shylock's words. 'Hath not a Jew eyes?' evokes the traditional medieval view of the Jews as spiritually blind, but what is politically subversive about Shylock's words is that he arrogates to his Jewish body the same properties that were attributed in the late Middle Ages to the insentient (but bleeding) *corpus Christi* and female virgin martyr. His words allude not only to the medieval myth of Jewish men menstruating ('If you prick us do we not bleed?') but also to the fantasy of the bleeding child-host. Scandalously, Shylock aligns himself with the eucharist, the most privileged signifier of Christian wholeness, and also with the female virgin martyr. His speech is redolent with sexual and gendered meanings that attest to the continued presence of the medieval in the early modern. And they point to a further 'perverse dynamic': that Christian culture relies on certain normative ideas of the body, sex, gender, sexuality in order to affirm its unity. In the 1290 Paris case, in virgin martyr hagiography, in *The Merchant of Venice*, 'sex' is used as a regulatory practice to define bodies that matter. A culturally legitimated script of the pure eucharist produces on the one hand what Judith Butler calls 'the domain of intelligible bodies' (those of the virgin martyrs) and on the other 'a domain of unthinkable, abject, unliveable bodies' (those of Jews).[59]

Notes

I would like to thank Anke Bernau, Juliette Dor, Simon Gaunt, Lisa Lampert, Katherine Lewis and Sarah Salih.

[1] *Les Grandes Chroniques de France*, ed. Jules Viard, 10 vols (Paris: Champion, 1920–53), vol. 8, pp. 144–5: 'En yce meismes an, en la kalende de juignet, il ot 1 juif à Paris, en la paroisse de saint Jehan en Greve, lequel fist tant par devers une femme crestienne, que elle li aporta le corps de Jhesu Crist en une oeste sacrée, laquelle elle avoit receue en la sepmaine peneuse, en la acommingant, et la bailla au juif. Quant le juif l'ot par devers soy, si mist la dicte oeste en plaine chaudiere de yaue chaude, le jour du vendredi aouré. Et quant ladicte oeste fu en l'yaue boullant, il la commença à poindre de son coutel; et lors devint l'yaue aussi comme toute vermeille. Et apres ce, il osta ladicte oeste de la chaudiere et la commença à batre d'une verge, laquelle chose fut toute prouvée contre le juif par l'evesque Symon Matiffart. Si avint que, du conseil et de l'assentement des preudeshommes qui à Paris estoient regens en theologie et en decret, ledit juif fu condampné a mourir et fu ars devant tout le peuple. Et estoit appellé le Bon Juif, et sa femme avoit à non Bellatine, laquelle avoit une fille de l'aage de XII ans ou environ, que ledit evesque Symon fist baptizier, et la fist demourer avec les Filles Dieu à Paris.' English translation mine. Simon Mattifart (or Matifas) de Bucy was bishop of Paris (1290–1304). Various Latin and French versions of the case survive, but none can be dated before 1299: Miri Rubin, *Gentile Tales: The Narrative Assault on Late Medieval Jews* (New Haven: Yale University Press, 1999), p. 40.

[2] Rubin, *Gentile Tales*, pp. 40–69.

[3] Ibid., p. 41.

[4] For a checklist of these versions, see Charlotte D'Evelyn and Frances A.

Foster, 'Saints' legends', 'Collections of saints' legends', 'English translations of the *Legenda Aurea*', 'Legends of individual saints', in J. Burke Severs and Albert E. Hartung (eds), *A Manual of the Writings in Middle English, 1050–1500*, The Connecticut Academy of Arts and Sciences (Hamden: Archon Books, 1970), pp. 413–29, 430–9, 556–9, 559–60, 561–635.

5   *Seinte Margarete*, in *Medieval English Prose for Women: Selections from the Katherine Group and* Ancrene Wisse, ed. and trans. Bella Millett and Jocelyn Wogan-Browne (Oxford: Clarendon Press, 1990; rev. edn 1992), pp. 44–85. All subsequent references are to this edition and translation, with page and line numbers in parentheses in the text.

6   On the obsession with torture in the Katherine group, see Sarah Salih, 'Performing virginity: sex and violence in the Katherine group', in Cindy L. Carlson and Angela Jane Weisl (eds), *Constructions of Widowhood and Virginity in the Middle Ages* (Basingstoke: Macmillan, 1999), pp. 95–112 (pp. 95–6). For a reading of later medieval English versions of St Margaret's life, see Katherine J. Lewis, ' "Lete me suffre": reading the torture of St Margaret of Antioch in late medieval England', in Jocelyn Wogan-Browne et al. (eds), *Medieval Women: Texts and Contexts in Late Medieval Britain: Essays for Felicity Riddy* (Turnhout: Brepols, 2000), pp. 69–82.

7   For a diagrammatic representation of the formulaic tortures in the three Katherine group *vitae*, see Jocelyn Wogan-Browne, 'The virgin's tale', in Ruth Evans and Lesley Johnson (eds), *Feminist Readings in Middle English Literature: The Wife of Bath and All her Sect* (London: Routledge, 1994), pp. 165–94 (p. 176).

8   *Seynt Margarete*, in *The Minor Poems of John Lydgate*, part 1, ed. Henry Noble MacCracken, EETS, es, 107 (London: Kegan Paul, Trench, Trübner & Co. and Oxford University Press, 1911), pp. 173–92. Line numbers are given parenthetically in the text.

9   I am grateful to Lisa Lampert for this suggestion. For a problematization of the category of the erotic, see Sarah Salih, 'When is a bosom not a bosom? Problems with "erotic mysticism" ', in this volume.

10 On the expulsion of the Jews from England, see Sophia Menache, 'The king, the church and the Jews: some considerations on the expulsions from England and France', *Journal of Medieval History*, 13 (1987), 223–36, and 'Matthew Paris's attitudes towards Anglo-Jewry', *Journal of Medieval History*, 23 (1997), 139–62. The coincidence of dates between the Paris case and the expulsion of the Jews from England is remarked upon by Rubin, *Gentile Tales*, p. 47: 'The English crown evicted its Jews in the very year in which "Dieu fut bouilli" in Paris.'

11 *Non-Cycle Plays and Fragments*, ed. Norman Davis, EETS, ss, 1 (Oxford: Oxford University Press, 1970), pp. 58–89. As Davis notes, p. lxxiii: '*The Play of the Sacrament* is the only thing of its kind in medieval English.' His account of the sources (pp. lxxiii–lxxv) mentions the Paris legend (but does

not give a specific source) and notes fourteenth-century Italian analogues, pointing out that the *Play* differs in several details from the continental versions. Not all critics agree that the *Play*'s 'Jews' are Jews: various allegorical referents have been proposed, including 'generic doubters' and Lollards; see Lisa Lampert, 'The once and future Jew: the Croxton *Play of the Sacrament*, Little Robert of Bury and historical memory', *Jewish History*, 15 (2001), 235–55 (236). One reason why the host-desecration tales do not reach England earlier than 1461 may be due to the deportation: as Rubin argues, the tales have real currency only in areas of 'areas of dense Jewish population'; *Gentile Tales*, p. 47. However, this does not explain why the myth then appears in England in 1461.

[12] Jacques Derrida, *Positions*, trans. Alan Bass (Chicago: University of Chicago Press, 1981), p. 26.

[13] Kathleen Davis, *Deconstruction and Translation* (Manchester: St Jerome Publications, 2001), p. 15.

[14] Derrida, *Positions*, p. 43.

[15] *The Book of Margery Kempe*, ed. Sanford Brown Meech and Hope Emily Allen, EETS, os, 212 (London: Oxford University Press, 1949), p. 124.

[16] Louise O. Fradenburg, 'Criticism, anti-Semitism, and the *Prioress's Tale*', *Exemplaria*, 1 (1989), 69–115 (77).

[17] Jocelyn Wogan-Browne, *Saints' Lives and Women's Literary Culture, c.1150–1300: Virginity and its Authorizations* (Oxford: Oxford University Press, 2001), p. 118. Fradenburg remarks on 'the intimacy of the connection between anti-semitism and medieval legends of the Virgin', noting that '[t]he performance of miracles for hitherto perfidious Jews is simply part of the pageant of Marian Motherhood, which stages the life of the pure on the edge of abjection'; 'Criticism, anti-Semitism', pp. 88–90. See also Kathleen Biddick, 'Genders, bodies, borders: technologies of the visible', in Nancy F. Partner (ed.), *Studying Medieval Women* (Cambridge, MA: Mediaeval Academy of America, 1993), pp. 87–116 (p. 102).

[18] Robert Mills, 'Can the virgin martyr speak?'; Wogan-Browne, 'The virgin's tale', pp. 178, 191, n. 47; Wogan-Browne, *Saints' Lives and Women's Literary Culture*, pp. 118–22.

[19] Gavin I. Langmuir, *History, Religion, and Antisemitism* (London: I. B. Tauris, 1990), p. 291.

[20] See Geraldine Heng, 'The romance of England: *Richard Coer de Lyon*, Saracens, Jews, and the politics of race and nation', in Jeffrey Jerome Cohen (ed.), *The Postcolonial Middle Ages* (New York: St Martin's Press, 2000), pp. 135–71 (pp. 148–9).

[21] *Corset: A Rhymed Commentary on the Seven Sacraments by Rober le Chapelain*, ed. Keith Val Sinclair, Anglo-Norman Text Society, 52 (London: ANTS, 1995), cited in Wogan-Browne, *Saints' Lives and Women's Literary Culture*, p. 83. Line numbers are given in parentheses in the text.

[22] Sinclair, *Corset*: 'Kar celui est paiour ke chien / Ke feit le mal encuntre le bien, / Et ki est pres de prestre sacré, / Quant il ne l'honure en Dé / Sachez:

mult piert al sacrement, / Kil deshonure a escïent, / Kar il fount sicome li Giu firent.' (For he is worse than a dog who does wrong against the good, and who is near to the sacred priest when he doesn't honour him in God. Know this: he who wittingly dishonours it, loses a great deal of the sacrament [of marriage], because he behaves as the Jews did.) (ll. 445–7).

[23] Marjorie Garber, *Dog Love* (New York: Touchstone, 1997), p. 39.

[24] Wogan-Browne, 'The virgin's tale', pp. 178, 191, n. 47; *Seinte Katerine*, ed. S. R. T. O. d'Ardenne and E. J. Dobson, EETS, ss, 7 (London: Oxford University Press, 1981), p. 18, l. 119; *Þe Liflade ant te Passiun of Seinte Iuliene*, ed. S. R. T. O. d'Ardenne, EETS, os, 248 (London: Oxford University Press, 1961), p. 57, l. 608.

[25] Millett and Wogan-Browne, *Medieval English Prose for Women*, p. 124, ll. 16, 32.

[26] Wogan-Browne, *Saints' Lives and Women's Literary Culture*, pp. 118–22. Drawing on the work of René Girard, Wogan-Browne convincingly argues that the occlusion of Jews as persecutors of virgins in these texts evidences a scapegoating mechanism in which the Jew can never figure but is instead displaced in Jewish ritual-murder stories.

[27] Sylvia Tomasch, 'Postcolonial Chaucer and the virtual Jew', in Cohen (ed.), *Postcolonial Middle Ages*, pp. 243–60 (p. 243). See also Bernard Glassman, *Anti-Semitic Stereotypes without Jews: Images of the Jews in England, 1290–1700* (Detroit: Wayne State University Press, 1975); Denise Despres, 'Immaculate flesh and the social body: Mary and the Jews', *Jewish History*, 12 (1998), 47–69; Sheila Delany (ed.), *Chaucer and the Jews: Sources, Contexts, Meanings* (London: Routledge, 2002); Heng, 'The romance of England'. For editions of explicitly anti-Semitic hagiographic narratives (the *vitae* of William of Norwich and the Jewish martyrs of Blois), see *Medieval Hagiography: An Anthology*, ed. Thomas Head (New York: Garland, 2000).

[28] Tomasch, 'Postcolonial Chaucer', p. 244.

[29] Jocelyn Wogan-Browne, 'Outdoing the daughters of Syon? Edith of Wilton and the representation of female community in fifteenth-century England', in Wogan-Browne et al. (eds), *Medieval Women*, pp. 393–409 (pp. 402–3). Quotations are from the vernacular Life, *S. Editha sive Chronicon Vilodunense im Wiltshire Dialekt*, ed. C. Horstmann (Heilbronn: Henninger, 1883), ll. 4762 and 4896. See also Willis Johnson, 'The myth of Jewish male menses', *Journal of Medieval History*, 24 (1998), 273–95. On Edith's chastity, see also Joanna Huntington in this volume.

[30] Wogan-Browne, 'Outdoing the daughters', p. 402.

[31] Ibid., p. 400.

[32] Horstmann, *S. Editha*, ll. 4755–75.

[33] *Book of Margery Kempe*, pp. 190, 191, 192.

[34] 'XXXV The Pinners: *The Crucifixion*', in *The York Plays*, ed. Richard Beadle (London: Arnold, 1982), pp. 315–23. I owe this suggestion to Sarah Salih.

[35] *Book of Margery Kempe*, p. 204.

36   Ibid., p. 250.

37   Kathleen Coyne Kelly, 'Useful virgins in medieval hagiography', in Carlson
     and Weisl (eds), *Constructions of Widowhood and Virginity*, pp. 135–64 (p.
     136). See also Kelly, *Performing Virginity and Testing Chastity in the Middle
     Ages* (London: Routledge, 2000), pp. 41–2.

38   For the distinction between the terms *corpus verum* and *corpus mysticum*,
     see Biddick, 'Genders, bodies, borders', p. 108.

39   Osbern Bokenham, *Vita S. Margaretae*, in *Legendys of Hooly Wummen*, ed.
     Mary S. Serjeantson, EETS, os, 206 (London: Oxford University Press,
     1938), pp. 7–38, ll. 249–51. Line numbers are given parenthetically in the
     text.

40   *The Minor Poems of the Vernon Manuscript*, ed. Carl Horstmann and F. J.
     Furnivall, 2 vols, EETS, os, 98, 117 (London: Kegan Paul, Trench,
     Trübner, 1892 and 1901), p. 204, ll. 227–8. For another example (from a
     fifteenth-century short Latin verse and its Middle English translation on the
     virtues of the consecrated host), of the allegorization of the wafer in terms
     that call to mind the virgin's body, see Siegfried Wenzel, *Verses in Sermons:
     'Fasciculus Morum' and its Middle English Poems* (Cambridge, MA:
     Mediaeval Academy of America, 1978), pp. 182–3, cited in Rubin, *Corpus
     Christi*, p. 102.

41   *Minor Poems of the Vernon Manuscript*, pp. 168–97, ll. 553–8, cited in
     Rubin, *Corpus Christi*, pp. 218–19.

42   Biddick, 'Genders, bodies, borders', p. 111.

43   Ibid., p. 90.

44   Rubin, *Corpus Christi*, pp. 199–200.

45   J. L. Bolton, *The Medieval English Economy 1150–1500* (London: Dent,
     1980; repr. 1988 with supplement), pp. 58–9. On the scapegoating of the
     Jews for the Black Death, see Seraphine Guerchberg, 'The controversy over
     the alleged sowers of the Black Death in the contemporary treatises on
     plague', in Sylvia Thrupp (ed.), *Change in Medieval Society: Europe North
     of the Alps, 1050–1500* (New York: Appleton-Century-Crofts, 1984), pp.
     208–24; Langmuir, *History, Religion, and Antisemitism*, pp. 267, 301.

46   Biddick, 'Genders, bodies, borders', p. 113.

47   This volume, pp. 80–1.

48   This volume, pp. 201–7.

49   Edited in *Sammlung Altenglischer Legenden*, ed. Carl Horstmann
     (Heilbronn: Henninger, 1878; repr. Hildesheim, 1969), pp. 183–90. Line
     references are given parenthetically in the text: translations mine. For a
     prose translation of the complete poem, see *Chaste Passions: Medieval
     English Virgin Martyr Legends*, ed. and trans. Karen A. Winstead (Ithaca,
     NY: Cornell University Press, 2000), pp. 61–9.

50   Tomasch, 'Postcolonial Chaucer', p. 249.

51   Rubin, *Gentile Tales*, p. 41.

52   Jacques Rossiaud, *Medieval Prostitution*, trans. Lydia G. Cochrane
     (London: Blackwell, 1988), p. 55.

[53] Vern L. Bullough and Bonnie Bullough, *Prostitution: An Illustrated Social History* (New York: Crown Publishers, 1978), p. 121.

[54] Leah Lydia Otis, *Prostitution in Medieval Society: The History of an Urban Institution in Languedoc* (Chicago: University of Chicago Press, 1985), pp. 72–3: 'In Paris, Fulk of Neuilly, a student of Peter the Chanter, whose preaching of repentance was aimed principally at usurers and public women, founded, in cooperation with Peter of Roissac, a community for repentant prostitutes, which was erected into an abbey in 1206. A similar community, based on the Augustinian rule and called the Filles-Dieu, was founded by the Parisian theologian William of Auvergne in 1226. Saint Louis [Louis IX, reign 1226–70] is said to have been a generous benefactor of this community.'

[55] See Hans-Joachim Neubauer, *The Rumour: A Cultural History*, trans. Christian Braun (London: Free Association Books, 1999), cited in the review of this book by Frank Cioffi, 'Blather', *London Review of Books*, 22 (22 June 2000), p. 20.

[56] William Shakespeare, *The Merchant of Venice*, in *The Norton Shakespeare*, ed. Stephen Greenblatt, Walter Cohen, Jean E. Howard and Katharine Eisaman Maus (New York: Norton, 1997), 3. 1. 50–4.

[57] Jonathan Dollimore, *Sexual Dissidence: Augustine to Wilde, Freud to Foucault* (Oxford: Clarendon Press, 1991), p. 122.

[58] John Foxe, *Actes and Monuments of matters most speciall and memorable, happening in the Church, with a Vniuersall history of the same* [1563], 3 vols, 4th edn (London: John Daye, 1583).

[59] Judith Butler, *Bodies that Matter: On the Discursive Limits of 'Sex'* (New York: Routledge, 1993), p. xi.

10

Can the Virgin Martyr Speak?

ROBERT MILLS

Feminist analysis of female virgin martyrs often confronts a seemingly intractable double bind. On the one hand, tortured, dismembered virgins feature heavily in a script that casts the virgin as victim. Tertullian's remark that 'every public exposure of an honourable virgin is [to her] a suffering of rape',[1] like the conventional critique of modern pornography, conflates spectacle *with* sexual violence,[2] an argument that simultaneously raises rape to the status of ever-present threat and denies the virgin any sort of public space in which to resist. Likewise, hagiography critic Brigitte Cazelles argues that the theatrical ordeal of female virgin martyrs 'reduces, rather than promotes, their role as active contributors to the cultural or spiritual welfare of society'; female sanctity is grounded, for her, 'in bodily pain, silence, and passivity'.[3] On the other hand, female saints' lives have also been read for the discourses of 'empowerment' they embody, for the ways in which they defy the tradition of relegating women to an inactive, speechless, painful existence. Virgin martyrs are consistently public, it is countered; they engage in openly political discourse with the people who are portrayed as their oppressors; they actively resist objectification and rape. As Jocelyn Wogan-Browne remarks, saints' lives 'do at least open up the possibility of resistant readings, which in particular contexts may constitute relative empowerment or recuperation'.[4]

This article will endeavour to negotiate the conflict between victimization and empowerment that appears to characterize the virgin martyr's condition with reference to a body of postcolonial writings that similarly attempt to assess the role of women's desire, agency and subject status in the discourses in which they are inscribed. In her 1985 article 'Can the subaltern speak?', Gayatri Chakravorty Spivak describes the circumstances surrounding the death of a young Bengali woman on her husband's funeral pyre (the practice of 'sati' or widow sacrifice).[5] Because the widow's attempt at 'speaking' outside normal patriarchal channels was not understood or supported, an absence of subject status that brings into focus the difficulty with which the voices of oppressed subjects can ever be recovered, Spivak concludes that 'the subaltern cannot speak'.[6] I wish to use Spivak's example of the immolated widow as a way of thinking through the medieval female virgin martyr, not because I think we should ignore the clear cultural and historical differences between these two categories of subject, but because the tortured virgin shares one quality in particular with the sati: her identity is predominantly an effect of discourse, rather than a clearly identifiable, self-evident reality. Moreover, the martyr's discursive formation is predicated on the opportunities afforded by her iconic death. The martyr-to-be is merely a Christian noblewoman, albeit chaste and pure; it is only *in death* that her virginal status is confirmed and her role as martyr fixed. Likewise the prospective sati is only a widow until she makes her sacrifice and turns into sati proper; the only true sati is a dead sati.[7] The question I wish to pose is whether death, in turn, makes martyrs, like satis, emblematically silenced subjects. Spivak's point about the subaltern is not that the sati never actually talks in various ways, but that speaking is 'a transaction between speaker and listener' and that, as such, subaltern talk does not achieve the level of a dialogic utterance.[8] Sati is different from martyrdom in that martyrdom's status as fiction is more immediately apparent (at least for the modern reader). In addition, familiarity with the genre would mean that medieval audiences approached the lives in full awareness of the virgin's martyr status from the beginning. But if, as Gail Ashton has implied, the prevailing tendency in virgin martyr legends is to make virgins 'powerless mirror images of patriarchal assumption', 'patriarchal dolls' who ventriloquize predominantly masculine concerns, speaker and listener become one, effectively silencing what Ashton has more optimistically termed the 'authentic female voice'.[9] And if, as Karen Winstead has argued, the legends invite more radical interpretations in certain specific contexts,[10] is this desire for resistant subjects wishful thinking, a rhetorical move that downplays the patriarchal violence of these texts? Or can the voice of the virgin martyr be satisfactorily represented by the modern hagiographic scholar? In what voices do female virgin martyrs speak – their own, those of their authors or readers, or voices continuous with the language of their oppressors?

The subject of martyrdom: circumvented rape

In the *Golden Legend* (*c.*1260), Jacobus de Voragine features the stories of a number of virgin martyrs, including that of St Agnes, a young woman who died *c.*305 during the age of Constantine.[11] Agnes, a 13-year-old virgin, is returning home from school when the Roman prefect's son catches sight of her and immediately falls 'in love'. Agnes rejects his protestations, explaining that she has already promised herself to another lover 'far nobler than you, of more eminent descent. His mother is a virgin, his father knows no woman, he is served by angels . . . his love is chastity itself, his touch holiness, union with him, virginity.' When the prefect's son hears her words, he is beside himself with grief; the doctors diagnose lovesickness. The young man's father seeks Agnes out and tries to persuade her to change her mind; hearing rumours that her betrothed is in fact Christ, the prefect begins to use threats. Agnes exclaims: 'Do whatever you like, but you will not obtain what you want from me' (p. 102). The prefect replies that she must choose between either sacrificing to the virgin goddess Vesta ('since your virginity means so much to you') or being placed in a brothel.

Unable to compel Agnes to obey his commands on account of her rank, the prefect decides to bring up the issue of the young woman's Christianity. Agnes still refuses to sacrifice to the pagan gods, asserting that her virtue cannot be tarnished 'because I have with me a guardian of my body, an angel of the Lord'. So the prefect orders her to be stripped naked and taken to a brothel; miraculously God makes Agnes's hair grow till it covers her bared flesh. When she enters the 'house of shame', it is filled with light and she transforms the place into a house of prayer. The prefect's son goes there with his friends and invites them to go in and 'take their pleasure with her'; terrified by the miraculous glow, they all run away. Ridiculing their cowardice, the youth rushes in 'to force himself upon Agnes' but, overwhelmed by the light, he is set upon by a devil and dies of strangulation. His father, the prefect, on a mission to find out the circumstances of his son's death, persuades Agnes to bring the son back to life. Agnes complies and the priests of the temples, seeing the young man resurrected and now preaching the words of Christ, accuse the saint of witchcraft. The prefect, impressed by the miracle, defers responsibility to Aspasius, his deputy. Aspasius has Agnes thrown into a fire but the flames separate and, while Agnes survives unscathed, the spectators on either side are burned to a crisp. Finally the deputy orders a soldier to thrust a dagger in Agnes's throat, at which point 'her heavenly spouse consecrated her his bride and martyr' (p. 103).

The Life of St Agnes was disseminated in England in the later Middle Ages in a number of vernacular versions, including those in the late thirteenth-century or early fourteenth-century *South English Legendary*[12] and Osbern Bokenham's *Legendys of Hooly Wummen* (*c.*1447).[13] Much hagiographic scholarship has focused in recent years on the rape motifs in legends of this sort. The argument runs that female saints' lives frequently display an obsession with sexuality (over half of Jacobus' tales of holy women stress their chastity);[14] moreover critics have demonstrated that the martyr legends often contain a gender-marked narrative structure centred around motifs of sexual coercion.[15] In the *Golden Legend* alone, at least thirteen virgin martyrs undergo some form of violent constraint akin to rape: Lucy, Agnes, Agatha and Daria are forced into brothels; attempts are made to compel Anastasia, Juliana, Margaret and Ursula to marry; Justina, the Virgin of Antioch and Theodora undergo sexual harassment in one form or another; finally, actual attempts at rape are carried out on Margaret, Lucy, Justina, Anastasia's maids and, as we have seen, Agnes. In each case, the rape or sexual assault is never completed, because the wicked seducers are thwarted by the constancy of the holy virgins. Nonetheless, as Kathryn Gravdal implies, the torture scenes also open up 'a licit space that permits the audience to enjoy sexual language and contemplate the naked female body', while at the same time covertly placing the blame for masculine desire on the virgin's doorstep.[16] In a manner paralleling modern courtroom discourse suggesting that the victim 'was asking for it',[17] tales of this sort, scholars argue, convey the virgin martyr's dilemma: the virgin, however virtuous, is depicted as so physically attractive that she literally leads the heathen seducer to sin.[18] Jacobus opens by describing Agnes's 'beautiful' (p. 102) countenance; vernacular accounts imply a comparable emphasis. For instance, in the *South English Legendary*, we are told that 'so vair womman nas non / As þis maide forþward was of fel & of bon' (ll. 5–6) (there was not such a good-looking woman as this maiden henceforth was in skin and bone); and later on 'Þe constable hure let strupe so naked so heo was ibore / Þat echman ssolde hure deorne lymes iseo hure to ssende' (ll. 42–3) (The constable caused her to be stripped as naked as when she was born so that, to shame her, everyone would see her private parts). In Bokenham's *Legendys*, the narrator exclaims that Agnes 'fayr were in hir vysage / Bodyly and endewyde with gret beute' (ll. 4117–18). Significantly, what later becomes an act of 'foul lust' (l. 4413) is initially described as the prefect's son's 'blynd loue' (l. 4192), a verbal slippage that temporarily shifts the focus away from the coercion of the female saint to the dilemma of an 'anguysshyd' male lover (l. 4193). Though the term 'rape', in modern parlance, can become similarly inflected with sexual or romantic connotations (as the phrase 'date rape' implies),[19] feminist critics maintain that rape can be better understood as an exercise in power.[20] What more explicit expression of unequal power-relations could there be than a representation of a man stripping a young woman naked and driving her into a brothel? Convinced by such arguments, Simon Gaunt concludes: 'The universal subtext of saints' lives about women is forced sex, in other words rape.'[21]

Can one make such universal claims? Is forced sex the only underlying meaning borne by these stories? And if it is, did its mode of presentation have entirely negative implications for medieval women, whether as readers or listeners themselves, or as the wives and daughters of readers and listeners? The sexual desires of the evil tyrants are always thwarted, after all, and the rapists frequently receive their comeuppance in the form of grisly punishment and damnation.[22] According to Bokenham, as Agnes sits in the brothel in prayer, the prefect's son 'suddeynly doun fel up-on hys face, / And þe deuyl hym stranglyd in þat place' (ll. 4426–7). Moreover, as Gravdal admits, the rape plot can also be interpreted as opening up a space for female heroism, transforming the virgin's martyrdom into a specifically feminine form of *imitatio Christi*.[23] Several of the stories in Bokenham's *Legendys* contain dedications to specific female patrons and the extant manuscript of the text was presented to a convent of nuns in Cambridge: that a significant proportion of Bokenham's audience were women suggests the possibility of meanings in the *Legendys* that are not simply complicitous with attempts to legitimize sexual violence.[24] How do we make room for these seemingly 'positive' readings in our understanding of virgin martyrs?

The focus on the martyr's speech is especially significant in legends such as Bokenham's Life of St Agnes. As Alison Elliott points out, the dramatic climax in martyrdom legends is not usually the moment of death itself but the scenes of confrontation between the saint and persecutor prior to death; these scenes often contain a theatrical dynamic.[25] A close examination of Bokenham's rendition highlights this verbal element well. When the prefect's son first tries to woo Agnes with ornaments and precious stones, she spurns his affections, exclaiming: 'Go hens fro me, of syn norsshere / And contraryous to euere good entent' (ll. 4141–2).[26] The virgin continues by playing on the son's jealousy and adopting erotic language to describe the union with her 'louere' (l. 4162):

> And takyn of his mouth many a kys haue I
> Swettere þan eythir mylk or hony;
> And fulle oftyn in armys he halsyd [embraced] hath me
> Wyth-out blemyssyng of myn uirgynyte,
> Hys body to myn now conioynyd is. (ll. 4172–6)[27]

It is precisely this answer that makes the young man 'wex ful heuy' (l. 4191) and become sick. Soon after, Agnes is summoned before the prefect but, rather than proceeding straight to the tortures, the prefect engages in a lengthy dialogue with her. When he mentions his 'sonys loue' (l. 4241), Agnes simply throws back 'skorn' (l. 4243); when he asks her to worship idols, Agnes calls him 'prefect vycyous' (l. 4275). When he threatens the brothel, Agnes, 'inflammyd with grace / And strengthyd with gostly stedefastnesse' (ll. 4302–3), stands in front of the prefect and exclaims:

> I sekerly [confidently] despise al þi thretyng
> In hys goodnesse fully trusting
> Þat neþir I to ydols shal sacryfyse do,
> Nere with sinners vnclennes be defoulyd, lo. (ll. 4312–15)

Hearing her own threats of damnation, the prefect 'wex nere made' (l. 4351), demonstrating the power of Agnes's maddening discourse.

The power of the saints' speech to disrupt the rape script becomes most apparent in the torture scenes. According to Elaine Scarry, one of the injurious effects of torture is to disable language in the victim[28] – not so in Bokenham's virgin martyr narratives, for the virgin continually punctuates the scenes of suffering with words addressed to her spectators (both within and outside the text), her tormentors and God. In the brothel, she gives praise when a white stole is sent to her to cover her nakedness; henceforth whoever enters the place exits praying. In this way, a den of corporeal sin becomes transformed into a place of spiritual conversation. Later, when she has been cast in the flames, Agnes uses language to escape more 'wykkyd mennys thretys' (l. 4558); her prayer literally puts out the flames (l. 4594). The adversarial content of the speech in these texts seems to resist the stereotype of passive femininity usually marked out for women in medieval romances, which routinely portray heroines as empty signs within a masculine homosocial discourse.[29] But it also contradicts the recommendations of secular virginity discourse that emphasize the verbal decorum with which virgins should comport themselves. Christine de Pisan, in *The Treasure of the City of Ladies*, argues that women who are chaste

> should display an expression of humility with the eyes lowered, and their speech should be kindly . . . Their speech should be amiable and courteous to all people; they should have a humble manner and not be too talkative . . . These maidens ought to take care not to get into arguments or disputes with anyone, neither serving-man nor chambermaid. It is a very ugly thing in a girl to be argumentative and to answer back, and she could lose her good name because of it.[30]

Agnes, according to this model, should behave in ways that are 'amiable and courteous'.[31] But instead the martyr responds to her sufferings by arguing, cursing and talking back; it is precisely through such means that she *keeps* her good name.

My question in this context is whether St Agnes's verbal dissidence can be taken as evidence that the virgin martyr speaks (at least, in a voice that can be identified as her 'own'). So long as scholars attempt to retrieve some sort of sovereign female consciousness from the text, a 'concealed voice' that can be realistically salvaged and reinscribed, the performative character of hagiographic speech acts will be mis-understood. Strategically these researches have potency, but they do not address the complicity of such scholarship in the production of what may turn out to be a very problematic way of thinking about gender. Indeed, an approach like Ashton's, which seeks to excavate the 'doubled discourse' of hagiography with reference to Irigarayan notions of mimesis and textual fissure, confronts precisely this difficulty. With her claims that the dialogue between saint and pagan tormentor is 'inherently fissured', and that it is possible to discover, beneath layers of patriarchal discourse, the speaking 'I' of a 'marginalised, vulnerable woman', Ashton's analysis runs the risk of eliding the disruptive feminine voices she discovers with the actions, experiences and words of *actual* female subjects, thereby ignoring the complex workings of gender in the context of hagiographic writing, reading and viewing.[32] Instead of excavating the 'authentic' male or female voice, it may ultimately be more productive to deconstruct the binary representational systems by which those gendered voices are constituted in the first place, to consider the ways in which dichotomous sexual difference acts as a screen for the projection of other categories of difference. In this respect, the theory of speech mapped out by Judith Butler provides a useful way of thinking through the issue of hagiographic voices: Butler suggests that a speech act is not a momentary occurrence 'but a certain nexus of temporal horizons', a product of citation whereby 'the contexts it assumes must not be quite the same as the ones in which it originates'.[33] It follows that the virgin martyr's voice is itself embedded in citational practice, a discursive performance that chimes with a chorus of other, not always harmonious, voices – voices that variously precede, succeed and exceed the text and condition the latter's reception and meaning. Some of the contemporary ideologies in which those voices are inscribed will be considered in due course; at this point it is simply worth noting that one of the major discourses 'recycled' in the context of the virgin's speech is the voice of God, as witnessed in Agnes's speech describing erotic union with Christ, which borrows imagery from the Song of Songs.[34]

Analyses of saintly speech also need to account for those moments in which attempts are made to censor or put an end to discursive performance. After all, Bokenham's Life of St Agnes demands not only that we read the saint's martyrdom through acts of speech but also that we perceive it in the context of an act that attempts to silence that speech: she is only consecrated martyr after her throat is stabbed. The passage describing the incident is remarkably terse:

> Thys seyng, Aspasye, þe prefectys vyker,
> The sedycyous peple to plese the entent,
> Comaundyd a swerd both bryht & clere
> Into hyr throte depe for to be sent,

> And þus þis holy mayde, þis innocent
> Cruelly martyrd for crystys sake,
> To hym as hys spouse he dede take. (ll. 4596–4602)

The maid is transformed into martyr and uncontested virgin only once her throat is cut.[35] In other words, earning the label 'martyr' seems to demand, by definition, a violent *cessation* of verbal activity. Taken out of context, this passage suggests that silencing is a symbolic component of the virgin martyr's death.

In actual fact, however, Bokenham's Life of St Agnes refuses to acknowledge the threat that death poses to speech: in a vision after her death, Agnes's parents see her pray one last time (ll. 4627–34), suggesting that Aspasius' attempts at censorship are woefully inadequate. Indeed, the narrative continues by telling the story of how Constance, daughter of Constantine, prays at Agnes's tomb and has a vision in which Agnes appears and exhorts her to 'do constaunthly' (l. 4662); Bokenham goes on to refer to the afterlife of the saint in the writings of Ambrose (which he suggests are his source) and he concludes by making a personal request for intercessory prayer (ll. 4708–35). The martyr's death does not put an end to the martyr's voice, and the act of silencing conversely endows her speech with permanence and authority.[36] These scenes raise a fundamental issue in the analysis of hagiographic writings. On the one hand, we can accept the terms of the fantasy by understanding martyred saints as products of *process*, reading martyrdom and virginity as ongoing activities, 'performances' punctuated by continuous speech acts.[37] On the other hand, we can reject the fantasmatic dimensions of the genre and understand saintly identities as products of *closure*, perceiving martyrdom and virginity as stable subject positions accomplished only through death and, it follows, silence.[38] Before attempting to address these points in more depth, let us consider the subject of sati.

The subject of sati: bodies in pain

In 1987, Roop Kanwar, an educated 18-year-old woman from a village in the state of Rajasthan in India, died on her husband's funeral pyre while hundreds of people looked on. Initially, the state government refused to respond, despite the banning of sati in modern India. But intense media interest and pressure from women's groups eventually combined to produce legislation prohibiting both the commission and glorification of sati. All the same, no one was convicted of participating in Roop Kanwar's sati. Indeed, subsequent to the issue of the new legislation, large pro-sati rallies occurred in the state capital, objecting to the government's intervention in traditional religious customs; meanwhile Roop Kanwar's village has been transformed into a lucrative pilgrimage site.[39]

The arguments that surround Hindu widow sacrifice hinge, as in medieval hagiographic scholarship, on questions of female agency. Was the sati voluntary? Or was the widow forced upon the pyre? Those who defend the practice of sati portray it as an individual decision, invested with the ingredients of self-sacrifice: they compare the widows with religious male martyrs, soldiers and ascetic monks.[40] (These associations are reminiscent of the discourse of 'becoming male' espoused in Christian patristic virginity discourse.[41]) Yet critics of sati expose the custom as murder: they argue that, even if she outwardly complied with the decision to throw herself in the flames, the woman's choices were constrained, both by the prospect of life as a mistreated widow and by a deluge of ideological indoctrination.[42] As with scholarship on medieval female saints, we find the subject of sati trapped between positions of victimhood ('she was forced to die') and positions of empowerment ('she chose to die').

Rajeswari Sunder Rajan suggests that the only way to break the critical impasse is to shift the emphasis from notions of sati-as-death (a model that places emphasis on the widow's *intentions*, whether sati is considered suicide or murder) to a concept of sati-as-burning (the idea that pain itself provides a ground for subjectivity, and that the focus be directed to the widow's *experience*). Describing an anti-sati poster produced by an anti-sati activist organization, she suggests that the graphic at its centre, depicting a woman rising upward from the flames, simultaneously communicates an experience of pain and an attempt to protest against it. Sunder Rajan concludes of the image:

> There is no naturalistic insistence on the mutilation of burning, but the posture and expression of the figure, though stylised, capture the essence of pain. The sati is not a dead woman, but a burning woman seeking to escape, not a spectacle but the subject of action and agency.[43]

Might the subject of martyrdom be read similarly, as an embodiment of both protest and pain? In the Bokenham Life, the focus is certainly on martyrdom as a discursive performance: the martyr is an agent who speaks and protests. Yet the narrator refuses to picture Agnes as a body-in-pain. The language used communicates permanence, not decay: the saint is introduced as a 'gemme of uirgynyte' (l. 4120). This suggests that fleshly pain, in this legend at least, is not a primary focus; the refusal to represent the virgin's suffering is especially apparent in the lines describing Agnes's death, which seem astonishingly blunt. The virgin's experience of pain, in Bokenham's Life of St Agnes, does *not* appear to be subject-constitutive.

We may do better comparing Sunder Rajan's analysis with an example more directly comparable to the visual content of the anti-sati poster. There is a gold cup in the British Museum made in the late fourteenth century and given to Charles VI of France (reigned 1380–1422) by Jean, duc de Berry (1340–1416), on the occasion of a visit to Tourraine in 1391 (Figs 3 and 4).[44] The cup relates, round its lid, the life and miracles of St Agnes, including her death at the hands of Aspasius; the bowl of the cup depicts the saint's burial and miracles connected with her tomb. In the last scene on the lid, Agnes kneels, eyes closed, amid a bundle of faggots as the prefect's deputy looks on; untouched by the flames, an executioner thrusts a spear towards her neck (Fig. 3). The British Museum cup certainly depicts Agnes as a subject of process: here the saint is not dead but dying; the artist captures the moment just before the neck is penetrated with the lance. (Indeed, the moment portrayed is reminiscent of passion iconography showing the penetration of Christ's side with the spear of Longinus; the speech-scroll that emerges from Agnes's mouth, exclaiming 'Into thy hands O Lord I commend my spirit', likewise opens up the scene to typological readings.) But it is debatable whether an image of this sort communicates the same message as the written legends, where it is predominantly injurious acts of speech that allow for the manufacture of empowering models of subjectivity. After all, in the process of being burned, Agnes is depicted as still and bound while the executioner is violently in motion. So it becomes necessary to interpret the martyr's silence and inaction as a form of strength if we are to understand the burning scene as a politically enabling image. It is only when we turn our attention to the rest of the cycle that we see a virgin as someone who acts and reacts, as in the scene in which Agnes resurrects the prefect's son (Fig. 4).

Other images of St Agnes, too, convey a similar dynamic, such as the cycle in the late twelfth-century Pamplona Bible (Figs 5 and 6). On one

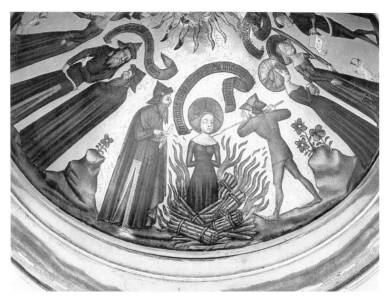

Figure 3 'The burning of St Agnes', scene from the lid of the Royal Gold Cup (*c*.1380). London, British Museum. © British Museum.

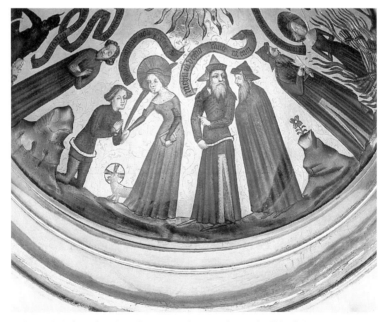

Figure 4 'The miracles of St Agnes', scene from the lid of the Royal Gold Cup (*c*.1380). London, British Museum. © British Museum.

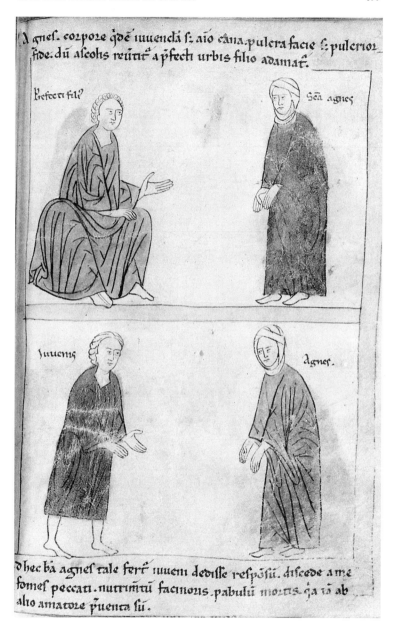

Figure 5 'St Agnes Cycle', Pamplona Bible (late twelfth century).
Augsburg, Universitätsbibliothek, Cod.I.2.4°15, fol. 249.

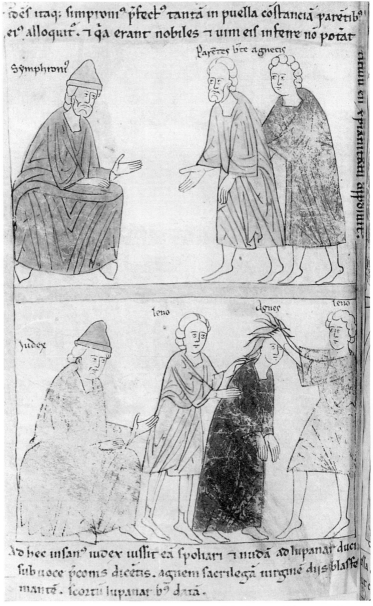

Figure 6 'St Agnes Cycle', Pamplona Bible (late twelfth century).
Augsburg, Universitätsbibliothek, Cod.I.2.4°15, fol. 249v.

folio, the saint is depicted conversing with the prefect's son, her head and body covered by garments; on the next, she is shown being led off to a brothel by two men, one of whom grabs her arm while the other tousles her hair (shorthand, in the medieval symbolic lexicon, for the threat of sexual violation).[45] According to Diane Wolfthal, such pictures projected, to medieval viewers, 'a collective image of how a rape victim should look'.[46] In an example closer in provenance to Bokenham's *Legendys*, a fifteenth-century window in the church of St Agnes at Eye in Suffolk, the saint is represented with drops of blood on her garments and a sword shoved through her neck.[47] Again, for the modern non-believer, it takes a leap of imagination to read the virgin martyr in terms analogous to Sunder Rajan's assessment of the anti-sati poster.

Medievalism, colonialism and the politics of speech

In order to bypass the methodological crisis posed by maintaining the stark division between victimization and empowerment, Sunder Rajan asks us to redefine subject-status itself, to view victim *as* subject. This communicates the fundamental point that there is not any necessary opposition between power and passivity. But her argument still asks us to choose between the contrasting models of process and closure that, I have suggested, also characterize medieval representations of martyrdom. Do we indeed need to choose? Does the answer simply depend on which element of the legends we bring into focus – the speech-authorizing deaths or the meaning-proliferating tortures? Can we imagine virgins as subjects and *at the same time* as objects, rather than letting the virgin-as-signifier disappear into a stark choice between victim and agent? The reason why I pose this dilemma is that, in certain contexts, virgin martyrs are inescapably both. Requiring feminist analysis to make a choice between subject-constitution ('the virgin resists objectification through language') and object-formation ('the virgin is a passive victim of patriarchal violence') invites interpretative paralysis, during which alternative desires and textual investments are potentially foreclosed. The risk – and possibility – is that we simply ventriloquize our own concerns when we make the virgin martyr speak.[48] This is not a plea for historicity, for reading the virgin martyr 'on her own terms' – the fictionality of the legends precludes such investigations.[49] But it does highlight the difficulties that arise from making political claims about medieval texts and images.

This is precisely what concerns Spivak in her article on the subaltern. Describing the arguments surrounding the abolition of sati rituals by the British in nineteenth-century India, Spivak asserts that the Hindu widow becomes subject both to the chivalric colonialist formula of 'white men saving brown women from brown men' and to the Indian nativist argument that 'the women actually wanted to die'. As she puts it: 'Between patriarchy and imperialism, subject-constitution and object-formation, the figure of the woman disappears, not into a pristine nothingness, but into a violent shuttling which is the displaced figuration of the "third-world woman" caught between tradition and modernization.'[50] In other words, even when the subaltern tries, to the death, to cry out, she remains caught in a trap between two ideologies; as a speech act, the sati fails because the words of the immolated widow cannot be properly interpreted. Problematizing a clear-cut division between colonizers and colonized, Spivak inserts 'brown women' as a category exploited by both.

Likewise, the agency of the virgin martyr cannot be idealized as a force totally separate from the order it opposes. Exploited by ideologies of patriarchal violence and simultaneously inserted into narratives of female resistance, the saint has a role to play in the discourses of both;[51] the sexual politics of virgin martyr legends are also tangled up in other networks of power, such as class, religious identity and race. Agnes is, after all, described in Bokenham's Life as a woman born of parents of 'hy nobylesse' (l. 4236); she has not escaped the privileges of social class and her parents are part of the same Roman establishment as the prefect himself. (Hence the prefect's initial hesitation in using 'opyn violence' (l. 4236) against her.) Moreover, one of the ways in which the saint declares her allegiance to Christ is to evoke the 'precyoushere ornamentys' (l. 4145) and 'shynyng gemmys' (l. 4153) he has given her – a rhetorical strategy which challenges the spiritual impoverishment of the prefect's son in distinctly material terms, as if to say 'my gems are better than your gems'.[52] The visual images closest in provenance to Bokenham's *Legendys* highlight this economic framework well: panels representing female saints on the south side of the rood screen at North Elmham in Norfolk depict them dressed in the fashions of fifteenth-century queens and noblewomen.[53]

Agnes is also, like the prefect with whom she does battle, a religious fundamentalist: 'I do reproue / For crystys sake, & wyl hym not han / Doum ydols to worshepe' (ll. 4262–4). For all her presentation as a violated victim in the overt content of the tale, Agnes zealously espouses a religion that, in Bokenham's day, comfortably inhabited the position of intolerant oppressor: Christianity's self-representation as victim should not obscure from view its simultaneous alignment *with* violence. Indeed, we should remember that, in certain saints' lives, the evangelizing tone was bound up with discourses of anti-Semitism, Islamophobia and the contemporary war against heresy. In the early thirteenth-century Katherine group, aristocratic female audiences were invited to define themselves against 'þe Gius' who put Christ to death;[54] the Auchinleck manuscript, compiled in the 1330s, contains lives of St Margaret and St Katherine which describe the saints' persecutors as 'sarraȝins so blake' endeavouring to make the virgins believe in 'Mahoun'.[55] Other texts in the Auchinleck manuscript imply a mixed secular audience, perhaps a noble household,[56] demonstrating the ways in which rich female readers were occasionally presented with saintly intercessors constructed with reference to racial as well as gendered categories.

Of course, in fifteenth-century England there was not a significant Jewish or Muslim population; it was heresy that offered the best opportunity for demarcating and safeguarding the Christian *communitas*.[57] Perhaps one of the associations that Bokenham's audience had with the 'sedycyous peple' (l. 4541) burned by the flames that leave Agnes miraculously unharmed were heretics, possibly Lollards: the punishment for relapsed heretics was burning at the stake and Bokenham makes it very clear that the same people who 'dede makyn anoon a ryht greth feer' (l. 4542) are those 'on ych syde brent' (l. 4544). After the Lollard heresy had been declared a capital offence in England in 1401, with the institution of the statute *De haeretico comburendo*, actual executions by fire took place several times in the south-east, in the first three decades of the fifteenth century. Though the East Anglian mystic Margery Kempe herself escaped such a fate, when she was arrested in Beverley on suspicion of Lollardy she was confronted with local housewives who ran out of their houses with their distaffs, crying 'Brennyth this fals heretyk'.[58] This raises the possibility that the eradication of heresy and motifs of burning were linked in the minds of Bokenham and his readers. I do not wish to suggest that, where we see fire, we should automatically think heresy: images of flames connote, amongst other things, purgatorial and infernal torment. But the facts that Agnes's fiery ordeal echoes a punishment recently imposed on heretics, and that her enthusiastic rejection of idols superficially chimes with the Wycliffite suspicion of images, are grounds for suggesting the

possibility of 'resistant' or heterodox readings. This may explain why
Bokenham goes to some effort to explain that Agnes stands 'in þe
myddys of þe feer' (l. 4550), that the flames 'in no wyse cam anneys ny'
(l. 4546) and that she was '[w]yth dew from heuen bathyd' (l. 4562); it
may also account for the relative absence of late medieval iconography
depicting Agnes's burning (the British Museum cup being a rare
exception). The iconic image of a saint in flames perhaps conveyed, all
too powerfully, the martyr-like associations that risked attaching
themselves to executed heretics.[59]

Speculation aside, it is clear from this discussion that the operations of
power in hagiographic representations can become notoriously blurred:
saints' lives often negotiate the division between self and other in ways
that disguise oppressors as victims and victims as oppressors. Once
again, such issues are brought into focus by an examination of
hagiographic art. Consider a panel from a painting by Meister Francke
depicting the tortures of St Barbara (a virgin martyr put to death in
Nicomedia in the third century CE). In Francke's painting, the saint's
beauty is a marker of social status as much as sexual desirability: her
immaculate complexion and blonde locks contrast wildly with the
scruffy louts responsible for her arrest and torture (Fig. 7). If we insist
that a painting like this is transparently about male desire and female
disempowerment, we risk overlooking the class prejudices of the image.
Modern fantasies of the archetypal pornographic consumer frequently
register upper-class fears about lower-class men; likewise, Francke's
painting presents the voyeuristic, sadistic gaze as an attribute of the
uncivilized, economically dispossessed male.[60] One of the overarching
fantasies of martyrdom iconography is that the sexually voracious
'pornographic' gaze is somewhere else, that it is 'other'; in comparable
paintings depicting the martyrdom of male saints, the torturers are
occasionally depicted as black or Jewish, while the people who commissioned such iconography were invariably white and well-to-do.[61]
Images of this sort are striking but they are by no means exceptional.
Looking to medieval visual culture reminds us that the horizons of
expectation aroused by medieval texts cannot easily be separated from
the extra-textual contexts in which they were conceivably understood.[62]
So to foreground 'empowerment' or 'victimization' as the hermeneutical
framework for exploring medieval hagiography is not necessarily to
engage in readings that are politically valuable or 'gender-positive'.

Medieval studies is traditionally reticent about admitting its stake
in positions of colonization; too often the ethical implications of

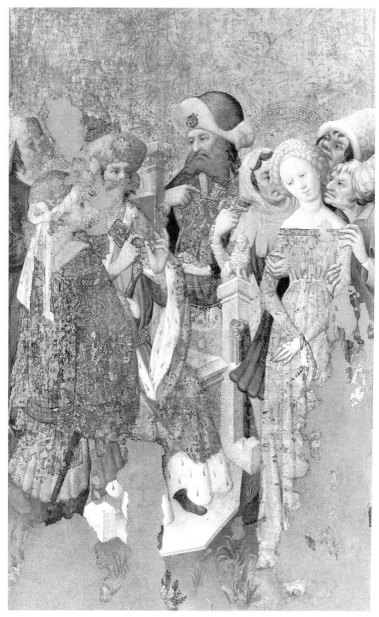

Figure 7 'Barbara's trial', panel from Meister Francke, *Martyrdom of Saint Barbara* (*c.*1410–15). National Museum of Finland, Helsinki.

recovering voices from the past have also been downplayed. It should be recalled that the Middle Ages as a historical construct was originally invented in a climate that was also a breeding ground for Orientalism. (Orientalism, in Edward Said's definition, is a systematic and continuous discursive formation aimed at creating binary distinctions between East and West and thereby 'dominating, restructuring, and having authority over the Orient'.[63]) To ignore the imperialistic foundations of medieval studies ultimately risks entering into a rhetorical collusion *with* those power structures, producing a dichotomizing tendency from which hagiography criticism is certainly not immune. As Kathleen Biddick has powerfully argued, feminist scholarship should resolutely resist falling into the neo-colonial trap. Critiquing the rhetoric of Caroline Walker Bynum's writings on mystics, Biddick writes: 'A historical study of medieval gender interrupts this foundational category of *Christianitas* by asking how a historical construction of gender in medieval Christendom was *simultaneously* a construction of other differences.'[64]

The usefulness of Spivak's account of gender in modern-day India is that it critiques the fetishization of immolated widows as victims or agents by demonstrating that they are caught in the divisions of an implacable double bind, a bind in which difference itself becomes displaced. Deploying Spivak's formula, it might in turn be argued that feminist hagiographic scholarship risks following a pattern of academics 'saving white women from brown men'. Excavating the 'resistance' in a given text or historical situation also requires that we simultaneously keep in view the sheer bigotry of certain medieval texts and images (particularly when read together). Looking *with* the martyred body in question entails highlighting not only the structures of objectification and heterosexual desire by which virgin martyrs are coerced and the routes of power and verbal dissidence by which they achieve transcendence, but also a number of more objectionable responses not accounted for in readings that simply foreground a gender-inflected 'rape script' or narratives of saintly 'empowerment'. As in modern societies, where women's political activity has been harnessed by right-wing movements and religious fundamentalists (the anti-abortion movement is a case in point), women's active participation in politics does not automatically stem from feminist concerns. Nor do the discourses that cluster around images of ostensibly powerful women always concern themselves explicitly with gender: the appropriation of Joan of Arc in the service of nationalist and xenophobic agendas in modern France highlights the difficulties that arise from imagining saints as sovereign, speaking 'subjects'.[65]

This is not to say that we should discard all attempts to discover representations of female militancy and power. But we may need to rethink our concept of hagiographic voices. When the virgin martyr speaks, the 'I' that we imagine she inhabits may not in fact be an 'I' at all (at least, in the singular, Cartesian sense of the term). Rather, what appears to be a speaking 'I', a subject of agency and power, may in fact be a nexus of multiplicity, a site of heteroglossia in which a body of contradictory discourses compete for our attention. Of course, this requires that our researches are historically situated – that, in our attempts to 'speak the saint', we consider the manifold ways in which female saints made meaning for their original makers, tellers and receivers. But we should also reflect on the operations of desire outside the text, the ways in which virgins continue to make meaning for critics today.[66]

Notes

I wish to thank Emma Campbell for her comments on an earlier draft and Ashley Tellis for first suggesting to me the parallel between Christian martyrdom and sati.

[1] Tertullian, *Liber de virginibus velandis*, *PL*, 2, col. 892. My translation.

[2] For an argument that pornography is the theory, and rape the practice, see Robin Morgan, 'Theory and practice: pornography and rape', in Laura Lederer (ed.), *Take Back the Night: Women on Pornography* (New York: William Morrow, 1980), pp. 125–47.

[3] Brigitte Cazelles, *The Lady as Saint: A Collection of French Hagiographic Romances of the Thirteenth Century* (Philadelphia: University of Pennsylvania Press, 1991), pp. 9, 54.

[4] Jocelyn Wogan-Browne, 'The virgin's tale', in Ruth Evans and Lesley Johnson (eds), *Feminist Readings in Middle English Literature: The Wife of Bath and All her Sect* (London: Routledge, 1994), pp. 165–94 (p. 180).

[5] Gayatri Chakravorty Spivak, 'Can the subaltern speak? Speculations on widow-sacrifice', *Wedge*, 7/8 (1985), 120–30. For the purposes of the discussion that follows, I have employed the insights of the 1988 version: Gayatri Chakravorty Spivak, 'Can the subaltern speak?', in Cary Nelson and Lawrence Grossberg (eds), *Marxism and the Interpretation of Culture* (Basingstoke: Macmillan, 1988), pp. 271–313, cited henceforth as Spivak, 'Can the subaltern speak?' In this article, I have used the term 'sati' to refer both to the practice of widow sacrifice and to the widow who performs it.

[6] Spivak, 'Can the subaltern speak?', p. 308. 'Subaltern' refers in Spivak's

writings to those subjects who have limited or no access to imperialistic narratives of domination; ibid., pp. 283–5.

[7] This parallels R. Howard Bloch's point that 'the only true virgin is a dead virgin'; Bloch, *Medieval Misogyny and the Invention of Western Romantic Love* (Chicago: University of Chicago Press, 1991), p. 108. In thinking through this issue, I have also found invaluable the insights of Sarah Salih, *Versions of Virginity in Late Medieval England* (Cambridge: Brewer, 2001), pp. 95–8.

[8] 'Subaltern talk: interview with the editors', in Donna Landry and Gerald Maclean (eds), *The Spivak Reader: Selected Works of Gayatri Chakravorty Spivak* (London: Routledge, 1996), p. 289.

[9] Gail Ashton, *The Generation of Identity in Late Medieval Hagiography: Speaking the Saint* (London: Routledge, 2000), pp. 41, 104, 148.

[10] For example, see Winstead's discussion of the Katherine group in *Virgin Martyrs: Legends of Sainthood in Late Medieval England* (Ithaca, NY: Cornell University Press, 1997), pp. 34–63.

[11] Jacobus de Voragine, *Legenda Aurea*, ed. Theodor Graesse (Dresden and Lipsius, 1846), pp. 113–17; English translation in Jacobus de Voragine, *The Golden Legend: Readings on the Saints*, trans. William Granger Ryan (Princeton: Princeton University Press, 1993), pp. 101–4. Further page references to the English translation are given after quotations in the text.

[12] *The South English Legendary*, ed. Charlotte d'Evelyn and Anna J. Mill, 3 vols, EETS, os, 235, 236, 244 (London: Oxford University Press, 1956 (vols 1, 2) and 1959 (vol. 3)), vol. 1, pp. 19–25. Further line references to this edition are given after quotations in the text.

[13] Osbern Bokenham, *Legendys of Hooly Wummen*, ed. Mary S. Serjeantson, EETS, os, 206 (London: Oxford University Press, 1938), pp. 110–29. Further line references to this edition are given after quotations in the text. There is an Anglo-Saxon life of St Agnes by Ælfric (*c.*988); *Ælfric's Lives of Saints*, ed. Walter W. Skeat, 2 vols, EETS, os, 94, 114 (London: Oxford University Press, 1966), vol. 1, pp. 170–94. Other vernacular versions of the St Agnes legend include the early fourteenth-century Anglo-Norman poem *La Vie Seinte Agneys*, written by Nicole Bozon, a Franciscan friar based in northern England: see *The Old French Lives of Saint Agnes and Other Vernacular Versions of the Middle Ages*, ed. Alexander J. Denomy (Cambridge, MA: Harvard University Press, 1938). Court records survive concerning a proposed performance of a play depicting the life of St Agnes in Winchester in 1409: see Jane Cowling, 'A fifteenth-century saint play in Winchester: some problems of interpretation', *Medieval and Renaissance Drama in England*, 13 (2001), 19–33. For an account of the transformation into the vernacular of the late fifth-century Latin *Gesta sanctae Agnetis* (which forms the basis for most subsequent medieval versions), see Anne B. Thompson, 'The legend of St Agnes: improvisation and the practice of hagiography', *Exemplaria*, 13/2 (2001), 355–97.

[14] The saints' chastity is explicitly stressed in 55 per cent of female lives in the

Golden Legend compared with 8 per cent of male; over a third (34 per cent) feature graphic scenes of sexual coercion compared with an almost negligible number for men. The male *vitae* generally place more emphasis on worldly affairs such as religious, secular or military office, preaching, conversions and miracle-working.

15 Rehearsals of this argument are too numerous to cite in full, but representative examples include Kathryn Gravdal, *Ravishing Maidens: Writing Rape in Medieval French Literature and Law* (Philadelphia: University of Pennsylvania Press, 1991), pp. 21–41; Catherine Innes-Parker, 'Sexual violence and the female reader: symbolic "rape" in the saints' lives of the Katherine group', *Women's Studies*, 24 (1995), 205–17; Corinne Saunders, *Rape and Ravishment in the Literature of Medieval England* (Cambridge: Brewer, 2001), pp. 120–51; and Diane Andrews Henningfeld, 'Contextualising rape: sexual violence in Middle English literature' (unpublished doctoral thesis, Michigan State University, 1994), pp. 136–59.

16 Gravdal, *Ravishing Maidens*, pp. 24, 35–40.

17 Sue Lees, *Carnal Knowledge: Rape on Trial* (London: Hamish Hamilton, 1996), pp. 129–58.

18 Gravdal, *Ravishing Maidens*, p. 35.

19 Lees, *Carnal Knowledge*, pp. 66–94.

20 Susan Brownmiller, *Against our Will: Men, Women and Rape* (Harmondsworth: Penguin, 1975), p. 256.

21 Simon Gaunt, *Gender and Genre in Medieval French Literature* (Cambridge: Cambridge University Press, 1995), p. 197.

22 See Wogan-Browne, 'The virgin's tale', p. 178.

23 Gravdal, *Ravishing Maidens*, pp. 23–4.

24 Sheila Delany, *Impolitic Bodies: Poetry, Saints and Society in Fifteenth-Century England: The Work of Osbern Bokenham* (Oxford: Oxford University Press, 1998), pp. 15–22.

25 Alison Goddard Elliott, 'The power of discourse: martyr's passion and Old French epic', *Medievalia et Humanistica*, NS, 11 (1982), 39–60. See also Maud Burnett McInerney, 'Rhetoric, power, and integrity in the passion of the virgin martyr', in Kathleen Coyne Kelly and Marina Leslie (eds), *Menacing Virgins: Representing Virginity in the Middle Ages and Renaissance* (London: Associated University Presses, 1999), pp. 50–70.

26 The *South English Legendary* is also keen to stress saintly impertinence: Agnes calls the prefect's son 'þou luþer deþes fode' (l. 23) (you evil food of death) and 'þou develles lime' (l. 37) (you agent of the devil). Despite the presence of aggressive verbal action in late medieval vernacular lives of St Agnes, Thompson points out that the speech scenes in the fifth-century Latin *gesta* were severely diminished in subsequent redactions, including Jacobus'; 'The legend of St Agnes', pp. 366–78.

27 For an argument that language comparable to this in the *Golden Legend* 'actually compromises Agnes's inviolate position because of its profane resonances', see Kathleen Coyne Kelly, 'Useful virgins in medieval

hagiography', in Cindy L. Carlson and Angela Jane Weisl (eds), *Constructions of Widowhood and Virginity in the Middle Ages* (London: Macmillan, 1999), pp. 135–64 (p. 157).

28   Elaine Scarry, *The Body in Pain: The Making and Unmaking of the World* (New York: Oxford University Press, 1985), p. 35.

29   Gaunt, *Gender and Genre*, pp. 71–121.

30   Christine de Pisan, *The Treasure of the City of Ladies, or The Book of the Three Virtues*, trans. Sarah Lawson (Harmondsworth: Penguin, 1985), pp. 160–1. For a comparable prescription in a religious text, see the thirteenth-century *Ancrene Wisse*, which declares that recluses must not recount 'any trivial stories or items of news, or sing or talk in a worldly manner between themselves'; *Medieval English Prose for Women: Selections from the Katherine Group and* Ancrene Wisse, ed. Bella Millett and Jocelyn Wogan-Browne (Oxford: Clarendon Press, 1990, rev. edn 1992), p. 142.

31   Indeed Christine de Pisan explicitly argues that virgins should 'eagerly read' the biographies of saints such as Agnes; *Treasure of the City of Ladies*, p. 161.

32   Ashton, *Generation of Identity*, p. 110. In this respect, I find the analysis of saintly speech more helpful in Françoise Meltzer, *For Fear of the Fire: Joan of Arc and the Limits of Subjectivity* (Chicago: University of Chicago Press, 2001). Though her focus is a woman whose trial records reveal historical voices ostensibly more 'recoverable' than those registered in the lives of early Christian martyrs, Meltzer resists the temptation to equate instants of enunciation with occasions of sovereign subjectivity.

33   Judith Butler, *Excitable Speech: A Politics of the Performative* (London: Routledge, 1997), pp. 14–15.

34   For an argument that passion cycles 'recycle' texts made familiar by liturgical usage, see Duncan Robertson, *The Medieval Saints' Lives: Spiritual Renewal and Old French Literature*, Edward C. Armstrong Monographs on Medieval Literature, 8 (Levington: French Forum, 1995), pp. 44–5. For arguments about speech and female subjectivity in saints' lives that parallel my own – formulated specifically in response to Ælfric's tenth-century Life of St Agnes – see Clare A. Lees and Gillian R. Overing, 'Before history, before difference: bodies, metaphor, and the Church in Anglo-Saxon England', *Yale Journal of Criticism*, 11 (1998), 315–34; Miranda Hodgson, 'Impossible women: Ælfric's sponsa Christi and "la mystérique"', *Medieval Feminist Forum*, 33 (2002), 12–21. Thanks to Clare Lees for providing these references.

35   This is a motif that appears with some frequency in the lives of other virgin martyrs too: in Bokenham's Life of St Christine, the judge orders the saint's 'tong out kut to be' (l. 3052); in his Life of St Lucy, the tormentors 'shouyn a swerd' (l. 9406) in the saint's throat.

36   Sarah Kay, 'The sublime body of the martyr: violence in early romance saints' lives', in Richard W. Kaeuper (ed.), *Violence in Medieval Society* (Woodbridge: Boydell, 2000), pp. 3–20 (pp. 18–19).

37 An approach taken by Salih, who draws an analogy between medieval virginity discourse and Judith Butler's theories of gender performativity in *Versions of Virginity*, pp. 31–8, 95–106.

38 For instance Ashton, whose work foregrounds the fact that Bokenham's virgins are 'passive, pious, silent vessels filled with virtue, itself a gift from God'; *Generation of Identity*, p. 31.

39 The details of Roop Kanwar's death are recounted in Rajeswari Sunder Rajan, *Real and Imagined Women: Gender, Culture and Postcolonialism* (London: Routledge, 1993), pp. 16–17.

40 Ibid., pp. 18–19.

41 Jerome, *Commentarium in Epistolam ad Ephesios*: 'But when she wishes to serve Christ more than the world, she shall cease to be woman, and shall be called man', *PL*, 26, col. 533. My translation. Sunder Rajan notes that the conflation of sati with Christian martyrdom is a 'familiar cognitive procedure'; *Real and Imagined Women*, p. 46.

42 Ibid., p. 19.

43 Ibid., p. 31.

44 O. M. Dalton, *The Royal Gold Cup in the British Museum* (London: British Museum, 1924).

45 Diane Wolfthal, *Images of Rape: The 'Heroic' Tradition and its Alternatives* (Cambridge: Cambridge University Press, 1999), p. 43.

46 Ibid., p. 43.

47 Cowling, 'A fifteenth-century saint play in Winchester', pp. 24–5. Other images of Agnes appear on fifteenth-century East Anglian rood screens: see Eamon Duffy, 'Holy maydens, holy wyfes: the cult of women saints in fifteenth- and sixteenth-century England', in W. J. Shields and Diana Wood (eds), *Women in the Church*, Studies in Church History, 27 (Oxford: Basil Blackwell, 1990), pp. 175–96.

48 An investment that is to some degree inescapable: this chapter itself, by engaging with feminist and postcolonial theory, is certainly not immune to the charge of ventriloquism and, indeed, anachronism.

49 For an analysis that does consider the historicity of the rape of virgins in early Christian persecutions, with the conclusion that the tortured virgin 'is more useful as a metonym, as an inviolate body that stands in for the Church, than as an actual, historical person', see Kelly, 'Useful Virgins', pp. 139–44.

50 Spivak, 'Can the subaltern speak?', p. 306.

51 Though the degree to which one discourse is emphasized over another is dependent on the particular contexts in which the legends arise. As Winstead demonstrates, the transformations of English virgin martyr legends between 1100 and 1450 'signal a struggle over the meaning of these powerful cultural symbols'; *Virgin Martyrs*, p. 5.

52 For an argument that the saintly struggles in the fourteenth-century *North English Legendary* are likewise portrayed in economic as well as sexual terms, ibid., pp. 79–80.

53 Reproduced in Eamon Duffy, *The Stripping of the Altars: Traditional Religion in England 1400–1580* (New Haven: Yale University Press, 1992), p. 171 and pl. 68.

54 For example, 'Seinte Margarete', in Millett and Wogan-Browne (eds), *Medieval English Prose for Women*, p. 48; for other examples of anti-Semitic sentiment in virgin martyr legends, see Wogan-Browne, 'The virgin's tale', pp. 178, 191, n. 47, and Ruth Evans in this volume. For a compelling account of the extent to which aristocratic female audiences of the thirteenth century were 'complicit in the oppositions of Christian aristocratic ladyhood and Jewishness', in the context of vernacular *Vengeance nostre seignur* cycles inserted into the manuscripts they read, see Jocelyn Wogan-Browne, *Saints' Lives and Women's Literary Culture c.1150–1300: Virginity and its Authorizations* (Oxford: Oxford University Press, 2001), pp. 118–22. For an argument that Jews provided 'a nexus of enmity and violence within which latter-day martyrdoms could be imagined and narrated', see Miri Rubin, 'Choosing death? Experiences of martyrdom in late medieval Europe', in Diane Wood (ed.), *Martyrs and Martyrologies*, Studies in Church History, 30 (Oxford: Blackwell, 1993), pp. 153–83 (pp. 165–8).

55 'Seynt Katerine', in *Altenglische Legenden: Neue Folge*, ed. Carl Horstman (Heilbronn: Henninger, 1881), pp. 242–58 (pp. 242, 252); see also 'Seynt Mergrete', in the same volume, which describes how Margaret complains that 'Fram þis foule Saraȝins / y may me nouȝt defende' (p. 227) and how the pagan tormentor Olibrius asks the virgin 'Wiltow leue on Mahoun / and þi god forsake?' (p. 233).

56 Thorlac Turville-Petre, *England the Nation: Language, Literature, and National Identity, 1290–1340* (Oxford: Clarendon Press, 1996), pp. 134–6.

57 Indeed, as Susan Schibanoff has pointed out in a survey of the links between orientalism and sexual difference in Chaucer's *Man of Law's Tale*, Islam was often constructed in this period as a sort of heresy, a 'fraudulent new version' of Christianity; Schibanoff, 'Worlds apart: orientalism, antifeminism and heresy in Chaucer's *Man of Law's Tale*', *Exemplaria*, 8 (1996), 59–96 (70).

58 *The Book of Margery Kempe*, ed. Barry Windeatt (Harlow: Longman, 2000), p. 258. On motifs of burning in the lives of other saints, see Ashton, *Generation of Identity*, pp. 146–7; on the imposition of burning as a penalty for relapsed heretics in fifteenth-century England, see Delany, *Impolitic Bodies*, p. 9.

59 For instance, in 1440, the relapsed heretic Richard Wyche was executed but began to attract the sort of devotion normally reserved for saints; ibid., p. 9.

60 I have found the views expressed in Laura Kipnis, *Bound and Gagged: Pornography and the Politics of Fantasy in America* (New York: Grove Press, 1996) helpful in thinking through the relationship between pornographic representation and class prejudice.

61 See, for instance, the late-thirteenth-century illumination in *Le Livre*

d'images de Madame Marie from northern France depicting the stoning of St Stephen (Paris, Bibliothèque Nationale, MS nouv. acq. fr. 16251, fol. 76), and the martyrdom scenes in the anonymous Valencian *Retable of St George* from *c*.1400 (London, Victoria and Albert Museum), depicting executioners with Moorish attributes.

62 See the catalogue of paintings in Ruth Mellinkoff, *Outcasts: Signs of Otherness in Northern European Art of the Late Middle Ages*, 2 vols (Berkeley: University of California Press, 1993).

63 Edward W. Said, *Orientalism: Western Conceptions of the Orient* (London: Penguin, 1978), pp. 2–3.

64 Kathleen Biddick, *The Shock of Medievalism* (Durham, NC: Duke University Press, 1998), p. 147.

65 Meltzer, *For Fear of the Fire*, pp. 15–16.

66 Wogan-Browne skilfully takes up the historical dimensions of this project in *Saints' Lives and Women's Literary Culture*, especially in ch. 7, 'The virgin speaks', pp. 223–56; Meltzer, *For Fear of the Fire*, brilliantly exposes the operations of fetishization and nostalgia in contemporary theoretical writings contemplating virginity discourse and the lives of early female saints.

11

'Saint, Witch, Man, Maid or Whore?' Joan of Arc and Writing History

ANKE BERNAU

You must understand me, you see, and know what it is to be weary, in this case, to be weary of a figure and its truth, of a strophe, a trope, and the folds of the said truth when it plays itself out with so many veils.[1]

The anonymous fifteenth-century *Journal d'un bourgeois de Paris* claims that before Joan of Arc was devoured by the flames, her executioner was careful to display 'her naked body to all the people', in order 'to take away any doubts from people's minds'. What was being revealed as proof were 'the secrets that could or should belong to a woman'.[2] This was not the first time that Joan's body had been inspected in order to determine the truth about her; in life, her virginity had been tested several times, both by her supporters and her detractors. Both sides declared her virginity to be intact.[3] Yet in the fifteenth and sixteenth centuries, English chronicles begin to tell a different story. Although its source is unknown, this alternative narrative is first mentioned in the Middle English 'Continuation G' of the prose *Brut* (1464–70) and is repeated by numerous later writers, such as William Caxton, Polydore Vergil, Edward Hall and Raphael Holinshed.[4] This story relates how, after her arrest, Joan claimed to be pregnant, thereby gaining a convenient reprieve. The pregnancy turned out to be feigned and the *Brut* concludes, rather laconically: '[and] þen she was brent in Roane'.[5]

Why this marked increase in hostility towards Joan in this period, and why was it expressed in a contestation of her virginity? Not only had a considerable amount of time passed since her death, but virginity was arguably becoming *less* significant as an ideal, through the rise of Protestantism. Despite this, it remained a potent and complex trope, both religiously and politically, throughout and beyond the Middle Ages.[6] Joan's virginity, her cross-dressing and the manner of her death link her closely to innumerable other narratives of virginity and holiness through which western Christianity had defined itself for centuries.[7] Although the reformation in England saw a shift in emphasis towards the Word and away from the cults of the Virgin and the saints, virginity remained a powerful symbol and behavourial ideal.[8] As Helen Hackett suggests in her study of Elizabeth I, the Protestant dismissal of virginity might even be 'predicated upon an even more elevated view of virginity: virginity is so special that it can only be attained by a tiny number of the exceptionally sinless, aided by God, and therefore remains the highest goal to which to aspire'.[9] Viewed in this light, the question of the truth of Joan's claims to virginity is shown to be significant to Protestants as well as Catholics. The virginal attributes of unity, purity, truth, authority and legitimacy not only paralleled the claims of historiographers in this period, but also lent themselves ideally to theories of the body politic and to the formulations of a growing awareness of an English national identity.[10] Using Pierre Nora's concept of the *lieu de mémoire* (memory place), Ruth Evans has argued that '[v]irginities were symbolic memory-places upon which the emerging nation of "England" was fastened'.[11] Virginity was therefore often a feature of royal ceremonial, and integral to royalty's self-representation. Thomas Hoccleve's fifteenth-century *Regement of Princes*, for instance, advises strongly that a good king should be chaste.[12] Hoccleve then offers the edifying example of a beautiful young man who, in a manner distinctly reminiscent of the legends of many female virgin martyrs, 'cracched . . . his face' with 'his naylës' and 'scocched it with knyuës' in order to help him 'vnclennesse eschue'.[13] The continence and purity of the king's body here provide a practical as well as symbolic model for the body politic. The iconography of virginity in general and of the Virgin Mary in particular was also drawn on in coronation ceremonies, pageants or even ballads dedicated to a queen, be she Protestant or Catholic,[14] and chaste or virginal women as symbols of national unity occur in writings up until the seventeenth century and beyond.[15] Virginity is always political and therefore never proclaims itself unproblematically or absolutely. As in Joan's case, virginity is determined socially as much as individually and its existence can be verified or denied in relation to particular ideological positions. Therefore virginity, by extension, becomes a sign of the validity (or not) of said positions.

The account of Joan's death from the *Journal d'un bourgeois de Paris* shows a fundamental ontological uncertainty about Joan's identity, an uncertainty echoed in Raphael Holinshed's *Chronicles of England, Scotland and Ireland*, where it is stated that Joan fought in a manner 'contrarie to all manhood (but she was a woman, *if she were that*)'.[16] This uncertainty is all too familiar to scholars of virginity. Yet the question here is not primarily what constitutes 'real' or 'true' virginity but, more fundamentally, what virginity signifies in a particular context. Virginity and representation – as well as the question of their respective legitimacy – are intimately enmeshed. I will be discussing here how the 'truth' of Joan's virginity has contingent implications for the truth claims of historiography, particularly a historiography involved in an increasingly nationalist agenda.[17] In other words: what does the writing about Joan's virginity tell us about the writing of national history?

All of the accounts express an intense preoccupation with the 'truth' of Joan's body and a concomitant anxiety about its capacity for deception. Even those few English writers in the sixteenth century who do not retell, in Richard Hardin's words, this 'one original English contribution to folklore about Joan', still present vitriolic accounts that cast doubt on Joan's virginity.[18] Edward Hall, for instance, suggests that she most likely remained chaste out of necessity, because of 'her foule face'.[19] While Caxton may not deride Joan in the way that some later writers do, omitting, for instance, her cross-dressing, his inclusion of the story of her claim of pregnancy nonetheless diminishes her status as 'La Pucelle de Dieu'. More explicitly, Hall, known as one of the most extreme of Joan's detractors, calls her a 'diabolicall blasphemeresse' and 'a persone scismatike and erronyous' (fol. 33v). Just in case that is not quite clear enough, he adds that she is a 'peuysh paynted Puzel', a 'craftie imagener' (fol. 33). Holinshed too emphasizes the duplicitous aspect of her appearance and her actions, claiming that she has 'great *semblance* of chastitie both of bodie and behaviour' (p. 600, col. b).[20] Thundering about her 'counterfeit contrition', he concludes that the story of her pregnancy proves that she is 'as false as wicked' (p. 604, col. b). Doubt is cast more explicitly on her claims to virginity when he comments, almost as an aside, '(if it were anie)' (p. 605, col. a). What emerges is the perception – shared by her supporters and her

detractors – that the truth of her body is connected to other truth
claims in a number of significant ways. The terms used to describe Joan
here all set out to imply that truth cannot be located in her and, more
forcefully, that she deliberately misleads. Yet if she is presented as
deceptive, heretical, *counterfeit* – values diametrically opposed to those
associated with virginity – one must recognize the implicit belief at
work that truth *can* be located in the body and that the body is a
foundational category in the production of truth claims. The question
of who – or even what – Joan *really* is and what it is that she *reveals*
haunts these chronicles and informs their hostile rhetoric.

   Brian Vickers has argued that, in the period from 1400 to 1700,
'rhetoric attained its greatest pre-eminence, both in terms of range of
influence and in value'.[21] Certainly rhetoric was inseparable from the
writing of history in the period considered here; in fact, 'history was
often thought of as a branch of rhetoric'.[22] A historiographer was
encouraged to demonstrate his rhetorical prowess and, in order to
convey his material most effectively, 'it was permissible . . . to invent'.[23]
Yet historiographers were increasingly occupied with the objectives
and methodology of their practice.[24] Caxton, for instance, is keen to
distinguish history from fable, a differentiation that itself has a
long history.[25] Forty years later, the humanist Polydore Vergil also
differentiates between history and fable, stating that 'it is a lawe
in historie that the writer shoulde never be soe bolde as to open
enie fallse thinge, nor soe demisse as not to utter enie trewthe'.[26]
History is therefore a '*full* rehersall and declaration of things don, not a
gesse or divination' (p. 26).[27] Although Hall's aim in his work is more
explicitly the praise and commemoration of 'princes, gouernoures and
noble menne' ('Preface', p. i), he is also careful to state that he has
'compiled and gathered (and not made) out of diuerse writers, as well
forayn as Englishe, this simple treatise' ('Preface', p. ii). While
Holinshed recognizes the problems of disparate source-materials, he
emphasizes the importance of desisting from an approach that would
'frame [the various sources] to agree to [his] liking' (vol. 3, 'Preface to
the Reader', p. ii). Moreover, he will aid the reader by using an
appropriate style: 'My speech is plaine, without any rhetoricall shew of
eloquence, hauing rather a regard to simple truth, than to *decking*
words' (ibid., p. i).[28] So while Holinshed recognizes diversity, 'proper'
language can nevertheless guide the reader of history. Although he
does not claim any absolute success, he does announce his intention to
correct the errors of others and to restore the 'full integritie' of, for

instance, 'names of persons, townes, and places' in his work (ibid., p. iii).

There are three concerns at work here which link the tropes of virginity, rhetoric and historiography. The first is a preoccupation with *wholeness*. As Richard Hakluyt stated, historiography's aim must be to 'incorporate into one body the torn and scattered limbs' of different sources.[29] Historiography in this period had both religious and political concerns: in the sixteenth century in particular it was central to the construction and articulation of an English identity which, in turn, was to be connected to a 'true' and 'original' religion. As Antonia Gransden has shown, in the Tudor period the 'need to prove continuity between past and present was arguably even greater in the religious than the political sphere' as the 'reformation threatened to disrupt the course of English religious history'.[30] At the same time, writers such as John Bale and John Foxe were making 'extravagant claims for the ancient purity of the English/British church'.[31] As Foxe says, 'God hath so placed us Englishmen here in one commonwealth, also in one church, as in one ship together'; nation and church become explicitly conjoined in his *Actes and Monuments* (1563).[32] Hagiography and history continued to share some of the same goals and rhetoric.[33] Texts such as Foxe's link saintliness and Englishness; while the Protestant martyrs are not necessarily virgins, the claim that Joan is a saint, or holy, places her within the same discursive field, particularly as she is also linked to a specific discourse of nation. Even if no explicit parallel is drawn, both the text and the nation's history, in their ideal state, are imagined to be like the prelapsarian, unfragmented body of the virgin. That body and the 'full integritie' it promises make it a foundational category in the production of knowledge; virginity, as a trope that appears to promise both wholeness *and* purity, signals, by extension, truth.[34]

Second, as both virginity (and its many narratives) and historiography claim to reveal truth, the rhetoric used to describe either is frequently apocalyptic. The concern of bringing truth to light and the fear of oblivion, or death, is an issue at the very heart of the historio-graphical project.[35] As Hall states, it is Oblivion, the 'cancard enemye' that swallows 'fame and renoune', 'auncie[n]t memory', 'conquestes and notable actes' ('Preface', p. i), which must be fought and overcome by the writing of histories. Vergil, in a similar vein and with similar language, laments the lack of sources that might reveal the origins of Britain, which are therefore 'full of darcknes', compared to which there is 'nothinge more obscure, more uncertaine, or unknowne' (p. 33). Historiography must banish obscurity and shine a light on the nation's origins, which will then enlighten the contemporary reader and offer knowledge on the truth of identity. Narratives of virginity also frequently draw on the language of revelation and light,[36] and Joan herself claimed to hear saintly voices (frequently said to be accompanied by a shining light)[37] that directly transmitted the Word of God to her. The connections between light, truth and purity are numerous in Christian thought.[38] Truth is having correct knowledge (1 Tim. 4:3; 2 Tim. 2:25) and so the truth claims of a virgin who insists that she communes with God and his saints are immensely powerful and cannot be dismissed lightly.

Yet virginity is a problematic concept, inherently difficult to define.[39] This leads to the third concern, with dissimulation, in particular with misleading rhetoric. The struggle between the respective truth claims, fuelled by the religious upheavals of the sixteenth century, leads writers to the assertion that certain types of language are more truthful than others. Bale divides language into two categories, figurative and plain, aligning the latter with Protestant attempts to make the truth of the *evangelium* accessible and clear. Significantly, the terms used by Joan's detractors to undermine her claims to purity (and therefore to God's support for her cause) are mirrored by the terms they use to describe the narratives that praise her. Hall, for instance, is most emphatic in his contempt for the types of discourse he associates with Joan: 'visions, traunses and fables, full of blasphemye, supersticion, and hypocrisy'. He 'maruell[s]' much that wise men did beleue her, and lerned clarkes would write suche phantasies' (fol. 35v). Holinshed also repeatedly qualifies the information he cites on Joan as being told by 'hir louers (the Frenchmen)' (p. 604, col. a) or by reminding the reader that this is what the 'French stories saie' (p. 600, col. b). When he recounts the results of the trial of rehabilitation of 1456, in which, he states, 'a quite contrarie sentence was there declared', it leads him to rage against those who read Joan favourably, such as John Tillet and Polydore Vergil (p. 605, col. a).[40] Joan's lack of purity is, for him, echoed in these writers who support her: '[W]hat puritie or regard of deuotion or conscience is in these writers, trow yee, who make no . . . difference betweene one stirred vp by mercie diuine, or naturall loue, and a damnable sorcerer suborned by satan . . .?' He does not leave any doubt as to what role these writers perform when he dismisses them as 'hir good oratours' (p. 605, col. a). Just as Hall describes Joan as 'painted' and her claims as 'reuelacions, dreames [and] phantasticall visions', sent by Satan to 'blynd the people' (fol. 32v), so Holinshed conflates the counterfeit nature of Joan with the counterfeit nature of the writings that support her and uphold her purity.[41] The falseness of the writings and the falseness of her body are made to reflect one another endlessly, with neither clearly preceding the other. The question arises: can Joan's virginity be confined to either its literal or figurative significations?

Virginity always stands for something other or more than itself – it is a metaphor par excellence. This is partly because it can be defined only through other terms. While virginity is perceived to symbolize stability in Christian thought, few tropes are actually so glitteringly multivalent: fountain, flower, treasure, garden, closed door, star . . . virginity is likened to them all, yet circumscribed by none.[42] Metaphor, like virginity, is closely linked to ideas of the 'proper' and 'improper'. In his highly influential *The Arte of Rhetorique* (1533), Thomas Wilson, following sixteenth-century practice, discusses metaphor before all other rhetorical tropes and figures. It is defined as 'an alternation of a worde, from the *proper* and *naturall* meaning, to that which is not proper, and yet agreeth thereunto by some likenesse'.[43] Joan's detractors particularly rely on her cross-dressing as a clear indication of her improper and 'unnatural' tendencies. Holinshed argues that while she may be a virgin, she has chosen to 'shamefullie' reject 'hir sex abominablie', by denying the clothing that is proper and natural to 'hir owne kind' (p. 604, col. b). Her misleading clothing can be paralleled to the 'misuse' of the adornments of rhetoric, where the mere semblance of truth is presented to the beguiled reader, who is blinded rather than made to see. Joan is accused of functioning like a metaphor: she has taken the '*proper* and *naturall* meaning' and made it to that 'which is not proper'. Citing Paul Ricoeur, Patricia Parker discusses the link between metaphor and usurpation. Metaphor is said to be 'doubly alien' in that it is 'a name that belongs elsewhere and one which takes the place of the word which "belongs"'.[44] Here, 'proper and metaphorical [come to be seen] as "rivals", or as legitimate and bastard brothers, with the metaphorical "alien" as changeling, picaro, or usurper'.[45] The possibilities of both 'legitimate' and 'illegitimate' are contained within the representational capacity of Joan's virginity, while in historiography the question of the 'proper' or legitimate relation of events was becoming more pressing. In both cases the question is: can the illegitimate twin be expelled from one's own rhetoric and, by extension, one's own claims?

While Joan and her supporters are represented as being promoters of deceptive writing, English historiographers are concerned to present their work in a manner reminiscent of what Derrida has called 'white mythology'. By this he means philosophy's claims that it is able to 'remove all figural referentiality from language in order to leave only pure Logos' – claims that Derrida challenges.[46] Escaping rhetoric, however, proves to be impossible. When, for instance, Alain de Lille in his *De planctu naturae* (*c.*1180) expresses the desire to resist the metaphors of colour – 'cosmetics, adorning, clothing' – in order to return to a state of purity, he nonetheless expresses this turning away 'in insistently approaching rhetoric through the rhetorical device of a metaphor'.[47] This is something the historiographers discussed here share, while claiming for their representation an unambiguous referentiality. Yet even where a potential lack of clarity or a diversity of interpretations is admitted, as in Holinshed, it is always also implied that the discerning reader will be led to recognize the truth by the plain – pure? – language of the writer in the end.

As Françoise Meltzer points out, citing Derrida, 'by twinning the voice with the desire for light, the move of apocalyptic discourse is delimited as masculine. The voice, its breath . . . its teleological uncoverings, are phallogocentric. Revelation itself initially poses as the uncovering "of the secret and the *pudenda*".'[48] The term *pudenda*, while ostensibly gender neutral, is nevertheless primarily indicative of female genitalia. This brings us back to the revealing of Joan's body at her execution, as well as before, during the examinations of her virginity, which are meant to resolve the secret or enigma that she embodied. These writers, in seeking to uncover Joan – to reveal the *pudenda* that fixes meaning – align themselves with a masculinist project; in the fight for the light, the tone and rhetoric adopted are consciously gendered as masculine. The ubiquitous associations found in medieval writing of the 'blank page as the female body, subject to manipulation and penetration as the reader strips aside the veil of rhetorical ornament to penetrate to a deeper meaning' are familiar.[49] In medieval Latin literary theory, the truth of a text was frequently perceived as hidden or 'veiled'.[50] The veil itself has long been associated with the feminine, rather ambiguously as a sign of both chastity and seduction.[51] Equally, 'woman' has, in the apocalyptic tradition as well as in the figure of Joan for her contemporaries, been read as both 'veiled, as mystery, [as] enigma hiding truth' and as a figure of danger.[52] Therefore, while Joan's cross-dressing was seen by her detractors as a revelation of her 'true' (that is, dangerously deceptive) nature, it was also perceived as a hiding away of her 'true' nature (*who* or *what* is she?) and as 'unnatural'.[53] In addition, the act of cross-dressing highlights the tensions involved in any attempt to subsume the virgin under the heading of 'the feminine' or 'woman'.

Yet, as Parker shows, writers in the early modern period, particularly also in England, increasingly expressed 'a desire for a more "masculine" or virile style . . . a style that would have . . . a "manly" strength and vigor'.[54] Not only are the types of discourse associated with Joan and her followers aligned with fables and even lies, but her supporters are said to be emasculated as a result of their faith in her. Certainly the gender implication of the distinction between 'good' (true) and 'bad' (false) writing is explicitly brought into play against Joan's supporters when Hall exclaims: 'What more rebuke can be imputed to a renoumed regyon, then to affirme, wryte [and] confesse, that all notable victories, and honourable co[n]questes . . . were gotten and achiued by a shepherdes doughter, a chamberlaine in an hostrie, and a beggars brat' (fol. 33v). By polarizing these writings according to two clearly delineated and gendered categories, Joan's virginity and her claims are again coercively aligned with the feminine. The unease evinced by these attempts at domestication simultaneously reveals the impossibility of assigning the virgin a fixed place in any binary structure.

Within Tudor accounts of Joan, writing, action, the body politic and truth are shown to be intricately interwoven within an implicitly gendered framework. Joan and her untruthful words/body mislead the French body politic (characterized by the different estates and their respective roles), including the king, causing wise men (who should know better) to 'confesse' that their 'notable victories' and 'honourable conquestes' ('masculine' actions) are all due to a woman, and a common woman at that. As a result, the body politic is not only emasculated but also threatened with obscurity, since, as Hall shows, history is meant to commemorate the actions of (noble) *men* and those who are so deceived as to write in support of Joan are therefore clearly not writing history. This is backed up by Hall's ongoing references to the English as manful, puissant and courageous, while the French are braggarts, cowards and, in line with the privileging of 'masculine' deeds over 'effeminate' words, prone to flattery and empty promises (fol. 30).[55]

Authoritative English voices are both gendered and nationalized. In his otherwise cohesive narrative of the battles between the French and

the English/Burgundians during Joan's involvement, Holinshed interrupts himself only once. The account is abruptly suspended *in medias
res*, with the information that in this same year 'among diuerse notable
men of learning and knowledge', one Richard Fleming, English-born,
'a doctor of diuinitie professed in London, did flourish'. In favour with
both Henry VI and God, Fleming is introduced as the founder of
Lincoln College, Oxford, and is said to have written '[d]iuerse bookes',
two of which are mentioned especially by Holinshed. The first is '[a]
protestacion against the Spaniards, the Frenchemen, and the Scots',
and the second an 'Etymologie of England' (p. 603, col. b). The story
of the battle is then taken up once again, with different sources being
cited, all of which are introduced with the comment that Joan's capture
will allow the reader to decipher her real worth 'plainelie'. The brief
insertion about Fleming, thus placed, has the effect of juxtaposing
English learning (which specifically engages with England's enemies,
Englishness and English language) against the 'plain' verdict on Joan
that is delivered by a number of sources, all of whom may differ in
some aspects but end univocally, with the shared conclusion of Joan's
capture. But, as argued above, virginity can never be 'plainly deciphered'. The complexities involved in utilizing familiar and shared
Christian symbols in the service of separate national and religious aims
are made startlingly clear when Hall attacks the French writers who
defend Joan after her trial of rehabilitation: 'Iho[n] Buchet, and diuerse
Frenche writers affirme her to be a sainct in heauen. But because, it is
no poynt of oure faith, no man is bound to beleue hys iudgement,
although he were an Archedeken' (fol. 33v). Hall's defensive explanation of Joan's rehabilitation negotiates the discrepancies of the writers'
views without denying the legitimacy of making such claims per se.
While one could argue that this is a straightforward example of anti-
Catholic rhetoric, that would be only partially true. After all, just a
little while before, he argued that Joan's perfidy was clearly shown by
the *Catholic* clergy's condemnation of her.[56] While terms (such as 'holy'
or 'saint') remain the same, in that they possess a shared meaning
within Christianity, they are also used for distinct and antagonistic
truth claims within Christianity. If virgins can be said to signify either
true or false beliefs (Joan does not have to be believed to be a saint
because 'it is no point of our faith'), then the outcome of Joan's
disputed virginity has significant repercussions for the truth claims of
the historiographers who discuss her. The English historiographers
cannot just dismiss Joan's virginity as irrelevant, precisely because both

the claims of the historiographical project and Joan's virginity aspire to an absolute truth. As Joan embodies claims of truth *and* untruth, of original *and* counterfeit, how can she be written and read, bearing in mind the contiguity between Joan's virginity and historiography? The questioning of categories that virginity effects does not allow the English historiographers the 'full integritie' that they seek for their writing. Joan's elusive virginity can be read as a metaphor for historiography itself, connected as it is to nation, politics, religion, truth, rhetoric and ambiguity.

So how do the English historiographers 'solve' the problem of Joan's virginity? On the whole, they do not. The one who tries to do so most emphatically is Hall, who concludes his account of Joan by locating the truth of history and historiography not in historical writers or historiographical methods, but in the ideals of female behaviour. His historiography becomes determined by his appeal to what he posits as a universal view of the 'good woman'; a view so eternal and authoritative that, as he tells it, it is shared by Christians, pagans, ancients and moderns, defying (even denying) differences of time, faith or nation. This view of woman forms a closed, unbroken circle: time has not changed or fragmented this truth and so it can and must serve as a foundation for the writing of the 'truth of Joan' and, by extension, the truth of history. Hall explains that 'all auncient writers, aswell deuine, as prophane, alledge these three thynges, beside diuerse other, to apparteine to a good woman': 'shamefastnesse', 'pitie' and 'womanly behauor'. He goes on to 'prove' that Joan's behaviour does not conform to any of these three maxims; the verdict is therefore irrefutable: as it is plain that as she cannot be considered a good woman, 'it must nedes, consequently folowe, that she was no saynct' (fol. 34v). Hall still relies on sources and authority here, on 'auncient writers', but for once they appear to speak with one voice. The English version of history – of Joan – is confirmed and proven through an appeal to the unchanging prescriptions of 'proper' feminine conduct. Historiographical methodology is replaced by the reading of gender performance as a determinant of truth. Even if Joan's physical intactness cannot be disproved, her immoral behaviour is said to demonstrate that she lacks the moral virtues integral to true female virginity and sanctity: obedience, humility, silence.[57] As soon as this doubt can be cast, her physical integrity is seriously devalued. The historical event is placed within a static framework that defies time or change: that of female purity. We have come full circle. Yet it is not the body itself that provides answers, merely the reading of that body, which has been shown to be fraught with difficulty, even while 'truth' and 'woman' cannot, it seems, be disconnected. These problems are heightened in relation to virginity, which remains elusive and therefore resistant to appropriation. This in turn ensures the contingency of any reading of Joan and, by extension, of historiography, belying the effectiveness of the display of Joan's body with which this chapter began. For what exactly is to be seen? What is revealed? While the display of 'the secrets that *could* or *should* belong to a woman' is supposed to 'take away any doubts from people's minds', the phrasing itself reiterates the doubt.[58] If these secrets are to be the guarantors of truth, what is to be revealed is nonetheless still veiled, in the folds of a text always written in an ambiguous subjunctive.

As Gransden (among others) has pointed out, '[t]he idea that the renaissance swept away the medieval tradition of historiography has long been discounted'.[59] The medieval antiquarian and rhetorical traditions and the idea of 'history as the manifestation of God's will on earth' were all drawn on heavily throughout the sixteenth century.[60] At the same time, historical narrative became increasingly popular; the new printing technology and the availability of classical as well as contemporary continental sources shaped historiographical practices. Looking at how Joan's virginity is treated by a range of sixteenth-century English writers highlights some of the problems of categorization, not least, I would argue, those of periodization. Kathleen Coyne Kelly and Marina Leslie have pointed out that '[t]o chart the history of virginity as a steady, evolutionary progression from a religious ideal in the Middle Ages toward a more secularized ideal in the Renaissance would obscure the extreme instability of the concept of chastity in both periods', particularly as 'medieval and early modern attitudes toward virginity are not generalizable and evolutionary, but specific, change-able, and often conflicted'.[61] While I agree with this assertion, I would add that the discourses of and on virginity are not only 'specific, changeable, and often conflicted' *within* distinct periods, but that they always point *beyond* the trope itself towards a questioning of other categories. Writing about virginity, it would seem, is never just that, and writing about Joan's virginity is not just about religious or political differences, but also an ongoing discussion of *writing itself*, of representational practices.[62] Who is writing whom? Do these historio-graphers write Joan's virginity, or are the discursive explorations of her virginity just as much about historiography per se? It is no surprise that

Joan's virginity becomes an issue at a time of change: virginity resists redefinition by these English writers who cannot banish the potent implications of the trope. How does one erase the past contexts from a term while still actively using the familiar associations constructed by them as a basis for shared meaning?

Virginity offers sameness and 'defends against the pollution brought on by change'.[63] This quality is in some ways clearly a desirable one for these English historiographers who were anxious to write the origins of the nation and the Church as having always already been there. It is also precisely the quality which bears the greatest threat for that project, as the element of the miraculous inherent in Joan '*is* the manifestation of that force which emanates unilaterally from God, a force figured as contrasting with, and bypassing, human creative activity and the historical processes by which human production and reproduction make the world'.[64] In discussing virginity, these writers are struggling with what Nora sees as the difference between history and the *lieu de mémoire*:

> Unlike historical objects, *lieux de mémoire* have no referents in reality . . . they are pure signs. This is not to say that they are without content, physical presence, or history – on the contrary. But what makes them *lieux de mémoire* is precisely that which allows them to escape from history.[65]

Poised uneasily between the demands of this world and the next, and entangled in generic uncertainties, historiography in this period both desires and rejects Joan's virginity and what virginity represents, revealing in its discussion of Joan its own limitations and vulnerability. Drawing on a rhetoric with religious overtones while writing history in the form of a coherent human narrative with specific claims, these writers cannot 'purify' their texts of the traces of other discourses that have shaped, constructed and proclaimed the ideal of female virginity; its dense, overlapping layers of meaning are wrapped around no core.

Nora argues that while the purpose of *lieux de mémoire*

> is to stop time, to inhibit forgetting, to fix a state of things, to immortalize death, and to materialize the immaterial . . . it is also clear that [they] thrive only because of their capacity for change, their ability to resurrect old meanings and generate new ones along with new and unforeseeable connections.[66]

Joan's virginity – virginity in general – as *lieu de mémoire* is just that, both a warding-off of change and infinitely mutable. Joan's virginity is important and at the same time elusive because of the contingent meanings and connotations that the trope brings with it. While Joan ultimately may not have been of paramount interest to these writers, their impassioned yet inconclusive denunciation of her inadvertently reveals an uncertainty in their narratives. The practice of historiography itself and the changing – often conflicting – demands and circumstances in which historiographers found themselves in the fifteenth and sixteenth centuries are highlighted by their discussion of Joan's virginity and its claims to universality and timelessness. In these texts virginity is an example of the uncanny, the enigma that continues to haunt history, which, as Michel de Certeau shows, returns to that which 'it cannot understand' and that it 'winds around without reaching'.[67]

Notes

I would like to thank John Arnold, Ruth Evans and Sarah Salih for their helpful comments on this chapter. Thanks also to Jane Marie Pinzino, who accepted a version of it as part of a session sponsored by the International Joan of Arc Society at the International Medieval Congress, Leeds (2001).

[1] Hélène Cixous and Jacques Derrida, *Veils*, trans. Geoffrey Bennington (Stanford: Stanford University Press, 2001), p. 39.

[2] *A Parisian Journal, 1405–99*, trans. Janet Shirley (Oxford: Oxford University Press, 1968), pp. 263–4.

[3] *Procès de Condamnation et de Réhabilitation de Jeanne d'Arc dite La Pucelle*, ed. Jules Quicherat, 5 vols (Paris, 1841–9; New York: Johnson, repr. 1965), vol. 3, p. 102. Kathleen Coyne Kelly, *Performing Virginity and Testing Chastity in the Middle Ages* (London: Routledge, 2000), pp. 17–18.

[4] The *Brut* functions as a single name under which are grouped a number of prose works in Anglo-Norman, Middle English and Latin, which continue the chronicle tradition of Geoffrey of Monmouth. In this chapter I will be looking at the representation of Joan in William Caxton's continuation to his edition of John Trevisa's translation of Ranulf Higden's *Polychronicon* (1495), Polydore Vergil's *Anglica Historia* (1512–55; first printed 1534, Basle), Edward Hall's *Chronicle* (1542, burnt; repr. 1548 and 1550) and Raphael Holinshed's *Chronicles of England, Scotland, and Ireland* (1577, 1587). For ease of reference, I will be referring throughout this chapter to 'Holinshed', even though the *Chronicles* is a compendium and it is unclear how much of the passage on Joan was actually written by Holinshed himself; see Richard F. Hardin, 'Chronicles and mythmaking in

Shakespeare's Joan of Arc', *Shakespeare Survey*, 42 (1989/90), 25–35 (26–7), and Annabel Patterson, *Reading Holinshed's Chronicles* (Chicago: University of Chicago Press, 1994), pp. 3–4. While these are not the only historiographers of this period to mention Joan (see also Robert Fabyan, John Stow, John Bale, Richard Grafton), the similarities as well as differences between them demonstrate the range and limitations of the historical writing on Joan in England in this period.

[5] *The Brut, or the Chronicles of England*, ed. Friedrich W. D. Brie, 2 vols, EETS, os, 131, 136 (London: Oxford University Press, 1908), 136, p. 501. See also W. T. Waugh, 'Joan of Arc in English sources of the fifteenth century', in J. G. Edwards, V. H. Galbraith and E. F. Jacob (eds), *Historical Essays in Honour of James Tait* (Manchester: Subscribers, 1933), pp. 387–98 (p. 394).

[6] As Helen Hackett suggests of the Virgin Mary, '[t]he medieval Virgin can readily be described in Freudian terms as an "overdetermined" symbol, a composite figure overlaid with a multiplicity of superimposed meanings because she fulfilled a multiplicity of different desires'; *Virgin Mother, Maiden Queen: Elizabeth I and the Cult of the Virgin Mary* (London: Macmillan, 1995), p. 26. I would extend that to the trope of virginity in general.

[7] See also Kelly, *Performing Virginity*, p. 39. On Joan's cross-dressing, see Susan Crane, 'Clothing and gender definition: Joan of Arc', *Journal of Medieval and Early Modern Studies*, 26 (1996), 297–320, and Susan Schibanoff, 'True lies: transvestism and idolatry in the trial of Joan of Arc', in Bonnie Wheeler and Charles T. Wood (eds), *Fresh Verdicts on Joan of Arc* (New York: Garland, 1996), pp. 31–60.

[8] For a discussion of virginity and chastity in early modern conduct books, see, for instance, Nancy Weitz Miller, 'Metaphor and the mystification of chastity in Vives's *Instruction of a Christen Woman*', in Kathleen Coyne Kelly and Marina Leslie (eds), *Menacing Virgins: Representing Virginity in the Middle Ages and Renaissance* (London: Associated University Presses, 1999), pp. 132–45. On the continuing relevance of virginity in the Renaissance, see Peter Stallybrass, 'Patriarchal territories: the body enclosed', in Margaret W. Ferguson, Maureen Quilligan and Nancy J. Vickers (eds), *Rewriting the Renaissance: The Discourses of Sexual Difference in Early Modern Europe* (Chicago: University of Chicago Press, 1986), pp. 123–42, and Marie H. Loughlin, *Hymeneutics: Interpreting Virginity on the Early Modern Stage* (Lewisburg: Bucknell University Press, 1997).

[9] Hackett, *Virgin Mother*, p. 54.

[10] For use of the body-politic model in the early modern period, see David George Hale, *Body Politic: A Political Metaphor in Renaissance English Literature* (The Hague: Mouton, 1971). See also Philippa Berry, *Of Chastity and Power: Elizabethan Literature and the Unmarried Queen* (London: Routledge, 1989).

[11] Ruth Evans, 'Medieval virginities', in David Wallace and Carolyn Dinshaw

(eds), *Cambridge Companion to Medieval Women's Writing* (Cambridge: Cambridge University Press, forthcoming). Pierre Nora, 'Between memory and history', in Nora (ed), *Realms of Memory: Rethinking the French Past,* vol. 1, *Conflicts and Divisions*, trans. Arthur Goldhammer (New York: Columbia University Press, 1996), pp. 1–20. See also Joanna L. Chamberlayne, 'Crowns and virgins: queenmaking during the Wars of the Roses', in Katherine J. Lewis, Noël James Menuge and Kim M. Phillips (eds), *Young Medieval Women* (Stroud: Sutton, 1999), pp. 47–68, and Katherine J. Lewis, 'Becoming a virgin king: Richard II and Edward the Confessor', in Samantha J. E. Riches and Sarah Salih (eds), *Gender and Holiness: Men, Women and Saints in Late Medieval Europe* (London: Routledge, 2002), pp. 86–100. Of course it could be argued that virginity functioned in similar ways in the self-representation of other nations, not least France. This underlines my point that both the specific and the general are always present within virginity's symbolic potential.

¹² *Hoccleve's Works: The Regement of Princes*, ed. Frederick J. Furnivall, EETS, ES, 72 (London: Kegan Paul, Trench, Trübner, 1897), pp. 131–2, ll. 3627–9, 3655–7. On the use of references to virginity – particularly to the Virgin Mary – to authorize one's writings, see Antonia Gransden, *Historical Writing in England,* vol. 2, *c.1307 to the Early Sixteenth Century* (Ithaca, NY: Cornell University Press, 1982), p. 467. On the use of this in hagiography, see Anke Bernau, 'A Christian *corpus*: virginity, violence and knowledge in the Life of St Katherine of Alexandria', in Jacqueline Jenkins and Katherine J. Lewis (eds), *St Katherine of Alexandria: Texts and Contexts in Medieval Europe* (Turnhout: Brepols, forthcoming).

¹³ Hoccleve, *Regement of Princes*, p. 134, l. 3731. On virgin kings in hagiography see Dyan Elliott, *Spiritual Marriage: Sexual Abstinence in Medieval Wedlock* (Princeton: Princeton University Press, 1993), pp. 113–28, and Sarah Salih, *Versions of Virginity in Late Medieval England* (Cambridge: Brewer, 2001), pp. 18–19.

¹⁴ See Hackett, *Virgin Mother*, pp. 29–37, and Chamberlayne, 'Crowns and virgins', p. 56.

¹⁵ For a discussion of the familiar medieval prophecy of the 'healing virgin' as found in Geoffrey of Monmouth's *De prophetiis Merlini* and its relation to Joan of Arc, see Deborah Fraioli, 'The literary image of Joan of Arc: prior influences', *Speculum*, 56/4 (1981), 811–30, esp. 818–19. For the use of the chaste prophetess Sabrina as symbol of a Protestant British unity in the seventeenth century, see Philip Schwyzer, 'Purity and danger on the west bank of the Severn: the cultural geography of *A Masque Presented at Ludlow Castle, 1634*', *Representations*, 60 (1997), 22–48. It is well known that the female body was frequently used to represent topography, particularly also in emerging colonial discourses. One apposite example here is Sir Walter Ralegh's notorious remark that '*Guiana* is a Countrey that hath yet her Maydenhead'; *The Discoverie of the Large, Rich and Bewtiful Empire of Guiana* (London: Robert Robinson, 1596), p. 96. Many thanks to Richard Sugg for pointing out this example to me.

16 My emphasis. Raphael Holinshed, *Chronicles of England, Scotland and Ireland*, 3 vols (London: Henry Denham, 1587), vol. 3, p. 603, col. b.

17 The question of whether the term 'nationalism' can be applied to pre-Enlightenment periods and situations has been debated extensively and it does not lie within the scope of this chapter to summarize that debate. I would point readers to the following discussions: Kathleen Davis, 'National writing in the ninth century: a reminder for postcolonial thinking about the nation', *Journal of Medieval and Early Modern Studies*, 28 (1998), 611–37; Andrew Hadfield, *Literature, Politics and National Identity: Reformation to Renaissance* (Cambridge: Cambridge University Press, 1994), pp. 1–22; Anthony D. Smith, *Myths and Memories of the Nation* (Oxford: Oxford University Press, 1999), esp. pp. 97–123. For a discussion of gender and the writing of history, see Joan W. Scott, 'Gender: a useful category of historical analysis', *American Historical Review*, 91 (1986), 1053–75 (1074), and Susan Stanford Friedman, 'Making history: reflections on feminism, narrative, and desire', in Diane Elam and Robyn Wiegman (eds), *Feminism beside Itself* (New York: Routledge, 1995), pp. 11–53.

18 Hardin, 'Chronicles and mythmaking', p. 28. Most sixteenth-century writers used as the source for their information on Joan the writing of the Burgundian enemy of Charles VII and of Joan, Enguerand de Monstrelet. It is interesting that while Hall, Holinshed and Vergil all use Monstrelet, their respective versions of Joan are quite different; see Charles Lethbridge Kingsford, *English Historical Literature in the Fifteenth Century* (Oxford: Clarendon Press, 1913), p. 254, and Ingvald Raknem, *Joan of Arc in History, Legend and Literature* (Oslo: Universitetsforlaget, 1971), p. 52.

19 Edward Hall, *The Union of the Two Noble Families of Lancaster and York* (Menston, IL: Scolar Press, 1970), fol. 25. This edition is a reproduction of Richard Grafton's definitive 2nd edition of the work from 1550. Apart from where the 'Preface' is cited, all folio references are taken from the section of the work entitled 'The Troubleous Season of Kyng Henry the Sixt'.

20 My emphasis.

21 Brian Vickers, 'On the practicalities of Renaissance rhetoric', in Vickers (ed.), *Rhetoric Revalued: Papers from the International Society for the History of Rhetoric*, Medieval and Renaissance Texts and Studies, 19 (Binghamton, NY: Centre for Medieval and Early Renaissance Studies, 1982), pp. 133–41 (p. 133). Joseph M. Levine, for instance, points out that '[t]he Renaissance humanists taught that the best training of the statesman lay in a mastery of ancient rhetoric and political example, in the literature and history of antiquity': *Humanism and History: Origins of Modern English Historiography* (Ithaca, NY: Cornell University Press, 1987), p. 75.

22 Peter Burke, *The Renaissance Sense of the Past* (London: Arnold, 1969), p. 105.

23 Ibid., p. 106.

24 Ibid., p. 119. This also holds true for poets in the period.

25 See Alastair J. Minnis and A. B. Scott (eds), with the assistance of David

Wallace, *Medieval Literary Theory and Criticism, c.1100–c.1375: The Commentary Tradition* (Oxford: Clarendon Press, 1988), p. 43. Minnis notes that twelfth-century literary theory, drawing on 'authorities such as Cicero, Macrobius, and Isidore of Seville', made 'a clear distinction between history and fable. *Historia* was the literally true record of actual happenings (*gesta res, res factae*) which were removed in time from the recollection of our age, whereas *fabula* comprised untrue events, fictitious things (*res fictae*) which neither happened nor could have happened' (p. 113).

26 *Polydore Vergil's English History,* vol. 1, ed. Henry Ellis, Camden Society Series, orig. ser., 36 (London: J. B. Nichols, 1846), p. 30.

27 Vergil's desire for a 'full rehersall' in his work was prevented by political factors which 'caused [him] constantly to revise his *Anglica Historia* by modifying or removing contentious material'; Gransden, *Historical Writing*, p. 470.

28 My emphasis. Even more explicitly, William Harrison states in his 'Epistle Dedicatorie' to the first volume of the *Chronicles of England, Scotland, and Ireland* that he will present the information 'truelie and plainelie . . . rather than with vaine affectation of eloquence to paint out a rotten sepulchre'.

29 Richard Hakluyt, *The Principal Navigations, Voyages, Traffiques and Discoveries of the English Nation*, 8 vols (London: Dent, 1907), vol. 1, 'The preface to the second edition, 1598', p. 19. Cited in Hadfield, *Literature, Politics and National Identity*, p. 59.

30 Gransden, *Historical Writing*, p. 472.

31 Hadfield, *Literature, Politics and National Identity*, p. 19.

32 Cited in J. F. Mozley, *John Foxe and his Book* (London: SPCK, 1940), p. 143.

33 See Patterson, *Reading Holinshed's Chronicles*, p. 37, and Joerg O. Fichte, 'Foxe's *Acts and Monuments*: the spirit's triumph over the flesh', in Piero Boitani and Anna Torti (eds), *The Body and the Soul in Medieval Literature* (Cambridge: Brewer, 1999), pp. 167–79 (p. 169). Here what Gabrielle M. Spiegel says about (medieval) historiography is apposite: '[its] ethical function ties history to rhetoric, for it is the orator's duty to guide the historian's expression so he may achieve moral persuasiveness': *The Past as Text: The Theory and Practice of Medieval Historiography* (Baltimore: Johns Hopkins University Press, 1997), pp. 87–8.

34 At the same time this emphasis on regaining or reconstructing the unity of the nation's history reveals the very constructedness of 'unity', be it of the virgin body, the nation or the narrative.

35 Hadfield notes that the book of Revelation was 'the most frequently analysed Biblical text in the Reformation'; *Literature, Politics and National Identity*, p. 66. Katherine R. Firth points out that Foxe, in his *Acts and Monuments*, 'did place his nation, with other European nations, in a historical context bounded by the prophecies of the Revelation'; *The Apocalyptic Tradition in Reformation Britain, 1530–1645* (Oxford: Oxford University Press, 1979), p. 109.

[36] See, for instance, Aldhelm, who in his *De Virginitate* (late seventh century) claims that 'virginity is the sun, chastity a lamp, conjugality darkness'; *Aldhelm: Prose Works*, trans. Michael Lapidge and Michael Herren (Cambridge: Brewer, 1979), p. 75.

[37] See Marina Warner, *Joan of Arc: The Image of Female Heroism* (London: Vintage, 1991), p. 122.

[38] Christ is the truth (John 14:6) and the light of the world (John 8:12), a light that was borne by a spotless virgin.

[39] Françoise Meltzer recalls Freud's discussion of the 'profoundly ambivalent status of virginity' which makes it 'both totem and taboo, both sacredness and danger': *For Fear of the Fire: Joan of Arc and the Limits of Subjectivity* (Chicago: University of Chicago Press, 2001), p. 61.

[40] The Frenchman and royal secretary, Jean du Tillet, was a passionate defender of the Catholic faith.

[41] Interestingly, the same happens in France. When French chronicler, Girard du Haillan, questioned Joan's virginity in his history of the nation in 1570, another writer, François de Belleforest, stated that he was 'amazed that a Frenchman should yield to the fantasies of foreigners'; cited in Warner, *Joan of Arc*, p. 107.

[42] See also Anke Bernau, 'Virginal effects: text and identity in *Ancrene Wisse*', in Riches and Salih (eds), *Gender and Holiness*, pp. 36–48.

[43] My emphasis. Sir Thomas Wilson, *The Arte of Rhetorique*, ed. G. H. Mair (Oxford: Clarendon Press, 1909), p. 172. Cited in Hadfield, *Literature, Politics and National Identity*, p. 115.

[44] Patricia A. Parker, *Literary Fat Ladies: Rhetoric, Gender, Property* (London: Methuen, 1987), p. 36.

[45] Ibid., pp. 37–8. Joan is explicitly called a usurper by Hall, in his citation of the letter of 'the Kyng of England', p. 157.

[46] Andrew Cowell, 'The dye of desire: the colors of rhetoric in the Middle Ages', *Exemplaria*, 11 (1999), 115–39 (134). See Jacques Derrida, 'White mythology: metaphor in the text of philosophy', in Derrida, *Margins of Philosophy*, trans. Alan Bass (London: Prentice Hall, 1982), pp. 207–71.

[47] Cowell, 'Dye of desire', p. 133. Sheila Delany argues that 'the vocabulary of sophistry and craft bespeaks a long-standing mistrust of the rhetor, as well as mistrust of rhetoric as a technique of disguise, hence entrapment': *The Naked Text: Chaucer's* Legend of Good Women (Berkeley: University of California Press, 1994), p. 80.

[48] Meltzer, *For Fear of the Fire*, p. 101.

[49] Andrew Taylor, 'Reading the dirty bits', in Jacqueline Murray and Konrad Eisenbichler (eds), *Desire and Discipline: Sex and Sexuality in the Premodern West* (Toronto: University of Toronto Press, 1996), pp. 280–95 (p. 282).

[50] See Robert S. Sturges, 'The Pardoner, veiled and unveiled', in Jeffrey Jerome Cohen and Bonnie Wheeler (eds), *Becoming Male in the Middle Ages* (New York: Garland, 1997), pp. 261–77 (p. 272). Sturges also sees a continued use of the figure of the veil, particularly in Lacanian psychoanalysis, p. 272.

[51] See Marjorie Garber, *Vested Interests: Cross-Dressing and Cultural Anxiety* (New York: Routledge, 1992), p. 338. On the veil as a sign of women's sin and of virginity in the writings of Christian theologians, see Lynda L. Coon, *Sacred Fictions: Holy Women and Hagiography in Late Antiquity* (Philadelphia: University of Pennsylvania Press, 1997), pp. 36–41.

[52] Meltzer, *For Fear of the Fire*, pp. 101–2.

[53] See Holinshed on Joan as 'unnatural'; p. 604, col. b.

[54] Patricia Parker, 'Virile style', in Louise Fradenburg and Carla Freccero (eds), with the assistance of Kathy Lavezzo, *Premodern Sexualities* (New York: Routledge, 1996), pp. 201–22 (p. 201).

[55] That Holinshed shares this view is shown when he emphasizes that the duke of Bedford fought 'by dint of sword and stroke of battell to prooue his writing and cause true' (p. 602, col. a).

[56] After pointing out the problems involved in using the word 'French' as an umbrella term, Raknem concludes that 'most people in French France regarded [Joan] as a visionary and a God-sent saviour and saint, while the supporters of the English, the English themselves, and many of the *Catholic* clergy, were willing to swear that she was a sorceress and a fiendish agent' (my emphasis); *Joan of Arc*, p. 53.

[57] This definition of female virginity goes back to the early church fathers; see Joyce E. Salisbury, *Church Fathers, Independent Virgins* (London: Verso, 1991), pp. 27–8.

[58] My emphasis.

[59] Gransden, *Historical Writing*, p. 469.

[60] Ibid., p. 476.

[61] Kathleen Coyne Kelly and Marina Leslie, 'Introduction: the epistemology of virginity', in Kelly and Leslie (eds), *Menacing Virgins*, pp. 15–25 (p. 21).

[62] Hardin suggests that the intensification of Joan's vilification is to be linked to political upheavals in the late sixteenth century: 'Chronicles and mythmaking', p. 34. While this is a valid case, I am more interested in the rhetoric and aims of historiography itself and what its treatment of Joan reveals.

[63] Louise O. Fradenburg, 'Criticism, anti-Semitism, and the *Prioress's Tale*', *Exemplaria*, 1 (1989), 69–115 (88).

[64] Fradenburg, 'Criticism', p. 86. As Salih points out, '[s]aints and virgins occupy two kinds of time': *Versions of Virginity*, p. 31.

[65] Nora, 'Between memory and history', p. 19.

[66] Ibid., p. 15.

[67] Michel de Certeau, *The Writing of History*, trans. Tom Conley (New York: Columbia University Press, 1988), p. 40.

12

Virginity Now and Then: A Response to *Medieval Virginities*

JOCELYN WOGAN-BROWNE

R eading this collection, it is striking to see how much and by how many paths virginity has come to our attention in recent years. Indeed, as this volume's title rightly insists, it has been impossible for some time to think of virginity as a single definable entity: we all have virginities now. As a scholar of the older 'women's history' virginities, I am excited by all the new areas virginity research explores in the present collection, as well as by the directions in which it takes established areas of enquiry. Since medieval virginities inhabit different paradigms from our own, they have refused simply to be assimilated to our frameworks for enquiry and have taught us to look more widely at cultural, social and political constructions of virginity. Through the last decade or so of feminisms, bodies, genders, postmodernisms and postcolonialisms, virginity has both kept pace with developments in literary and cultural studies and bred its own areas of particular concern which in turn interact with other work. The wonderfully protean forms of virginity revealed in the present collection and the range and significance of the issues generated by the collection's use of virginity as a focus of enquiry exemplify the interdisciplinarity and intellectual vigour of medieval studies at their best.

The present volume reveals a new and important breadth in virginity studies, but it is significant that it does so by integrating women's studies, not by moving on or recontaining them. Like many other stories the modern scholarly narrative of virginity begins with women but rapidly develops implications for everyone. Much work on virginity at the end of the 1980s and the start of the 1990s was concerned with women in the cultural imaginary, women in representation, and women's records, with virginity conceived of primarily as a personal attribute and as a condition of particular pertinence to medieval women's religious lives. As discussion explored reifying and somatically based accounts of virginity and their social and institutional ideologies, it became clear that a significant history of medieval women could be written through the cultural and social history of professed virginity. This helped to intensify attention to medieval female communities and to create a history of Christianity more seriously inclusive of women, the more so as the relations of professed virginity with laywomen's conditions and status allowed the inclusion of honorary virginities and the lives of wives and widows. Female virginity and chastity became immensely important border zones in lay–monastic relations. The relations between virginity (professed or honorary) and female literacies also became a matter of particular concern. Did religious virginity confer more reading and writing time on medieval women? And if so, did these women, like their secular sisters, attend to a script of their own inculturation via romance (in this case the romance of the virgin with the Christ bridegroom) or to something more liberating? Such questions have produced a decade of intense work in which the religious reading of women has become a significant aspect of women's history, literary history and the history of the book. No doubt this has been driven partly by our investments in empowering and socio-economically transformative uses of literacy, and by pleasure in finding precedent traditions of female learning and eloquence (a particular pleasure for women academics, working in the second century in which universities have not been institutionally male). But these are fields with so many still unexamined or under-studied records that research in them should carry on, though, as in any lively scholarly area, modifications and developments in the framing of the enquiry will continue.

Here, essays by Kim Phillips and Robert Mills productively engage with concerns initially articulated in 'women's studies' virginity scholarship. Phillips turns to secular virginities and legal records and narratives, requiring us to contextualize modern valuations of religious virginity. While the mass of modern scholarship on medieval holy women retrieves lost histories and creates new agendas of research, it remains nonetheless completely unrepresentative, demographically speaking, of the Middle Ages. Consecrated virginity is the choice or fate of relatively few medieval women and the texts of such female virginities, *strictu sensu*, are correspondingly few.[1] Yet as a discourse and as a source of narrative exemplification, virginity informs a very large literature. We are right to attend to its cultural powers and significance, but, must indeed, as Phillips shows, be very careful about turning these too easily and too frequently into the empowerment of medieval women.

The essay by Mills, who has himself made notable contributions to discussions of the gendering of martyrdom and of scopic and other pleasures and pains, reviews the debate over female subjectivity and volition, the proprietorship of the self, and the representation of rape.[2] The presence of systemic misogyny in major genres such as the virgin martyr *passio* and secular romance was argued for by Kathryn Gravdal in her 1991 book, *Ravishing Maidens* (a most welcome move since the issue had been bypassed without difficulty by some earlier commentators).[3] Mills's articulation of this debate's impasses between liberating and constricting accounts of virgin martyrs is necessary and valuable, as is also his controversial experiment in resolving it by attention to the position of victim as itself a subject position. Virgins and widows are already importantly linked in west European traditions of Christian virginity, but Mills's consideration of sati focuses attention in a new way on culturally specific assumptions that the victim's position permits no audible articulation by the victim.

Seeing virginity as a performance rather than a condition is crucial to the expansion of virginity studies. The work of Sarah Salih, one of the present editors, has been decisive here in providing non-essentializing ways of distinguishing performances as women and performances as virgin, and hence of conceiving virginities as performable by any and everyone.[4] The breadth and flexibility this adds to virginity's already formidable capacity for interaction with other studies and discourses is richly developed in this volume. The issue of whether male virginity and chastity is an altogether different phenomenon from female and feminized virginity, for instance, is further developed: John Arnold's study makes male anxieties about the boundaries and powers of the self and its embodiment vividly present. Some of the narratives analysed by Arnold, with their desire for a kind of 'manumission from the corporeal' and from the will-power that has to be brought to bear on it, are as vivid in their way as John Donne's extraordinary Holy Sonnet, 'Batter my heart'. Virginity has particularly fascinating associations with cross-dressing, as Anke Bernau shows in her forthcoming book and in her study of Joan of Arc in this volume: we may perhaps take cross-dressing also as a figure for the new flexibility with which male and female scholars can now consider all genders without, as sometimes used to be the case, erasing or universalizing one or another of them.

Joanna Huntington's study of male virginity adds to the existing excellent work on late Anglo-Saxon virginities with a fascinating account of Edward the Confessor's developing virginity in his various *vitae* through to the 1163 life by Aelred of Rievaulx (the dominant source for the later vernacular and Latin documents).[5] Like other studies here (especially Bernau's), it also shows how powerful virginity can be as an organizing focus in historiography. Virginity's combination of the pristine and the labile – always already a place of foundation and fecundity, the longed-for but never fixable realm of originary purity, the uninscribed bearer of memory and identity – is well illustrated by the role of native virgin saints in the historiographical chorography of England. Here both a pantheon of virgins (renewed throughout the medieval period) and a number of separate, differently developing cults play important roles.[6] The way Edward's male, married, royal virginity grows in power as a founding historiographical locus is in some ways not untypical. But more specific to him is the way his virginity becomes the fulcrum around which the turn in insular history from Anglo-Saxon to post-conquest is construed, increasingly so in later representations.[7] (So too, the Virgin Mary's pivotal role in Christian history, set not against the paganism of the Danes, but the Jews; or Bede opposing the Ely virgin Etheldreda to Helen of Troy; or Osbert of Clare on Christian and vestal virgins in his treatise for the widowed Adelidis, abbess of Barking.[8])

The historiographical and political implications indissociable from the virginity of a figure such as Edward are also specially visible in the case of Joan of Arc, whose contested virginity Bernau examines here in and as historiography. Bernau is the author of a striking essay on the clerisy, St Katherine (virgin patroness of learning), and the violence of knowledge in another collection, an essay that is a subtle mediation and development of issues much discussed since Gravdal's *Ravishing Maidens*.[9] Here too, on Joan of Arc, Bernau shows a wide and various range of concerns in play around a particular virginity: the extraordinary turbulence and productivity of virginity's relations with history are vividly present.

Historiography's virginities often combine representation of virginity's centrality in the maintenance of social structures with a sense of its potential for the *unheimlich* and the transcendent. William of Malmesbury's highly embodied *translatio* for the regnal history of the English kings, for instance, proceeds from the dissolution of the embalmed body of Virgil's Pallas to England and Normandy's doubleness in the form of adult, female, conjoined twins, one burdened by the corpse of the other, in order to launch a recuperative English history based on the claim that nowhere else has so many incorrupt saints' bodies. Five saints, four of them virgin, 'all with skin and flesh inviolate and joints yet supple', evince divine favour and a future for the English.[10] Virginity here is at once the antithesis and the metonym of monstrosity and the grotesque, not more reassuring than it is disturbing in this vision of a nation validated by undecaying bodies. But virginity's originary and fecundating power is one of its most persistent associations, not only in the Virgin Mary, but in innumerable Christian saints and classical sources. As Juliette Dor shows, these iconographically and typologically hallowed sources of virginity can be dazzlingly extended to include the grotesque body as represented in the mysterious vulva-centred female figures – sheela-na-gigs – carved on churches in the British Isles from the twelfth to the seventeenth centuries.[11] The complexities here – if these figures display virginity, sexuality and fecundity, they signify partly by metonym and partly by inversion – challenge lazy reading or assumptions about any of our images of virginity.

Another kind of late medieval virginity is the focus for Jonathan Hughes's tour de force on alchemy and the discourses of sexuality, gender and courtly power in the late Middle Ages, where virginity's apparently counter-intuitive positioning is made to yield much new information and cultural analysis. Salih also opens up new territories by using virginity to explore relations between the erotic and the religious, arguing against the contemporary assumption that the one can be understood simply to code for the other. In responding to the question 'Is virginity at risk here?', medieval texts return multifarious answers, pursuing, disavowing, troubling and being troubled by the discrimination of sexual and spiritual experience. Salih's lucid analysis replaces totalizing psychoanalytic and theological approaches to medieval alterity and identity with a 'common post-Augustinian heritage'. She creates a more nuanced paradigm for a problem that has been of continuing interest for medieval mysticism and the history of sexuality since its recent articulations by Caroline Walker Bynum and Nancy F. Partner.[12]

Diachronic issues are also important. The periodization of virginity histories, the relations of medieval virginities with earlier and sub-sequent forms, are areas where medieval work needs to consider its relations with post- and pre-medieval disciplinary formations, with, for example, late antique virginities on the one hand and Reformation virginities on the other, or with, for that matter, nineteenth-century virginities and reprises of virginity and medievalism.[13] Does virginity become marriage under Protestantism? (Bernau's essay, positioned in the late medieval/early modern zone that is currently such a focus of attention, suggests that a straightforward polarization into displaced religious and secular political emergent virginities cannot be adequate.[14])

As well as demonstrating the sheer morphic suppleness of virginity, the present volume insists on postcolonial virgin awarenesses. Jane Cartwright's account of Welsh virginity and chastity testing can be partly located against an established concern with the interrelations of somatic and other cultural scripts where virginity theory and practice is problematized and virginity's social construction elicited.[15] Anthropo-logy and gynaecology are partner-discourses, and law and literature contribute. But Cartwright's use of her rich Welsh sources also attests a new regionalism and variousness in virginity studies: the essay is aware both of its own cultural specificity and of comparisons and contrasts with other cultures. Although this volume is largely concerned with the insular Middle Ages, it is vitally aware of the scope for regional, comparative and variously ethnic virginities.

The possibilities of virginity as a cross-cultural optic, an organizing trope for relations between different groups (already implicit in the linking of virginity and ethnography in medieval travel literature, for example) is also developed here.[16] The question of Jewish and Christian virginities and beliefs about each other's virginities is an area where more work seems particularly desirable and, in this volume, Ruth Evans explores the relations between virginity and anti-Semitism to reveal a startling and intriguing new conjunction: the role of the virgin martyr as eucharistic host, tormented and mysterious, as is the host itself in blood-libel and host-torture narratives and drama. Such work should inspire futher explorations of the pervasive medieval conceptual linking of virginity and Jewishness. This is not always an opposition of purity and abjected filth. The work of Anna Abulafia and others on the range of Christian engagement with Judaism (hideously but not always or only violent) can be extended through virginity studies.[17] The Anglo-Norman version of William of Newburgh's commentary on the Song of Songs (*Explanatio sacri epithalamii in matrem sponsi, c.*1190) is an example.[18] The commentary's account of Song 2:6 explains that climbing up by the desert in the Song signifies virginity, because virginity was abandoned and reviled under Jewish faith:

> kar uirginité adunc desert fu nomé
> kar deguerpi en la lei fu e reuilé.
> E maleite la tindrent e escumege (fol. 77v, ll. 12–14)[19]

for virginity was at that time called 'desert' [wasteland] because it had been forsaken and reviled in the faith and they held it to be anathema and accursed.

To die unmarried and without having borne fruit is to be cursed in the Jewish belief system, the commentary explains.[20] Nevertheless, it continues, Elias and Jeremiah were virgins and so too the Virgin Mary, who broke and removed the curse of the Jewish faith in giving her virginity to God. The Virgin is thus the column of smoke ('virge de fume') who comes up from the desert in purity greater than any previously given to human nature.

Song of Songs commentaries were at this time developing a historical level of interpretation and an understanding of the Song as history and prophecy.[21] How far did the efflorescence of Song commentary in the twelfth and thirteenth centuries create mutual awareness of culturally different virginities? And among what constituencies? Concern about barrenness and the failure of progeny is, after all, quite as intense in Christian family systems as in Jewish.

The telos of Christian history and virginity's capacity to transmit the sacred future is opposed by the Jews, according to an Anglo-Norman version of Grosseteste's Latin translation (from the Greek) of the lexicon of *Suidas*.[22] This is an account of evidence for the virginity of Mary, said to be known to, but traditionally hidden by, the Jews. When a death among the temple priests makes the wise young Jesus a candidate for election to office, Mary must swear to his paternity and maternity. Astonished by her claims, the priests send for a jury of 'matrones e norrices por encerthier e prouer si marie estoit uirge' (matrons and nurses to enquire into and test whether Mary was a virgin). No details are given (unlike the dramatic representations of the midwife Salomé in medieval cycle drama), but the priests 'furent certain de la uirginité' (were sure of her virginity) and they record Mary's virginity and Jesus's divine paternity in their temple book, electing 'iesu filius dei uiuentis et marie uirginis' (Jesus the son of the living God and Mary the virgin) to the next vacancy.[23] But when the Jews realize after the crucifixion that they have killed God's son, the priests' book is removed from the temple and hidden. Here at least error provokes conspiracy and cover-up, rather than the conspiracy of the always already wicked provoking error. Like the glimpse of cultural relativism in the Anglo-Norman version of William of Newburgh's commentary, the possibility of slightly more open responses can perhaps be seen here. (Also visible is the need to think the Virgin Mary back into virginity studies in further ways than as the vexed but compelling role model for women which her impossible combination of the inimitable and the normative makes her.)

In Grosseteste's *Suidas*, virginity's role in the production of history is once more important and problematic, this time in Christianity's preoccupation with effacing the structural use of anti-Semitism in the creation of its own identity.[24] I have cited here a couple of readily available instances from the sources I am familiar with, but there is presumably a whole history of awareness and suppression and changing intellectual positions to be traced here. A fuller history of Jewish virginities in the Christian Middle Ages, like the work of Susan Einbinder on Jewish martyrdoms in medieval Europe, would be of great interest.[25] Islamic virginities are, obviously, equally urgent, and increasingly feasible is the possibility of comparing Indian and medieval Chinese and Japanese virginities. So, too, there is room for more work on virginity polemics in Christian theologies and societies: for example, the theology and politics of Lollard contestation of older doctrinal valuations of virginity ('A vow of continence mad in our chirche of wommen, þe whiche ben fekill and vnperfyth in kynde, is cause of br[i]ngging of most horrible synne'); or the splendid comparative perspectives with continental virginities offered by, for example, the work of Constant Mews and others.[26]

These further virginities will be in as multiple and varied relations with other discourses, social constructs and people's life histories as the essays in this book suggest for (principally) medieval British and north-western European sources. The other and the normative, the liminal and the socially central, the pure and the fecund – all virginity's paradoxes remain generative. Rather than speculating further on the rich future possibilities for the field, which can safely be left to the new generations of scholars interested in virginity, I would like to conclude anecdotally with an account of one of the early realizations about virginity which was important to my own research and which I think suggestive of the significance and power of virginity beliefs.

This is the story of a paper I called 'A short history of the hymen', which I gave in various forms and workshops to Women in Medicine organizations in the UK in the early 1990s. My aim was to use the hymen's recurrent appearances and disappearances in the history of medical and other discourses as an instance of how powerfully cultural narratives determine what is perceived as the object of knowledge and, for that matter, our sense of self. My argument rested on the fact that, as is now well recognized in virginity scholarship, the hymen is not a constant of bodily knowledge, but appears and disappears at various periods from the Greeks to twentieth-century medicine.[27] Not only does its visibility to specific enquiry depend on who needs whom to have a hymen for what purpose, but so, too, do general and scientific beliefs about its presence or absence, nature and appearance.[28] Cultural need, not anatomical fact, has driven the morphology of the hymen, and women have needed hymens not because anatomy was destiny but because of men's claims to proprietorship of their sexuality and fertility: hymens need to be little imperforate seals ready to be torn open in the violent production of blood as a sign that no rival proprietor had precedence. With their instructions on the fabrication of hymens or, what is usually as or more important, the hymeneal blood that is the sign of the hymen, medieval examples from the Trotula and associated gynaecological texts were particularly useful in underlining this point.[29] Although these hymen recipes sounded very uncomfortable, the ability to make one's own hymen seemed potentially not so much to confirm as to subvert patriarchal body models. So anatomically unreifiable is the hymen that it could disappear periodically from body models and from theoretical knowledge. Yet, at other times, it had to be literally made up, produced on demand.

Looking at modern medical accounts, I found the hymen as evanescent and problematic as at any other stage of its history. In contemporary medicine, the hymen was still a now-you-see-it, now-you-don't phenomenon, and not only around the moment of what the medical books liked to call 'rupture'. Few textbooks mentioned it at all, but some detailed it extensively. So was it or was it not part of the modern medical body's morphology?[30]

At that time (1991) the study of anatomy was installed in the organization of medical education as the basis, the 'real'. Even if it was something of a taxonomic chore, necessarily preliminary to the treatment of live patients, it supposedly taught you what the body, quite simply and objectively, *was*. Medical textbooks of the late 1980s and early 1990s in fact continued to construct the body on a neo-Cartesian model as a machine, which had to work properly in its various parts and mechanisms. Their prefaces were reminiscent of medieval encyclopedias: *Fachprosa* has no less strategic and copious a prologue rhetoric than more literary genres. Thus the 1995 edition of their greatest representative, *Gray's Anatomy* (first published in 1858), offered a historical *cursor mundi* from 'the origin of life on earth' (with some beguiling allusions to dinosaurs in its illustrations) to 'final steps to modern man [sic]'.[31] Vesalian anatomy's severance of form and function and the degeneration of anatomy into mere taxonomy would be updated and corrected in *Gray's*, the preface explained, to a functionalist model based on Descartes, for it was now recognized that 'machines work' and hence 'all living structures are constantly changing at one level or another' (p. 3).

It says much for the probity of the editors of *Gray's* that the hymen made it into the volume at all since, according to their description, it 'has no established function' (p. 1876). The ability of *Gray's* to offer lucid, concise accounts against the grain of its own assumptions makes one see why the book has its classic status. One also of course sees how important its assumptions have been in forming the professional culture of medicine.

Gray's offered several valuable realizations for the enquiring virginity scholar. The first was in its characteristically precise and clear account of the hymen:

> **Hymen vaginae**. This is a thin fold of mucous membrane situated just within the vaginal orifice; the internal surfaces of the fold are normally folded to contact each other and the vaginal orifice appears as a cleft between them. The hymen varies greatly in shape and area; when stretched, it is annular and widest posteriorly; sometimes it is semilunar, concave towards the pubes; occasionally it is cribriform or fringed. It may be absent or form a *complete*, *imperforate* hymen [italics mine]. When it is ruptured, small round *carunculae hymenales* are its remnants. It has no established function. (p. 1876)

Two *folds*, not a discrete, normatively imperforate seal. Even if *Gray's* saw the imperforate hymen as the only *complete* one, this body model was already in radical disjunction from the cultural narrative of the hymen. But *Gray's* had more to show. Thanks to my reifying conception of a hymen as a discrete body-part with which one was reluctantly but inevitably born, I had been looking at the wrong discourse. *Gray's* account of the hymen was located in an account of the embryology, not the anatomy, of the womb. The hymen thus became not simply an anatomical given, but the outcome of embryonic growth. A female embryo grows a womb, downwards and outwards, and grows too, the hymenal folds at its outer vaginal portals, which should normally be separable enough to avoid a later painful retention of the menses.

All this was exciting news. One was not, and never had been, a hollow space sealed off with a membrane, an empty, passive vessel of lack, awaiting the painful marking of ownership. The hymen is actually a rather clever thing to have grown, and a happy healthy one has built-in drainage. The fantasy of male proprietorship and the cultural need for violent rupture in which (as with Plutarch's 12-year-old Roman brides) men can be credited with the initiation not only of sexuality and socialization of women but also of the onset of their menstrual cycle, could be dispensed with. (And men perhaps released from their cultural roles in heterosexual relations as commodity brokers, proprietors and rupturers?)

These liberating possibilities emerged, however, against the grain of medical discourse. As I read on through the textbooks, it was clear that most shared the *Gray's* model of the body as a machine and of anatomy as an account of functioning parts (not, as Thomas Laqueur, Marie-Christine Pouchelle and others have emphasized, for pre-eighteenth century humoral models, an economy of fluids[32]). And in this model, the female machine was sadly defective. The organization of medical narratives considering the hymen's context involved a preliminary lengthy account of the normative male body. Then came an account of the weaker, deviant, dysfunctional female version of the model. Thus in *Last's Anatomy*, 1990 edition:

The Female Urogenital Triangle

All the male formations and structures are present in the female, but modified greatly for functional reasons. The essential difference is the *failure* in the female of midline fusion of the genital folds. The male scrotum is *represented* by the labia majora of the vulva, and the corpus spongiosum of the male urethra is *represented* by the labia minora [italics mine].[33]

So we have not *presence* of the labia majora but *absence* of the scrotum. Self-representation on the part of the labia majora or the labia minora is unthinkable in this language, however 'value-free' it may imagine itself to be. *Last's Anatomy* doesn't allow much space to ask, 'Is a failed fusion of the genital folds a lost scrotum or is it a successful vagina?' Worse was to come:

> the perineal membrane of the male is represented in the female by **only** a **narrow** shelf of membrane [*how typically inadequate*] . . . **Lacking** the **rigid** support of the **complete** perineal membrane of the male, the perineal body is more mobile in the female [*so, probably more flighty and unreliable?*] . . . The female urethra [has] a **few**, **poorly developed** pit-like glands, said to be homologous with the prostate but bearing no relation to the structure of that gland [*Of course not, how could they be as good as the male paradigm?*] . . . Should the sphincter urethrae **fail** [*a possibility not contemplated in the preceding account of male systems*], the urine escapes to the exterior (stress incontinence). The smooth muscle of the bladder neck is **not strong enough to withstand much pressure (coughing, sneezing, skipping etc.)** [*Should women then perhaps lie permanently on Victorian daybeds lest they damage themselves in their fragile, incontinent beings?*] The anterior U-shaped fibres demand a **fixture** against which to compress the urethra, and **surgical relief** [*Surgical* what?] provides such a **firm structure** (usually postoperative scar tissue) behind the urethra [*So it's scientifically applied scar tissue women need to operate in a world of men, especially if they want to skip, sneeze or cough?*]. (*Last's Anatomy*, pp. 354–6; bold and italics mine)

Considered as an image of women's bodies professionally inculcated into young men (and smaller numbers of young women) in medical training until recently, this is a profoundly alarming narrative. One might want to ask one's doctor the date of his training, which anatomy textbook he trained on, and in what edition, before consenting to surgery.

Consider too, the even more alarming case of anatomical illustrations in these texts. The accompanying Figures 8a and 8b show a pair of nineteenth-century representations of the urogenital systems. The smooth semi-realism of a rather attractive lily-like penis, curving, not floppy, virile and tensile, is set against a howling vagina. This terrifying

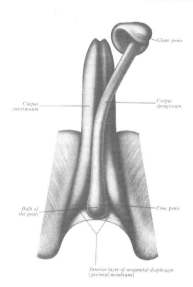

Figure 8a *Gray's Anatomy*, 14.11. 'Ventral aspect of the constituent erectile masses of the penis in erect position. The glans penis and the distal part of the corpus spongiosum are shown detached from the corpora cavernosa penis and turned to the left.'

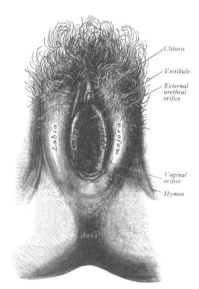

Figure 8b *Gray's Anatomy*, 14.31. 'Female external genitalia, with the labia majora and labia minora separated.'
(Both reprinted from Williams et al., *Gray's Anatomy*, 37/E, © 1989 Elsevier Ltd.)

black mouth surmounted by a beak-like clitoris and a Medusa crown of hideously vigorous serpents of pubic hair perhaps suggests why so much surgical control must be exerted over women's bodies elsewhere in the medical narratives. And *this* terrifying site is where the hymen lives. This is a scary story for everyone, the more so since these illustrations are from the exemplary *Gray's Anatomy*, 1995 edition.[34] Occurring only here in the volume, the modern editors' abandonment of the conventions of photographic and diagrammatic anatomical illustration perhaps serves as a kind of modesty veil: an old vagina is somehow more polite than a modern one? Or a post-virginal vagina is less embarrassing than the sight of a young unused one? However that may be, at this crucial moment in the representation of women by older to younger men, a recycled nineteenth-century engraving of monstrosity is what is on offer.

Trying to understand medieval and modern constructions of hymeneal virginity both in the literal sense of twelfth- and thirteenth-century gynaecological recipes and in wider figurative senses revealed the cultural force of the phenomenon under investigation in unforgettable ways.[35] Medical schools now often incorporate attention to the social and human context of medicine in their training. But other damaging cultural valuations and constructions of virginity remain widespread. In its construction as sign the hymen can never finally be fixed, can never give total assurance, and greater violence than *Last's Anatomy*'s provision of 'surgical relief' is often perpetrated on women in the face of these anxieties. Not only is the hymen reified by being made present, as in the Trotula recipes for its creation, but it is reified in absence by being cut away. One Somali justification for female excision and infibulation is that it is necessary because of 'the inability of women to find other ways of establishing virginity'.[36] So too some African procedures suture the vulva or remove all the surrounding glands lest the virgin's secretions destroy her new husband's spermatozoa. (This seems a particularly harsh analogue to European traditions of the venomous virgin, well-known from Mandeville's accounts of the 'cadeberiz' or 'foles of wanhope'– those sexual kamikaze pilots who go before the bridegroom in order to protect him from virginal venom.[37]) Other cultures focus anxiety on the sexual pleasure of women: the clitoridectomies notoriously performed on nineteenth-century women in Britain, or the 'treatments' of hysteria, lesbianism, masturbation and other 'female deviance', that continued into the 1950s in the USA and the UK.[38] The figures for worldwide genital mutilation currently run to an estimated 130 million women and girls per year, with two million more at risk.[39]

This particular aspect of virginity in our post-colonial condition was sharply framed for me around the time I wrote the paper referred to above. On the one hand, I encountered a priest friend, miserably walking in our inner-city park, and struggling to come to terms with what he felt to be a failure in which he was not unimplicated, even if not responsible for it: yet another young girl from the area of his congregation had been sent home to Somalia to her grandmother to be mutilated.[40] On the other hand, at a luncheon party attended by an ex-military man with colonial experience, I spoke about genital mutilation and the need to stop it. 'How's your Urdu?' enquired my colonel auditor – pleasantly enough, but he had made a fair point. Catholic sympathy, in the broadest and best sense, on the one hand: the perceptions of the administrator of a colonized and (for the colonizers) difficult-to-enter culture on the other. At 'home' in Britain, or among the colonized 'others', the politics of who does what to whom in the name of the custody of women's bodies and virginities does not permit simple answers.[41]

A volume on medieval virginities is in one sense remote from these issues (though not further away than my Urdu-less indignation or closer than my sense that, nevertheless, systematic mutilation of citizens might warrant *some* kind of protest, even by those outside the culture concerned).[42] But the present collection's sophisticated, nuanced attention to the cultural construction of virginities and their implications constitutes both a properly academic contribution and the best contribution academics can make professionally in these matters. Thinking hard about all our virginities and who has what kind of stake in them is valuable cultural work.

Notes

[1] Eileen Power estimates that, between 1250 and 1540, there 'cannot have been more than 3,500 nuns altogether in England, decreasing to 1900 in 1534': M. M. Postan (ed.), *Medieval Women* (Cambridge: Cambridge University Press, 1975), p. 89. The work so often invoked to represent virginity in modern scholarship, the 'Letter on virginity for the encouragement of virgins', better known as *Hali Meiðhad*, is often cited as if it were one of a vast reservoir of such texts. In fact the virginity letter or treatise as such has very few discrete examples in Middle English, rather

more in its background of Latin letters (see Robert Raymo, 'Works of religious and philosophical instruction', in Albert E. Hartung (gen. ed.), *Manual of the Writings in Middle English* (Hamden: Connecticut Academy of Arts and Sciences, 1983–), vol. 7, pp. 2255–378, 2467–582; Barbara Newman, 'Flaws in the golden bowl: gender and spiritual formation in the twelfth century', *Traditio*, 45 (1989/90), 111–46, repr. in her *From Virile Woman to WomanChrist: Studies in Medieval Religion and Literature* (Philadelphia: University of Pennsylvania Press, 1995), pp. 19–45.

2 'A man is being beaten', in Rita Copeland, David Lawton and Wendy Scase (eds), *New Medieval Literatures*, vol. 5 (Oxford: Oxford University Press, 2002), pp. 115–54; ' "Whatever you do is a delight to me!": masculinity, masochism, and queer play in representations of male martyrdom', *Exemplaria*, 13 (2001), 1–37.

3 Kathryn Gravdal, *Ravishing Maidens: Writing Rape in Medieval French Literature and Law* (Philadelphia: University of Pennsylvania Press, 1991). The notion that secular or sacred romance always encodes rape fantasies was (in my view rightly) resisted in debate about the precise subject status of represented virgin martyrs and possible ways of reading the romance of their passions. But it is salutary to remember how recently the represented condemnations by virgin martyrs of their torturers could be seen as the misandry of resistant women (see, for example, Thomas J. Heffernan, *Sacred Biography: Saints and their Biographers in the Middle Ages* (New York: Oxford University Press, 1988).

4 Drawing on Judith Butler's work on the discursive production of the body, Salih looked at virginity as an embodied performance and 'a rearticulation of the heterosexual hegemony [which] can be understood as a distinct gender'. Virgin martyrs are accordingly not only virgins as distinct from women, but 'virgins who were once women, and who could be women again if they [weren't] careful'; 'Performing virginity: sex and violence in the Katherine group', in Cindy L. Carlson and Angela Jane Weisl (eds), *Constructions of Widowhood and Virginity in the Middle Ages* (Basingstoke: Macmillan, 1999), pp. 95–112 (pp. 98, 109). See also her *Versions of Virginity in Late Medieval England* (Cambridge: Brewer, 2001). In subsequent work Salih has argued that we cannot assume even the virgin bride of Christ automatically to connote a heterosexual model of desire and union; 'Queering *sponsalia Christi*: virginity, gender, and desire in the early Middle English anchoritic texts', in Copeland, Lawton and Scase (eds), *New Medieval Literatures*, vol. 5, pp. 155–75.

5 Recent work explores still further contexts and meanings: notable are Catherine Cubitt, 'Virginity and misogyny in tenth- and eleventh-century England', *Gender and History*, 12 (2000), 1–32; Clare A. Lees, 'Engendering religious desire: sex, knowledge, and Christian identity in Anglo-Saxon England', *Journal of Medieval and Early Modern Studies*, 27 (1997), 17–46; Monika Otter, 'Closed doors: an epithalamium for Queen Edith, widow and virgin', in Carlson and Weisl (eds), *Constructions of Widowhood and*

Virginity, pp. 63–92; Paul Hayward, 'Suffering and innocence in Latin sermons for the Feast of the Holy Innocents, *c*.400–800', *Studies in Church History*, 31 (1994), 67–80 (79) (for the growing Anglo-Saxon tendency to 'see the martyred infants as examples of active virginity', not just as murdered royal children).

6　Jocelyn Wogan-Browne, *Saints' Lives and Women's Literary Culture, c.1150–1300: Virginity and its Authorizations* (Oxford: Oxford University Press, 2001), ch. 2.

7　See, for example, Matthew Paris, *La Vie seint Aedward le Rei*, ed. Kathryn Young-Wallace, Anglo-Norman Text Society, 41 (London: ANTS, 1983); 'St Edward the Confessor', in *Supplementary Lives in Some Manuscripts of the Gilte Legende*, ed. Richard Hamer and Vida Russell, EETS, os, 315 (Oxford: Oxford University Press, 2000), pp. 3–38, esp. p. 26.

8　See Wogan-Browne, *Saints' Lives*, ch. 6.

9　'A Christian *corpus*: virginity, violence and knowledge in the Life of St Katherine of Alexandria', in Jacqueline Jenkins and Katherine J. Lewis (eds), *St Katherine of Alexandria: Texts and Contexts in Western Medieval Europe* (Turnhout: Brepols, 2003).

10　William of Malmesbury, *Gesta Regum Anglorum: The History of the English Kings*, ed. and trans. R. A. B. Mynors, R. M. Thomson and Michael Winterbottom (Oxford: Clarendon Press, 1998–9), p. 387; Robert M. Stein, 'Making history English: cultural identity and historical explanation in William of Malmesbury and Lamon's *Brut*', in Sylvia Tomasch and Sealy Gilles (eds), *Text and Territory: Geographical Imagination in the European Middle Ages* (Philadelphia: University of Pennsylvania Press, 1998), pp. 97–115.

11　Given Irish immigration to the southern hemisphere in the nineteenth century, the *OED*'s definition of 'sheila' seems pertinent: 'Sheila: Australia and New Zealand colloq., also shaler, sheelah etc [Orig. uncertain]. It may represent a generic use of the (originally Irish) personal name Sheila, the counterpart of Paddy.' Did some resonance of sheela-na-gig underpin the generic quality of what is now often found as a personal name as well as a generic term for woman/girlfriend? Are Australian sheilas not merely bonza but sheela-na-gigs?

12　See further Lara Farina, *Reading for Pleasure: Erotic Discourse and Early English Religious Writing* (London: Palgrave, forthcoming).

13　There is now an enormous literature on the history of virginity: a few items from across the chronological range are: Kate Cooper, *The Virgin and the Bride: Idealized Womanhood in Late Antiquity* (Cambridge, MA: Harvard University Press, 1996); Helen King, *Hippocrates' Woman: Reading the Female Body in Ancient Greece* (London: Routledge, 1998); Jo Ann McNamara, *A New Song: Celibate Women in the First Three Christian Centuries* (New York: Haworth Press, 1983); Giulia Sissa, *Greek Virginity*, trans. Arthur Goldhammer (Cambridge, MA: Harvard University Press, 1990); the early medieval studies referred to in n. 5 above; Carlson and

Weisl (eds), *Constructions of Widowhood and Virginity*; Kathleen Coyne
Kelly and Marina Leslie (eds), *Menacing Virgins: Representing Virginity in
the Middle Ages and Renaissance* (London: Associated University Presses,
1999); Salih, *Versions of Virginity*; Karen A. Winstead, *Virgin Martyrs:
Legends of Sainthood in Late Medieval England* (Ithaca, NY: Cornell
University Press, 1997); Wogan-Browne, *Saints' Lives*; Mary Bly, *Queer
Virgins and Virgin Queens on the Early Modern Stage* (Oxford: Oxford
University Press, 2000); Richard Burt and John Michael Archer (eds),
Enclosure Acts: Sexuality, Property and Culture in Early Modern England
(Ithaca, NY: Cornell University Press, 1994); Helen Hackett, *Virgin
Mother/Maiden Queen: Elizabeth I and the Cult of the Blessed Virgin Mary*
(Basingstoke: Macmillan, 1995); Wendy Beth Heller, *Chastity, Heroinics
and Culture: Women and the Opera of Seventeenth Century Venice* (Ann
Arbor: University of Michigan Press, 1997); Sally Mitchell, *The Fallen
Angel; Chastity, Class and Women's Reading 1835–1880* (Bowling Green:
Bowling Green University Popular Press, 1981); Sally Cline, *Women,
Celibacy and Passion* (London: Deutsch, 1993).

[14] See also here the subtle essay of John Rogers, 'The enclosure of virginity:
the poetics of sexual abstinence in the English revolution', in Burt and
Archer (eds), *Enclosure Acts*, pp. 229–50.

[15] See Kathleen Coyne Kelly, *Performing Virginity and Testing Chastity in the
Middle Ages* (London: Routledge, 2000).

[16] For discussion of an ethnography of chastity and virginity focused through
a virgin male, see Wogan-Browne, ' "Bet . . . to rede . . . on holy seyntes
lyves": romance and hagiography again', in Carol M. Meale (ed.), *Readings
in Medieval English Romance* (Cambridge: Brewer, 1994), pp. 83–97.

[17] Anna Sapir Abulafia, *Christians and Jews in Dispute: Disputational
Literature and the Rise of Anti-Judaism in the West, c.1000–1150* (Aldershot:
Ashgate, 1998). Ruth Nissé, 'The *Liberte Aseneth* and Jewish conversions in
thirteenth-century England' (forthcoming).

[18] The commentary is self-described in its prologue as 'un lung chaunt d'amur'
(fol. 57, l. 6), claims high learning and many subtle matters for itself (fol. 57,
l. 10), and is extant only in a vernacular collection (Oxford, Bodleian
Library, MS Rawlinson poet. 23): see further Tony Hunt, 'Anecdota
Anglo-Normannica', *Yearbook of English Studies*, 15 (1985), 1–17 (4–5),
and Hunt, 'The Song of Songs and courtly literature', in Glyn S. Burgess
and Robert Taylor (eds), *Court and Poet* (Liverpool: ARCA, 1981), pp.
189–96.

[19] Oxford, Bodleian Library, MS Rawlinson 234, fols 57–105 (this passage fol.
77v, ll. 10–32 to fol. 78, ll. 1–6, accents added). See further Ruth J. Dean
with Maureen B. M. Boulton, *Anglo-Norman Literature: A Guide to Texts
and Manuscripts*, Anglo-Norman Text Society, occasional publications ser.,
3 (London: ANTS, 1999), no. 461.

[20] See also Kelly, *Performing Virginity*, p. 19.

[21] See Rachel E. Fulton, 'Mimetic devotion, Marian exegesis, and the Song of
Songs', *Viator*, 27 (1996), 85–116.

22 'An Anglo-Norman version of Grosseteste: part of his *Suidas* and *Testamenta XII Patriarcharum*', ed. Ruth J. Dean, *PMLA*, 51 (1936), 607–13.

23 Ibid., 612.

24 See further James Carroll, *Constantine's Sword: The Church and the Jews: A History* (Boston: Houghton Mifflin, 2001).

25 Susan Einbinder, 'Jewish women martyrs: changing models of representation', *Exemplaria*, 12 (2000), 105–27, and see her translations in *Medieval Hagiology: An Anthology*, ed. Thomas Head (New York and London: Routledge, 2001), pp. 537–60.

26 *Selections from English Wycliffite Writings*, ed. Anne Hudson (Cambridge: Cambridge University Press, 1978), p. 28, ll. 154–6; Constant Mews (ed.), *Listen Daughter: The* Speculum Virginum *and the Formation of Religious Women in the Middle Ages* (New York: Palgrave, 2001).

27 See Wogan-Browne, 'The virgin's tale', in Ruth Evans and Lesley Johnson (eds), *Feminist Readings of Middle English Literature: The Wife of Bath and All her Sect* (London: Routledge, 1994), pp. 165–94 (pp. 168, 187, n. 16); for a full study see Kelly, *Performing Virginity*, ch. 1, 'Hymenologies: the multiple signs of virginity'.

28 For the parallel phenomenon of re-virginalizing (in medieval religious virginities, Harlequin romances, and the career of Diana, princess of Wales), see Wogan-Browne, 'Virginity always comes twice', in Louise D'Arcens and Juanita Ruys (eds), *'Maistresse of My Wit': The Modern Study of Medieval Women* (Turnhout: Brepols, forthcoming).

29 See *Collectio Salernitana*, ed. Salvatore de Renzi, 5 vols (Naples: Filiatre-Sebezio, 1852–9); see, for example, vol. 4, pp. 20–1; vol. 5, pp. 194–5.

30 This appears to be partly a matter of the genre of textbook: so, for instance, the hymen is not present in Lord Zuckerman with Deryck Darlington and F. Peter Lisowski, *A New System of Anatomy: A Dissector's Guide and Atlas* (Oxford: Oxford University Press, 1961: 2nd edn, 1981), but in N. G. Kase, A. B. Weingold et al., *The Principles and Practice of Clinical Gynaecology* (Edinburgh: Churchill & Livingstone, 1990) it is given a full morphology and diagrammed in annular, septate, crescentic, cribriform and porous with carunculae as well as coitally lacerated forms.

31 *Gray's Anatomy*, ed. Peter L. Williams et al. (Edinburgh: Churchill Livingstone, 1995), pp. 1–10.

32 Thomas Laqueur, *Making Sex: Body and Gender from the Greeks to Freud* (Cambridge, MA: Harvard University Press, 1990), ch. 2; Marie-Christine Pouchelle, *The Body and Surgery in the Middle Ages*, trans. Rosemary Morris (Oxford: Polity Press, 1990); Danielle Jacquart and Claude Thomasset, *Sexuality and Medicine in the Middle Ages*, trans. Matthew Adamson (Oxford: Polity Press, 1988).

33 R. J. Last, *Last's Anatomy: Regional and Applied* (Edinburgh: Churchill Livingstone, 1990), 8th edn by R. M. H. McMinn, p. 354.

34 The original illustrations for *Gray's* (first published in London in 1858) were drawn by H. Van Dyke Carter, demonstrator of anatomy at St

George's Hospital, London (see further, Charles Mayo Goss (ed.), *Anatomy of the Human Body* (Philadelphia: Lea & Ferbiger, 1973), pp. vii–ix): they have been replaced (in different ways) in subsequent English and American editions which are edited independently of each other. What is striking in the English editions as late as 1995 is that all the other illustrations of the volume have become photographs or updated diagrams.

[35] The reaction of audiences of medical women (whose persistence in their tough and demanding work seemed more than ever essential, given the evident need for feminist gynaecologists if women were to be able to assess the medical value of their doctors' advice) was usually strong. Most felt they had subscribed to a culturally determined model of the hymen, in spite of their professional knowledge of *Gray's*: medical degrees had in England hitherto paid little attention to the discursive production of the body in their own discipline, though this began to shift in the later 1990s.

[36] Lillian Passmore Sanderson, *Against the Mutilation of Women: The Struggle to End Unnecessary Suffering* (London: Ithaca Press, 1981), p. 53.

[37] *Mandeville's Travels, Translated from the French of Jean d'Outremeuse, Edited from MS. Cotton Titus C. XVI in the British Museum*, ed. P. Hamelius, EETS, os, 153 (London: Oxford University Press, 1919), pp. 190–1. On venomous virgins more generally, see Margaret Hallissy, *Venomous Woman: Fear of the Female in Literature* (Westport, CT: Greenwood, 1987); *Placides et Timéo ou, li secrés as philosophes*, ed. C. A. Thomasset (Paris: Textes Littéraires Françaises, 1980), pp. 111–12, 302–3. On pharaonic and Sunna circumcision, see Ellen Gruenbaum, 'The limits to cultural relativism', in Gruenbaum, *The Female Circumcision Controversy: An Anthropological Perspective* (Philadelphia: University of Pennsylvania Press, 2001), pp. 2–3.

[38] Elizabeth A. Sheehan, 'Victorian clitoridectomy: Isaac Baker Brown and his harmless operative procedure', in Roger N. Lancaster and Micaela di Leonardo (eds), *The Gender/Sexuality Reader* (New York: Routledge, 1997); N. Toubia and S. Izett, *Female Genital Mutilation: An Overview* (Geneva: WHO, 1998), p. 21.

[39] Anika Rahman and Nahid Toubia, *Female Genital Mutilation: A Guide to Laws and Policies Worldwide* (New York: Zed Books, 2000), p. 6.

[40] Female genital mutilation has been a criminal offence since 1985 in the UK and is often therefore carried out abroad.

[41] See further, for example, Gruenbaum, 'Limits to cultural relativism', pp. 27–31; Bettina Shell-Duncan and Ylva Hernlund, 'Female "circumcision" in Africa: dimensions of the practice and debates', in Shell-Duncan and Hernlund (eds), *Female 'Circumcision' in Africa: Culture, Controversy, and Change* (Boulder, CO: Rienner, 2000), pp. 1–38, esp. pp. 25–38.

[42] For details of which countries have criminalized female genital mutilation and which have prosecuted under it, see Rahman and Toubia, *Female Genital Mutilation*, under individual country names.

Bibliography

Manuscripts

Aberystwyth, NLW, MS Mostyn 2288
Aberystwyth, NLW, MS Mostyn 88
Aberystwyth, NLW, MS Mostyn 159
Aberystwyth, NLW, MS Peniarth 17
Aberystwyth, NLW, MS Peniarth 51
Aberystwyth, NLW, MS Peniarth 60
Aberystwyth, NLW, MS Peniarth 77
Augsburg, Universitätsbibliothek, Cod.I.2.4°15
Cambridge, Trinity College, MS 0.2.5
Cambridge, Trinity College, MS B.11.7
Cambridge, Trinity College, MS R.14.45
Cambridge, Trinity College, MS R.15.52
Cardiff, Central Library, MS 3.242
London, College of Arms, MS 20/25
London, BL, MS Add 15, 047
London, BL, MS Cotton Domitian A.IX
London, BL, MS Egerton 2572
London, BL, MS Harley 543
London, BL, MS Harley 2407
London, BL, MS Harley 3528
London, BL, Harley Charter 43.A.14
London, BL, MS Royal 12 Exv
London, BL, MS Sloane 4

London, BL, MS Sloane 2463
London, College of Arms, MS 20/25
London Wellcome Institute Library, MS Western 632
Norwich, Norfolk Record Office, Will of Olive Dade
Norwich, Norfolk Record Office, Will of Katherine Gardener
Norwich, Norfolk Record Office, Will of Rose Wellys
Norwich, Norfolk Record Office, Will of Christian Worlich
Oxford, Bodleian Library, MS Ashmole 53
Oxford, Bodleian Library, MS Bodley 483
Oxford, Bodleian Library, MS Bodley Roll 1
Oxford, Bodleian Library, MS Bodley Ashmole 1416
Oxford, Bodleian Library, Bodley Ashmole Roll 26
Oxford, Bodleian Library, MS Douce 37
Oxford, Bodleian Library, MS Rawlinson 234
Oxford, Bodleian Library, MS Rawlinson poet. 23
Oxford, Jesus College, MS 111
Paris, Bibliothèque Nationale, MS fr. 14765
Paris, Bibliothèque Nationale, MS nouv. acq. fr. 16251
Public Record Office, CI 45/24
York, Borthwick Institute for Historical Research, CP F 189
York, Borthwick Institute for Historical Research, PR 1
York, Borthwick Institute for Historical Research, PR 2
York, Borthwick Institute for Historical Research, PR 3
York, Borthwick Institute for Historical Research, PR 4
York, Borthwick Institute for Historical Research, PR 4c
York, Borthwick Institute for Historical Research, PR 5
York Merchant Adventurers' Hall, Fossgate Deed 1
York Merchant Adventurers' Hall, St Edward Walmgate Deed 10
York Merchant Adventurers' Hall, Testamentary Business 1
York Merchant Adventurers' Hall, Walmgate Quitclaim 3

Reference

Brunel, Pierre (ed.), *Dictionnaire des mythes littéraires* (Paris: Éditions du Rocher, 1988).

Chevalier, Jean, and Alain Gheerbrant (eds), *Dictionnaire des symboles* (Paris: Laffont, Bouquins, 1982).

Green, Miranda J., *Dictionary of Celtic Myth and Legend* (London: Thames and Hudson, 1992).

Gray's Anatomy, ed. Peter L. Williams et al. (Edinburgh and New York: Churchill Livingstone, 1995).

Latham, Ronald E. (ed.), *Dictionary of Medieval Latin from British Sources* (London: Oxford University Press for the British Academy, 1975–97).

Lewis, Charlton T., and Charles Short, *A Latin Dictionary* (Oxford: Oxford University Press, 1879).

MacKillop, James, *Dictionary of Celtic Mythology* (Oxford: Oxford University Press, 1998).

Quicherat, Jules (ed.), *Procès de Condamnation et de Réhabilitation de Jeanne d'Arc dite La Pucelle*, 5 vols (Paris, 1841–9; New York: Johnson, repr. 1965).

Severs, J. Burke, and Albert E. Hartung (eds), *A Manual of the Writings in Middle English, 1050–1500*, The Connecticut Academy of Arts and Sciences (Hamden: Archon Books, 1967–).

Simek, Rudolf, *Dictionary of Northern Mythology* (Cambridge: Brewer, 1993).

Stephens, Meic (ed.), *The New Companion to the Literature of Wales* (Cardiff: University of Wales Press, 1998).

Thompson, Stith, *Motif-Index of Folk-Literature*, 6 vols (Bloomington: Indiana University Press, 1932–6).

Welch, Robert (ed.), *The Oxford Companion to Irish Literature* (Oxford: Clarendon Press, 1996).

Printed Primary Sources

Ælfric's Lives of Saints, ed. Walter W. Skeat, 2 vols, *EETS*, os, 94, 114 (London: Oxford University Press, 1966).

Aelred of Rievaulx, *Spiritual Friendship*, trans. Mary Eugenia Laker, intro. Douglass Roby (Kalamazoo: Cistercian Publications, 1977).

—— 'The "De Institutis Inclusarum" of Aelred of Rievaulx', ed. C. H. Talbot, *Analecta sacri ordinis Cisterciensis*, 7 (1951), 167–217.

—— *De sanctimoniali de Wattun*, PL, 195, cols 789–96.

—— 'The Nun of Watton', trans. John Boswell, in Boswell, *The Kindness of Strangers: The Abandonment of Children in Western Europe from Late Antiquity to the Renaissance* (Harmondsworth: Penguin, 1989), pp. 452–8.

—— *Vita S. Edwardi regis et confessoris*, PL, 195, cols 737–90.

—— *Life of St. Edward the Confessor*, trans. Jerome Bertram, 2nd edn (Southampton: St Austin Press, 1997).

—— *Aelred of Rievaulx: Treatises and Pastoral Prayer*, ed. M. Basil Pennington (Kalamazoo: Cistercian Publications, 1971).

Alain de Lille, *The Art of Preaching*, trans. Gillian R. Evans (Kalamazoo: Cistercian Publications, 1981).

Albertus Magnus, *Book of Minerals*, trans. Dorothy Wycoff (Oxford: Clarendon Press, 1967).

—— [pseud.], *De secretis mulierum*, trans. Helen Rodnite Lemay (Albany: State University of New York Press, 1992).

Aldhelm, *Aldhelmi Opera*, ed. Rudolfus Ehwald, Auctores Antiquissimi, 15 (Munich: Monumenta Germaniae Historica, 1984).

—— *Aldhelm: Prose Works*, trans. Michael Lapidge and Michael Herren (Cambridge: Brewer, 1979).

Altenglische Legenden: Neue Folge, ed. Carl Horstmann (Heilbronn: Henninger, 1881).

Anchoritic Spirituality: Ancrene Wisse *and Associated Works*, trans. Nicholas Watson and Anne Savage, preface by Benedicta Ward (New York: Paulist Press, 1991).

Ancient Deeds Belonging to the Corporation of Bath, XIII–XVI Centuries, ed. C. W. Shickle (Bath: Bath Records Society, 1921).

Ancrene Riwle, trans. M. B. Salu (Exeter: University of Exeter Press, 1990).

Ashby, George, *George Ashby's Poems*, ed. Mary Bateson, EETS, ES, 76 (London: Oxford University Press, 1899).

Ashmole, Elias, *Theatrum Chemicum Britannicum* (London, 1652).

Augustine of Hippo, *The City of God Against the Pagans*, trans. George E. McCracken, Philip Levine and William M. Green, 7 vols, Loeb Classical Library (London: Heinemann; Cambridge, MA: Harvard University Press, 1966).

—— *Concerning the City of God Against the Pagans*, trans. Henry Bettenson (Harmondsworth: Penguin, 1972).

Bacon, Roger [attrib.], *The Mirror of Alchimy, Composed by the Thrice-Famous and Learned Fryer, Roger Bachon*, ed. Stanton J. Linden (New York: Garland, 1992).

Bede, *A History of the English Church and People*, trans. Leo Sherley-Price (Harmondsworth: Penguin, 1955).

—— *Ecclesiastical History of the English People*, ed. Bertram Colgrave and R. A. B. Mynors (Oxford: Clarendon Press, 1969).

Bernard of Clairvaux, *On the Song of Songs I: Sermons 1–20*, trans. Killian Walsh (Kalamazoo: Cistercian Publications, 1981).

Bestiary: Being an English Version of the Bodleian Library, Oxford MS Bodley 764, trans. Richard Barber (Woodbridge: Boydell, 1999).

Blacman, John, *Henry the Sixth: A Reprint of John Blacman's Memoir*, ed. M. R. James (Cambridge: Cambridge University Press, 1919).

Bokenham, Osbern, *Legendys of Hooly Wummen*, ed. Mary S. Serjeantson, EETS, OS, 206 (London: Oxford University Press, 1938).

The Book of St Gilbert, ed. Raymonde Foreville and Gillian Keir (Oxford: Clarendon Press, 1987).

Borough Customs, ed. Mary Bateson, 2 vols, Selden Society, 18, 21 (London: Quaritch, 1904–6).

Brevia Placitata, ed. G. J. Turner and Theodore F. T. Plucknett, Selden Society, 66 (London: Quaritch, 1951).

Britton, ed. Francis Morgan Nichols, 2 vols (Oxford, Clarendon Press, 1865; repr. Holmes Beach: Gaunt, 1983).

The Brut, or the Chronicles of England, ed. Friedrich W. D. Brie, 2 vols, EETS, os, 131, 136 (London: Oxford University Press, 1908).

Caesarius Heisterbacensis, *Dialogus miraculorum*, ed. Joseph Strange, 2 vols (Cologne, 1851).

—— *The Dialogue on Miracles*, trans. H. von E. Scott and C. C. Swinton Bland, 2 vols (London: Routledge, 1929).

Camden Miscellany, 17, ed. Seiriol J. A. Evans, Camden Society, 3rd ser., 64 (London: Royal Historical Society, 1940).

Camden Miscellany, 24, ed. G. L. Harriss and M. A. Harriss, Camden Society, 4th ser., 9 (London: Royal Historical Society, 1972).

Capgrave, John, *John Capgrave's Lives of St Augustine and St Gilbert of Sempringham and a Sermon*, ed. J. J. Munro, EETS, os, 140 (London: Kegan Paul, Trench, Trübner, 1910).

Chaste Passions: Medieval English Virgin Martyr Legends, ed. and trans. Karen A. Winstead (Ithaca, NY: Cornell University Press, 2000).

Christine de Pisan, *The Treasure of the City of Ladies, or The Book of the Three Virtues*, trans. Sarah Lawson (Harmondsworth: Penguin, 1985).

Collectio Salernitana, ed. Salvatore de Renzi, 5 vols (Naples: Filiatre-Sebezio, 1852–9).

Cothi, Lewys Glyn, *Gwaith Lewys Glyn Cothi*, ed. Dafydd Johnston (Cardiff: University of Wales Press, 1995).

Court Rolls of the Manor of Hales, 1270–1307, ed. John Amphlett, Sydney Graves Hamilton and R. A. Wilson, 3 vols, Worcestershire Historical Society (Oxford: Parker, 1910–33).

Court Rolls of the Manor of Wakefield, ed. William Percy Baildon, Yorkshire Archaeological Society, 36 (Leeds, 1906).

Dafydd ab Edmwnd, *Gwaith Dafydd ab Edmwnd*, ed. Thomas Roberts (Bangor: Welsh MSS Society, 1914).

Dafydd ap Gwilym, *Gwaith Dafydd ap Gwilym*, ed. Thomas Parry (Cardiff: University of Wales Press, 1979).

—— *Dafydd ap Gwilym: His Poems*, trans. Gwyn Thomas (Cardiff: University of Wales Press, 2001).

Daniel, Walter, *The Life of Aelred of Rievaulx by Walter Daniel*, trans. F. M. Powicke (London: Nelson & Sons, 1950).

Denys le pseudo-Aréopagite, *Œuvres complètes*, trans. Maurice de Candillac (Paris: Aubier-Montaigne, 1943).

Duanaire Finn, ed. Gerard Murphy, Irish Texts Society, 28 (London: Simpkin Marchall, 1933).

An English Chronicle of the Reigns of Richard II, Henry IV, Henry V and Henry VI, ed. J. S. Davies, Camden Society, original ser., 64 (London: Camden Society, 1861).

English and Scottish Ballads, ed. Francis James Child (London: Samson Low, 1861).

Flamel, Nicolas, *Nicolas Flamel, His Exposition of the Hieroglyphicall Figures*, ed. Laurinda Dixon (New York: Garland, 1994).

Fleta, ed. H. G. Richardson and G. O. Sayles, Selden Society, 72 (London: Quaritch, 1953).

Fortescue, John, *Works of Sir John Fortescue*, ed. Thomas Fortescue, Lord Clermont, 2 vols (London: privately printed, 1869).

Foxe, John, *Actes and Monuments of matters most speciall and memorable, happening in the Church, with a Vniuersall history of the same* [1563], 3 vols, 4th edition (London: John Daye, 1583).

Galen, *Galeni Opera*, 8 vols, ed. C. G. Kuhn (Leipzig: Knobloch, 1823).

Gerald of Wales, *Giraldus Cambrensis Opera*, ed. J. S. Brewer, Rolls Series, 21 (London: Longman, 1862).

—— *The Jewel of the Church*, ed. and trans. John J. Hagen (Leiden: Brill, 1979).

—— *The Journey Through Wales/The Description of Wales*, trans. Lewis Thorpe (Harmondsworth: Penguin, 1978).

Gerson, Jean, *Early Works*, trans. Brian Patrick McGuire (New York: Paulist Press, 1998).

[*Glanvill:*] *The Treatise on the Laws and Customs of the Realm of England Commonly Called Glanvill*, ed. G. D. G. Hall, 2nd edn, with material by Michael Clanchy (Oxford: Clarendon Press, 1993).

Glyn, Guto'r, *Gwaith Guto'r Glyn*, ed. Ifor Williams and John Llywelyn Williams (Cardiff: University of Wales Press, 1961).

Les Grandes Chroniques de France, ed. Jules Viard, 10 vols (Paris: Champion, 1920–53).

Grosseteste, Robert, 'An Anglo-Norman version of Grosseteste: part of his *Suidas* and *Testamenta XII Patriarcharum*', ed. Ruth J. Dean, *PMLA*, 51 (1936), 607–13.

Hakluyt, Richard, *The Principal Navigations, Voyages, Traffiques and Discoveries of the English Nation*, 8 vols (London: Dent, 1907).

Hall, Edward, *The Union of the Two Noble Families of Lancaster and York* (Menston, IL: Scolar Press, 1970).

Heinrich von dem Türlîn, *Diu Crône*, ed. G. H. F. Scholl (Stuttgart: Litterarischer Verein, 1852).

Henry de Bracton, *On the Laws and Customs of England*, ed. George E. Woodbine and trans. Samuel E. Thorne, 4 vols (Cambridge, MA: Belknap, 1968).

Herodotus, *The Histories*, trans. Aubrey de Sélincourt (Harmondsworth: Penguin, 1972).

Hildegard of Bingen, *On Natural Philosophy and Medicine*, ed. and trans. Margret Berger (Cambridge: Brewer, 1999).

[*Historia:*] Huw Pryce, 'A new edition of the *Historia Divae Monacellae*', *Montgomeryshire Collections*, 82 (1994), 23–40.

Hoccleve, Thomas, *Hoccleve's Works III: The Regement of Princes*, ed. Frederick J. Furnivall, EETS, ES, 72 (London: Kegan Paul, Trench, Trübner & Co, 1897).

Holinshed, Raphael, *Chronicles of England, Scotland and Ireland*, 3 vols (London: Henry Denham, 1587).

Ingulph's Chronicle of the Abbey of Crowland with the First Continuations, ed. Henry T. Riley (London: Bohn, 1854).

Jacobus de Voragine, *Legenda Aurea*, ed. Theodor Graesse (Dresden and Lipsius, 1846).

—— *The Golden Legend*, trans. W. G. Ryan, 2 vols (Princeton: Princeton University Press, 1993).

Jerome, *Commentarium in Epistolam ad Ephesios*, *PL*, 26, cols 459–554.

—— *Select Letters of St Jerome*, ed. and trans. F. A. Wright, Loeb Classical Library (London: Heinemann, 1933).

Julian of Norwich, *A Revelation of Divine Love*, ed. Marion Glasscoe (Exeter: University of Exeter Press, 1986).

Kempe, Margery, *The Book of Margery Kempe*, ed. Sanford Brown Meech and Hope Emily Allen, EETS, OS, 212 (London: Oxford University Press, 1949).

—— *The Book of Margery Kempe*, ed. Barry Windeatt (Harlow: Longman, 2000).

The Lady as Saint: A Collection of French Hagiographic Romances of the Thirteenth Century, ed. Brigitte Cazelles (Philadelphia: University of Pennsylvania Press, 1991).

[*Lai du Cor:*] *The Anglo-Norman Text of Le Lai du Cor*, ed. C. T. Erickson, Anglo-Norman Text Society, 24 (Oxford: Blackwell, 1973).

The Life of Christina of Markyate: A Twelfth-Century Recluse, ed. and trans. C. H. Talbot, Medieval Academy Reprints for Teaching, 39 (Toronto: University of Toronto Press, 1998).

The Life of King Edward Who Rests at Westminster: Attributed to a Monk of Saint-Bertin, trans. Frank Barlow (1st edn, London: Nelson & Sons, 1962; 2nd edn, Oxford: Clarendon Press, 1992).

Þe Liflade ant te Passiun of Seinte Iuliene, ed. S. R. T. O. d'Ardenne, EETS, OS, 248 (London: Oxford University Press, 1961).

[*Lives:*] Baring-Gould, Sabine, and John Fisher, *Lives of the British Saints*, 6 vols (London: Cymmrodorion, 1907–13).

Lives of Edward the Confessor, ed. Henry R. Luard, Rolls Series, 3 (London: Longman, Brown, Green, Longmans & Roberts, 1858).

Llyfr Iorwerth, ed. Aled Rhys Wiliam (Cardiff: University of Wales Press, 1960).

Lull, Ramon, *Il Testamentum Alchemico Attributo a Raimundo Lullo: Edizione del testo latino e catelano del manuscritto Oxford, Corpus Christi College 244*, ed. Michaela Pereira and Barbara Spaggiari (Florence: Tavarnuzze, 1999).

Lydgate, John, *The Minor Poems of John Lydgate*, part 1, ed. Henry Noble MacCracken, EETS, ES, 107 (London: Kegan Paul, Trench, Trübner & Co. and Oxford University Press, 1911).

The Mabinogion, trans. Gwyn Jones and Thomas Jones (London: Everyman, 1949).

Malory, Thomas, *Works of Sir Thomas Malory*, ed. Eugène Vinaver, 3 vols, 3rd edn (Oxford: Oxford University Press, 1947).

—— *Works*, ed. Eugène Vinaver (Oxford: Oxford University Press, 1971).

Mandeville's Travels, Translated from the French of Jean d'Outremeuse, Edited from MS. Cotton Titus C. XVI in the British Museum, ed. P. Hamelius, EETS, OS, 153 (London: Oxford University Press, 1919).

Mannyng, Robert, of Brunne, *Handlyng Synne*, ed. Idelle Sullens (Binghamton, NY: Medieval and Renaissance Texts and Studies, 1983).

Margaret of Oignt, *The Writings of Margaret of Oignt, Medieval Prioress and Mystic*, ed. Renate Blumenfeld-Kosinski (Cambridge: Brewer, 1997).

Math Uab Mathonwy Pedwaredd Gainc y Mabinogi, ed. Ian Hughes (Aberystwyth: Adran y Gymraeg, Prifysgol Cymru, 2000).

[*Meddygon Myddveu:*] *Le Plus Ancien Texte des Meddygon Myddveu*, ed. Pol Diverres (Paris: Maurice le Dault, 1913).

Medieval English Prose for Women: Selections from the Katherine Group and Ancrene Wisse, ed. and trans. Bella Millett and Jocelyn Wogan-Browne (Oxford: Clarendon Press, 1990, rev. edn 1992).

Medieval Hagiography: An Anthology, ed. Thomas Head (New York: Garland, 2000).

Melusine, Compiled by Jean D'Arras, Englisht about 1500, ed. A. K. Donald, EETS, ES, 68 (London: Kegan Paul, Trench, Trübner & Co., 1895).

The Minor Poems of the Vernon Manuscript, ed. Carl Horstmann and F. J. Furnivall, 2 vols, EETS, OS, 98, 117 (London: Kegan Paul, Trench, Trübner, 1892 and 1901).

The Mirror of Justices, ed. W. J. Whittaker, Selden Society, 7 (London: Quaritch, 1895).

Non-Cycle Plays and Fragments, ed. Norman Davis, EETS, SS, 1 (Oxford: Oxford University Press, 1970).

Norton, Thomas, *Thomas Norton's Ordinal of Alchemy*, ed. John Reidy, EETS, OS, 272 (London: Oxford University Press, 1975).

Novae Narrationes, ed. Elsie Shanks and S. F. C. Milsom, Selden Society, 80 (London: Quaritch, 1963).

Odo of Cluny, *De Vita Sancti Geraldi Auriliacensis Comitis*, PL, 133, cols 639–703.

The Old French Lives of Saint Agnes and Other Vernacular Versions of the Middle Ages, ed. Alexander J. Denomy (Cambridge, MA: Harvard University Press, 1938).

Osbert of Clare, *The Letters of Osbert of Clare, Prior of Westminster*, ed. E. W. Williamson (1929; repr. Oxford: Oxford University Press, 1998).

—— 'La vie de S. Édouard le Confesseur par Osbert de Clare', ed. Marc Bloch, *Analecta Bollandiana*, 41 (1923), 5–131.

Paris, Matthew [attrib.], *La estoire de Seint Aedward le rei*, ed. Montague R. James (Oxford: Roxburghe Club, 1920).

—— *La Vie seint Aedward le Rei*, ed. Kathryn Young-Wallace, Anglo-Norman Text Society, 41 (London: ANTS, 1983).

A Parisian Journal, 1405–99, trans. Janet Shirley (Oxford: Oxford University Press, 1968).

Penllyn, Tudur, *Gwaith Tudur Penllyn ac Ieuan ap Tudur Penllyn*, ed. Thomas Roberts (Cardiff: University of Wales Press, 1958).

Philippe de Commynes, *Memoirs: The Reign of Louis XI, 1461–83*, trans. Michael Jones (Harmondsworth: Penguin, 1972).

Pius II, *The Commentaries of Pius II Bks 97–99*, trans. Florence A. Cragg-Smith, Smith College Studies in History, 35 (Northampton, MA: Dept of History of Smith College, 1937–57).

Placides et Timéo ou, li secrés as philosophes, ed. C. A. Thomasset (Paris: Textes Littéraires Françaises, 1980).

Placita Corone, ed. J. M. Kaye, Selden Society, supplementary ser., 4 (London: Quaritch, 1966).

Pliny, *Natural History*, ed. and trans. David Edward Eichholz (London: Heinemann, 1962).

Political, Religious and Love Poems, ed. Frederick J. Furnivall, EETS, os, 15 (London: Oxford University Press, 1866).

Raleigh, Walter, *The Discoverie of the Large, Rich and Bewtiful Empire of Guiana* (London: Robert Robinson, 1596).

Richard of Cirencester, *Speculum historiale de gestis regum Angliae*, ed. John E. B. Mayor, Rolls Series, 30, 2 vols (London: Longmans, Green & Co., 1863–9).

Ripley, George, *George Ripley's Compound of Alchemy (1591)*, ed. Stanton J. Linden (Aldershot: Ashgate, 2001).

Rober le Chapelain, *Corset: A Rhymed Commentary on the Seven Sacraments by Rober le Chapelain*, ed. Keith Val Sinclair, Anglo-Norman Text Society, 52 (London: ANTS, 1995).

The Roll of the Shropshire Eyre of 1256, ed. Alan Harding, Selden Society, 96 (London: Quaritch, 1980).

Rolls of the Justices in Eyre being the Rolls of Pleas and Assizes for Lincolnshire, 1218–19, ed. Doris Mary Stenton, Selden Society, 53 (London: Quaritch, 1934).

Rotuli Parliamentorum.

Saints' Lives, ed. Thomas Head (New York: Garland, 2000).

Sammlung Altenglischer Legenden, ed. Carl Horstmann (Heilbronn: Henninger, 1878; repr. Hildesheim, 1969).

S. Editha sive Chronicon Vilodunense im Wiltshire Dialekt, ed. C. Horstmann (Heilbronn: Henninger, 1883).

Seinte Katerine, ed. S. R. T. O. d'Ardenne and E. J. Dobson, EETS, ss, 7 (London: Oxford University Press, 1981).

The Sekenesse of Wymmen*: A Middle English Treatise on Diseases of Women*, ed. M. R. Hallaert, *Scripta*, 8 (Brussels: Omirel, 1982).

Select Cases in the Court of King's Bench, ed. George Osborne Sayles, 6 vols, Selden Society, 55, 57, 58, 74, 76, 82 (London: Quaritch, 1936–65).

Selections from English Wycliffite Writings, ed. Anne Hudson (Cambridge: Cambridge University Press, 1978).

Shakespeare, William, *The Norton Shakespeare*, ed. Stephen Greenblatt, Walter Cohen, Jean E. Howard and Katharine Eisaman Maus (New York: Norton, 1997).

Six Town Chronicles of England, ed. Ralph Flenley (Oxford: Clarendon Press, 1911).

Soldiers of Christ: Saints and Saints' Lives from Late Antiquity and the Early Middle Ages, ed. Thomas F. X. Noble and Thomas Head (London: Sheed & Ward, 1995).

Soranus' Gynecology, trans. Owsei Temkin (Baltimore: Johns Hopkins University Press, 1956).

The South English Legendary, vol. 1, ed. Charlotte D'Evelyn and Anna J. Mills, EETS, os, 235 (London: Oxford University Press, 1956).

The Statutes of the Realm, 12 vols (London: Record Commission, 1810–22; repr. 1963).

Supplementary Lives in Some Manuscripts of the Gilte Legende, ed. Richard Hamer and Vida Russell, EETS, os, 315 (Oxford: Oxford University Press, 2000).

Tertullian, *Liber de virginibus velandis*, *PL*, 2, cols 887–914.

—— *The Writings of Tertullian*, vol. 3, ed. Alexander Roberts and James Donaldson, trans. S. Thelwell (Edinburgh: Clark, 1895).

Three Lives of the Last Englishmen, trans. Michael Swanton (New York: Garland, 1984).

Trioedd Ynys Prydein, ed. and trans. Rachel Bromwich (Cardiff: University of Wales Press, 1978).

The Trotula: A Medieval Compendium of Women's Medicine, ed. and trans. Monica H. Green (Philadelphia: University of Pennsylvania Press, 2001).

Ulrich von Zatzikhoven, *Lanzelet*, ed. Kenneth Grant Tremayne Webster and Roger Sherman Loomis (New York: Columbia University Press, 1951).

Vergil, Polydore, *Polydore Vergil's English History*, vol. 1, ed. Henry Ellis, Camden Society, original ser., 36 (London: Nichols, 1846).

William of Malmesbury, *Gesta Regum Anglorum: The History of the English Kings*, trans. Roger A. B. Mynors, completed by Rodney M. Thomson and Michael Winterbottom, 2 vols (Oxford: Clarendon Press, 1998–9).

—— *The Vita Wulfstani of William of Malmesbury*, ed. Reginald R. Darlington, Camden Society, 3rd ser., 40 (London: Royal Historical Society, 1928).

Wilson, Thomas, *The Arte of Rhetorique*, ed. G. H. Mair (Oxford: Clarendon Press, 1909).

Þe Wohunge of ure Lauerd, ed. W. Meredith Thompson, EETS, os, 241 (London: Oxford University Press, 1958).

Woman Defamed and Woman Defended: An Anthology of Medieval Texts, ed. Alcuin Blamires with Karen Pratt and C. W. Marx (Oxford: Clarendon Press, 1992).

Women in England c.1275–1525: Documentary Sources, ed. and trans. P. J. P. Goldberg (Manchester: Manchester University Press, 1995).

The York Plays, ed. Richard Beadle (London: Arnold, 1982).

Yr Areithiau Pros, ed. D. Gwenallt Jones (Cardiff: University of Wales Press, 1934).

Secondary Sources

Abbott, Elizabeth, *A History of Celibacy: From Athena to Elizabeth I, Leonardo da Vinci, Florence Nightingale, Gandhi, and Cher* (New York: Scribner, 2000).

Abulafia, Anna Sapir, *Christians and Jews in Dispute: Disputational Literature and the Rise of Anti-Judaism in the West, c.1000–1150* (Aldershot: Ashgate, 1998).

Aers, David, and Lynn Staley, *The Powers of the Holy: Religion, Politics and Gender in Late Medieval English Culture* (University Park: Pennsylvania State University Press, 1996).

Ailes, M. J., 'The medieval male couple and the language of homosociality', in D. M. Hadley (ed.), *Masculinity in Medieval Europe* (London: Longman, 1999), pp. 214–37.

Allen, Sally G., and Joanna Hubbs, 'Outrunning Atlanta: feminine destiny in alchemical transmutation', *Signs: Journal of Women in Culture and Society*, 6 (1980), 210–19.

Andersen, Jørgen, *The Witch on the Wall: Medieval Erotic Sculpture in the British Isles* (Copenhagen: Rosenkilde & Bagger; London: George Allen & Unwin, 1977).

Asad, Talal, 'On ritual and discipline in medieval Christian monasticism', *Economy and Society*, 16 (1987), 159–203.

Ashton, Gail, *The Generation of Identity in Late Medieval Hagiography: Speaking the Saint* (London: Routledge, 2000).

Astell, Ann W., *The Song of Songs in the Middle Ages* (Ithaca, NY: Cornell University Press, 1990).

Ayers, Brian, 'Excavations within the north-east bailey of Norwich castle', *East Anglian Archeology*, 28 (1985), 49–58.

Baker, J. H., *An Introduction to English Legal History*, 3rd edn (London: Butterworths, 1990).

Bakhtin, Mikhail, *Rabelais and his World*, trans. Hélène Iswolsky (Cambridge, MA: MIT Press, 1968).

Baldwin, John W., 'Five discourses on desire: sexuality and gender in northern France around 1200', *Speculum*, 66 (1991), 797–819.

Balzaretti, Ross, 'Michel Foucault, homosexuality and the Middle Ages', *Renaissance and Modern Studies*, 37 (1994), 1–12.

Barlow, Frank, *Edward the Confessor*, 2nd edn (New Haven: Yale University Press, 1997).

Barron, Caroline M., 'The "golden age" of women in medieval London', *Reading Medieval Studies*, 15 (1989), 35–58.

Bartlett, Robert, 'Rewriting saints' lives: the case of Gerald of Wales', *Speculum*, 58 (1983), 598–613.

Bartrum, P. C., 'Tri Thlws ar Ddeg Ynys Brydain', *Études celtiques*, 10 (1962/3), 434–77.

Beattie, Cordelia, 'Meanings of singleness: the single woman in late medieval England' (unpublished doctoral thesis, University of York, 2001).

Beckwith, Sarah, 'A very material mysticism: the medieval mysticism of Margery Kempe', in David Aers (ed.), *Medieval Literature: Criticism, Ideology and History* (Brighton: Harvester Press, 1986), pp. 34–57.

—— 'Problems of authority in late medieval English mysticism: language, agency and authority in *The Book of Margery Kempe*', *Exemplaria*, 4 (1992), 171–99.

Bennett, Judith M., *Women in the Medieval English Countryside: Gender and Household in Brigstock before the Plague* (New York: Oxford University Press, 1987).

Benton, John F., 'Trotula, women's problems and the professionalization of medicine in the Middle Ages', *Bulletin of the History of Medicine*, 59 (1985), 30–53.

Bernau, Anke, 'Virginal effects: text and identity in *Ancrene Wisse*', in Samantha J. E. Riches and Sarah Salih (eds), *Gender and Holiness: Men, Women and Saints in Late Medieval Europe* (London: Routledge, 2002), pp. 36–48.

—— 'A Christian *corpus*: virginity, violence and knowledge in the Life of St Katherine of Alexandria', in Jacqueline Jenkins and Katherine J. Lewis (eds), *St Katherine of Alexandria: Texts and Contexts in Western Medieval Europe* (Turnhout: Brepols, 2003).

Berry, Philippa, *Of Chastity and Power: Elizabethan Literature and the Unmarried Queen* (London: Routledge, 1989).

Bertholot, Marcellin, *Collection des anciens alchimistes grecs* (Paris: Berthelot, 1888).

Biddick, Kathleen, 'Genders, bodies, borders: technologies of the visible', in Nancy F. Partner (ed.), *Studying Medieval Women* (Cambridge, MA: Mediaeval Academy of America, 1993), pp. 87–116.

—— *The Shock of Medievalism* (Durham, NC: Duke University Press, 1998).

Bildhauer, Bettina and Robert Mills (eds), *The Monstrous Middle Ages* (Cardiff: University of Wales Press, forthcoming).

Binski, Paul, 'Reflections on *La estoire de Seint Aedward le rei*: hagiography and kingship in thirteenth-century England', *Journal of Medieval History*, 16 (1990), 333–50.

—— *Westminster Abbey and the Plantagenets: Kingship and the Representation of Power 1200–1400* (New Haven: Yale University Press, 1995).

Bitel, Lisa M., *Land of Women. Tales of Sex and Gender in Early Ireland* (Ithaca, NY: Cornell University Press, 1996).

Bloch, R. Howard, *Medieval Misogyny and the Invention of Western Romantic Love* (Chicago: University of Chicago Press, 1991).

Blumenfeld-Kosinski, Renate, *Not of Woman Born: Representations of Caesarian Birth in Medieval and Renaissance Culture* (Ithaca, NY: Cornell University Press, 1990).

Bly, Mary, *Queer Virgins and Virgin Queens on the Early Modern Stage* (Oxford: Oxford University Press, 2000).

Bolton, J. L., *The Medieval English Economy 1150–1500* (London: Dent, 1980, repr. 1988 with supplement).

Boureau, Alain, *The Lord's First Night: The Myth of the droit de cuissage*, trans. Lydia G. Cochrane (Chicago: University of Chicago Press, 1998).

Brown, Peter, *The Body and Society: Men, Women and Sexual Renunciation in Early Christianity* (New York: Columbia University Press, 1988).

Brownmiller, Susan, *Against our Will: Men, Women and Rape* (Harmondsworth: Penguin, 1975).

Brundage, James A., 'Rape and marriage in the medieval canon law', *Revue de droit canonique*, 28 (1978), 62–75.

—— 'Rape and seduction in the medieval canon law', in Vern L. Bullough and Brundage (eds), *Sexual Practices and the Medieval Church* (Buffalo, NY: Prometheus, 1982), pp. 141–8.

Bugge, John, *Virginitas: An Essay in the History of a Medieval Ideal* (The Hague: Martinus Nijhoff, 1975).

Buhler, Curt F., 'Prayers and charms in certain Middle English scrolls', *Speculum*, 39 (1964), 270–8.

Bullough, Vern L., and Bonnie Bullough, *Prostitution: An Illustrated Social History* (New York: Crown Publishers, 1978).

Burke, Peter, *The Renaissance Sense of the Past* (London: Arnold, 1969).

Burt, Richard, and John Michael Archer, *Enclosure Acts: Sexuality, Property and Culture in Early Modern England* (Ithaca, NY: Cornell University Press, 1994).

Butler, Judith, *Bodies that Matter: On the Discursive Limits of 'Sex'* (New York: Routledge, 1993).

—— *Excitable Speech: A Politics of the Performative* (London: Routledge, 1997).

Bynum, Caroline Walker, *Jesus as Mother: Studies in the Spirituality of the High Middle Ages* (Berkeley: University of California Press, 1982).

—— *Holy Feast and Holy Fast: The Religious Significance of Food to Medieval Women* (Berkeley: University of California Press, 1987).

—— *Fragmentation and Redemption: Essays on Gender and the Human Body in Medieval Religion* (New York: Zone Books 1992).

Caciola, Nancy, 'Mystics, demoniacs, and the physiology of spirit possession in medieval Europe', *Comparative Studies in Society and History*, 42 (2000), 268–306.

Cadden, Joan, 'Medieval, scientific and medical views of sexuality: questions of propriety', *Mediaevalia et Humanistica*, NS, 14 (1986), 157–71.

Camille, Michael, 'Gothic signs and the surplus: the kiss on the cathedral', *Yale French Studies*, 88 (1991), 151–70.

—— *Images on the Edge: The Margins of Medieval Art* (London: Reaktion, 1992; repr. 1995).

—— 'Manuscript illumination and the art of copulation', in Karma Lochrie, Peggy McCracken and James A. Schultz (eds), *Constructing Medieval Sexuality* (Minneapolis: University of Minnesota Press, 1997), pp. 58–90.

—— *Mirror in Parchment: The Luttrell Psalter and the Making of Medieval England* (London: Reaktion, 1998).

Carlson, Cindy L., 'Like a virgin: Mary and her detractors in the N-Town cycle', in Carlson and Jane Weisl (eds), *Constructions of Widowhood and Virginity in the Middle Ages* (New York: St Martin's Press, 1999), pp. 199–217.

—— and Angela Jane Weisl (eds), *Constructions of Widowhood and Virginity in the Middle Ages* (Basingstoke: Macmillan, 1999).

—— 'Introduction: constructions of widowhood and virginity', in Carlson and Weisl (eds), *Constructions of Widowhood and Virginity in the Middle Ages* (Basingstoke: Macmillan, 1999), pp. 1–21.

Carr, Anthony David, *Medieval Anglesey* (Llangefni: Anglesey Antiquarian Society, 1982).

Carroll, James, *Constantine's Sword: The Church and the Jews: A History* (Boston: Houghton Mifflin, 2001).

Cartwright, Jane, 'Y Forwyn Fair, Santesau a Lleianod: Agweddau ar Wyryfdod a Diweirdeb yng Nghymru'r Oesoedd Canol' (unpublished doctoral thesis, University of Wales, Cardiff, 1996).

—— 'The desire to corrupt: convent and community in medieval Wales', in Diane Watt (ed.), *Medieval Women in their Communities* (Cardiff: University of Wales Press, 1997), pp. 20–48.

—— 'Dead virgins: feminine sanctity in medieval Wales', *Medium Ævum*, 71 (2002), 1–28.

Caviness, Madeline H., *Visualizing Women in the Middle Ages: Sight, Spectacle and Scopic Economy* (Philadelphia: University of Pennsylvania Press, 2001).

Chamberlayne, Joanna L., 'Crowns and virgins: queenmaking during the Wars of the Roses', in Katherine J. Lewis, Noël James Menuge and Kim M. Phillips (eds), *Young Medieval Women* (Stroud: Sutton, 1999), pp. 47–68.

Chaplais, Pierre, 'The original charters of Herbert and Gervase, abbots of Westminster (1121–1157)', in Patricia M. Barnes and C. F. Slade (eds), *A Medieval Miscellany for Doris Mary Stenton*, Pipe Roll Society, NS, 36, (London: Pipe Roll Society, 1962), pp. 89–110.

Charles-Edwards, T. M., 'Nau Kynywedi Teithiauc', in Dafydd Jenkins and Morfydd E. Owen (eds), *The Welsh Law of Women* (Cardiff: University of Wales Press, 1980), pp. 23–39.

Charles-Edwards, T. M., Morfydd E. Owen and Paul Russell (eds), *The Welsh King and his Court* (Cardiff: University of Wales Press, 2000).

Cioffi, Frank, 'Blather', *London Review of Books*, 22 (22 June 2000), p. 20.

Cixous, Hélène, and Jacques Derrida, *Veils*, trans. Geoffrey Bennington (Stanford: Stanford University Press, 2001).

Cline, Sally, *Women, Celibacy and Passion* (London: André Deutsch, 1993).

Clover, Carol J., *Men, Women and Chainsaws: Gender in the Modern Horror Film* (Princeton: Princeton University Press, 1992).

Cohen, Jeffrey Jerome (ed.), *Monster Theory: Reading Culture* (Minneapolis and London: University of Minnesota Press, 1996).

—— *Of Giants: Sex, Monsters, and the Middle Ages* (Minneapolis: University of Minnesota Press, 1999).

Constable, Giles, 'Aelred of Rievaulx and the Nun of Watton: an episode in the early history of the Gilbertine Order', in Derek Baker (ed.), *Medieval Women*, Studies in Church History, Subsidia, 1 (Oxford: Blackwell, 1978), pp. 205–26.

Coon, Lynda L., *Sacred Fictions: Holy Women and Hagiography in Late Antiquity* (Philadelphia: University of Pennsylvania Press, 1997).

Cooper, Kate, *The Virgin and the Bride: Idealized Womanhood in Late Antiquity* (Cambridge, MA: Harvard University Press, 1996).

Cowell, Andrew, 'The dye of desire: the colors of rhetoric in the Middle Ages', *Exemplaria*, 11 (1999), 115–39.

Cowling, Jane, 'A fifteenth-century saint play in Winchester: some problems of interpretation', *Medieval and Renaissance Drama in England*, 13 (2001), 19–33.

Crane, Susan, 'Clothing and gender definition: Joan of Arc', *Journal of Medieval and Early Modern Studies*, 26 (1996), 297–320.

Cubitt, Catherine, 'Virginity and misogyny in tenth- and eleventh-century England', *Gender and History*, 12 (2000), 1–32.

Cullum, P. H., 'Clergy, masculinity and transgression in later medieval England', in D. M. Hadley (ed.), *Masculinity in Medieval Europe* (London: Longman, 1999), pp. 178–96.

Dalton, O. M., *The Royal Gold Cup in the British Museum* (London: British Museum, 1924).

Davidson, H. R. Ellis, *Viking and Norse Mythology* (London: Chancellor, 1996).

Davies, Robert Rees, *Lordship and Society in the March of Wales 1282–1400* (Oxford: Clarendon Press, 1978).

—— 'The twilight of Welsh law, 1284–1536', *History*, 51 (1966), 143–64.

—— 'The status of women and the practice of marriage in late medieval Wales', in Dafydd Jenkins and Morfydd E. Owen (eds), *The Welsh Law of Women* (Cardiff: University of Wales Press, 1980), pp. 93–114.

Davis, Kathleen, 'National writing in the ninth century: a reminder for postcolonial thinking about the nation', *Journal of Medieval and Early Modern Studies*, 28 (1998), 611–37.

—— *Deconstruction and Translation* (Manchester: St Jerome Publications, 2001).

Dawes, Jean D., and J. R. Magilton, *The Cemetery of St Helen-on-the-Walls, Aldwark* (London: Council for British Archaeology, 1980).

Dean, Ruth J., with Maureen B. M. Boulton, *Anglo-Norman Literature: A Guide to Texts and Manuscripts*, Anglo-Norman Text Society, occasional publications ser., 3 (London: ANTS, 1999).

de Certeau, Michel, *The Writing of History*, trans. Tom Conley (New York: Columbia University Press, 1988).

Delany, Sheila, *The Naked Text: Chaucer's* Legend of Good Women (Berkeley: University of California Press, 1994).

—— *Impolitic Bodies: Poetry, Saints and Society in Fifteenth-Century England: The Work of Osbern Bokenham* (Oxford: Oxford University Press, 1998).

—— (ed.), *Chaucer and the Jews: Sources, Contexts, Meanings* (London: Routledge, 2002).

Derrida, Jacques, *Positions*, trans. Alan Bass (Chicago: University of Chicago Press, 1981).

—— *Margins of Philosophy*, trans. Alan Bass (London: Prentice Hall, 1982).

Despres, Denise, 'Immaculate flesh and the social body: Mary and the Jews', *Jewish History*, 12 (1998), 47–69.

Dillon, Myles, *The Cycles of the Kings* (London: Geoffrey Cumberlege; New York: Oxford University Press, 1946).

Dinshaw, Carolyn, *Getting Medieval: Sexualities and Communities, Pre- and Postmodern* (Durham, NC: Duke University Press, 1999).

Dixon, Laurinda S., *Alchemical Imagery in Bosch's Garden of Delights* (Ann Arbor: UMI Research, 1981).

—— 'The curse of chastity: the marginalization of women in medieval art and medicine', in Robert R. Edwards and Vickie Ziegler (eds), *Matrons and Marginal Women in Medieval Society* (Woodbridge: Boydell, 1995), pp. 49–74.

Dollimore, Jonathan, *Sexual Dissidence: Augustine to Wilde, Freud to Foucault* (Oxford: Clarendon Press 1991).

Duffy, Eamon, 'Holy maydens, holy wyfes: the cult of women saints in fifteenth- and sixteenth-century England', in W. J. Shiels and Diana Wood (eds), *Women in the Church*, Studies in Church History, 27 (Oxford: Blackwell, 1990), pp. 175–96.

—— *The Stripping of the Altars: Traditional Religion in England 1400–1580* (New Haven: Yale University Press, 1992).

Dutton, Marsha L., 'Aelred, historian: two portraits in Plantagenet myth', *Cistercian Studies Quarterly*, 28 (1993), 113–44.

Dyer, Christopher, *Standards of Living in the Later Middle Ages: Social Change in England c.1200–1520* (Cambridge: Cambridge University Press, 1989).

Edwards, Huw M. (ed.), *Gwaith Prydydd Breuan, Rhys ap Dafydd ab Einion, Hywel Ystorm, a Cherddi Dychan Dienw o Lyfr Coch Hergest* (Aberystwyth: Centre for Advanced Welsh and Celtic Studies, 2000).

Einbinder, Susan, 'Jewish women martyrs: changing models of representation', *Exemplaria*, 12 (2000), 105–27.

Eliade, Mircea, *The Forge and the Crucible: The Origins and Structures of Alchemy*, trans. Stephen Corrin (New York: Harper & Row, 1971).

Elliott, Alison Goddard, 'The power of discourse: martyr's passion and Old French epic', *Medievalia et Humanistica*, NS, 11 (1982), 39–60.

Elliott, Dyan, *Spiritual Marriage: Sexual Abstinence in Medieval Wedlock* (Princeton: Princeton University Press, 1993).

—— 'The physiology of rapture and female spirituality', in Peter Biller and A. J. Minnis (eds), *Medieval Theology and the Natural Body* (Woodbridge: York Medieval Press, 1997), pp. 141–73.

—— *Fallen Bodies: Pollution, Sexuality and Demonology in the Middle Ages* (Philadelphia: University of Pennsylvania Press, 1999).

Epp, Garrett P. J., 'Ecce homo', in Glenn Burger and Steven F. Kruger (eds), *Queering the Middle Ages* (Minneapolis: University of Minnesota Press, 2001), pp. 236–52.

Evans, Ruth, 'Medieval virginities', in David Wallace and Carolyn Dinshaw (eds), *Cambridge Companion to Medieval Women's Writing* (Cambridge: Cambridge University Press, forthcoming).

Farina, Lara, *Reading for Pleasure: Erotic Discourse and Early English Religious Writing* (London: Palgrave, forthcoming).

Ferguson, Margaret W., 'Foreword', in Kathleen Coyne Kelly and Marina Leslie (eds), *Menacing Virgins: Representing Virginity in the Middle Ages and Renaissance* (London: Associated University Presses, 1999), pp. 7–14.

Ferroul, Yves, 'Abelard's blissful castration', in Jeremy J. Cohen and Bonnie Wheeler (eds), *Becoming Male in the Middle Ages* (New York: Garland, 1997), pp. 129–49.

Fichte, Joerg O., 'Foxe's *Acts and Monuments*: the spirit's triumph over the flesh', in Pierre Boitani and Anna Torti (eds), *The Body and the Soul in Medieval Literature* (Cambridge: Brewer, 1999), pp. 167–79.

Firth, Katherine R., *The Apocalyptic Tradition in Reformation Britain, 1530–1645* (Oxford: Oxford University Press, 1979).

Foucault, Michel, 'The battle for chastity', in *Ethics, Subjectivity, and Truth: Essential Works of Foucault*, vol. 1, ed. Paul Rabinow (New York: New Press, 1997), pp. 185–97.

Fradenburg, Louise O., 'Criticism, anti-Semitism, and the *Prioress's Tale*', *Exemplaria*, 1 (1989), 69–115.

—— ' "Be not far from me": psychoanalysis, medieval studies and the subject of religion', *Exemplaria*, 7 (1995), 41–54.

—— 'Analytical survey 2: we are not alone: psychoanalytic medievalism', in Rita Copeland, David Lawton and Wendy Scase (eds), *New Medieval Literatures*, vol. 2 (Oxford: Clarendon Press, 1998), pp. 249–76.

Fraioli, Deborah, 'The literary image of Joan of Arc: prior influences', *Speculum*, 56 (1981), 811–30.

Franklin, Peter, 'Politics in manorial court rolls: the tactics, social composition, and aims of a pre-1381 peasant movement', in Zvi Razi and Richard Smith (eds), *Medieval Society and the Manor Court* (Oxford: Clarendon Press, 1996), pp. 162–98.

Frantzen, Allen J., *Before the Closet: Same-Sex Love from* Beowulf *to* Angels in America (Chicago: University of Chicago Press, 1998).

Frasetto, Michael (ed.), *Medieval Purity and Piety: Essays on Medieval Clerical Celibacy and Religious Reform* (New York: Garland, 1998).

Freeman, Elizabeth, 'Nuns in the public sphere: Ælred of Rievaulx's *De Sanctimoniali de Wattun* and the gendering of authority', *Comitatus*, 27 (1996), 55–80.

Freud, Sigmund, *The Complete Psychological Works*, standard edition, trans. James Strachey (London: Hogarth, 1953–74).

—— *On Sexuality: Three Essays on the Theory of Sexuality and Other Works*, vol. 8, The Pelican Freud Library, trans. James Strachey, ed. Angela Richards (Harmondsworth: Penguin, 1977).

Friedman, Susan Stanford, 'Making history: reflections on feminism, narrative, and desire', in Diane Elam and Robyn Wiegman (eds), *Feminism beside Itself* (New York: Routledge, 1995), pp. 11–53.

Fulton, Rachel E., 'Mimetic devotion, Marian exegesis, and the Song of Songs', *Viator*, 27 (1996), 85–116.

Garber, Marjorie, *Vested Interests: Cross-Dressing and Cultural Anxiety* (New York: Routledge, 1992).

—— *Dog Love* (New York: Touchstone, 1997).

Gaunt, Simon, *Gender and Genre in Medieval French Literature* (Cambridge: Cambridge University Press, 1995).

—— 'A martyr to love: sacrificial desire in the poetry of Bernart de

Ventadorn', *Journal of Medieval and Early Modern Studies*, 31 (2001), 477–506.

Glassman, Bernard, *Anti-Semitic Stereotypes without Jews: Images of the Jews in England, 1290–1700* (Detroit: Wayne State University Press, 1975).

Goldberg, P. J. P., *Women, Work, and Life Cycle in a Medieval Economy: Women in York and Yorkshire, c.1300–1520* (Oxford: Oxford University Press, 1992).

Gombrich, E. H., *Art and Illusion: A Study in the Psychology of Pictorial Representation*, 4th edn (London: Phaidon, 1972).

Goss, Charles Mayo (ed.), *Anatomy of the Human Body* (Philadelphia: Lea & Ferbiger, 1973).

Gransden, Antonia, *Historical Writing in England*, vol. 2, *c.1307 to the Early Sixteenth Century* (Ithaca, NY: Cornell University Press, 1982).

Gravdal, Kathryn, *Ravishing Maidens: Writing Rape in Medieval French Literature and Law* (Philadelphia: University of Pennsylvania Press, 1991).

Green, Miranda, *The Gods of the Celts* (Stroud: Sutton, 1986).

—— *Celtic Goddesses: Warriors, Virgins and Mothers* (London: British Museum Press, 1995).

Griffiths, R. A., *The Reign of King Henry VI: The Exercise of Royal Authority 1422–1461* (London: Benn, 1981).

Groot, Roger D., 'The crime of rape *temp.* Richard I and John', *Journal of Legal History*, 9 (1988), 324–34.

Gross, Anthony, *The Dissolution of the Lancastrian Kingship: Sir John Fortescue and the Crisis of Monarchy in Fifteenth-Century England* (Stamford: Watkins, 1996).

Gruenbaum, Ellen, *The Female Circumcision Controversy: An Anthropological Perspective* (Philadelphia: University of Pennsylvania Press, 2001).

Guerchberg, Seraphine, 'The controversy over the alleged sowers of the Black Death in the contemporary treatises on plague', in Sylvia Thrupp (ed.), *Change in Medieval Society: Europe North of the Alps, 1050–1500* (New York: Appleton-Century-Crofts, 1984), pp. 208–24.

Guilaine, Jean, *La Mer partagée: La Méditerranée avant l'écriture, 7000–2000 avant Jésus-Christ* (Paris: Hachette, 1994).

Hackett, Helen, *Virgin Mother, Maiden Queen: Elizabeth I and the Cult of the Virgin Mary* (Basingstoke: Macmillan, 1995).

Hadfield, Andrew, *Literature, Politics and National Identity: Reformation to Renaissance* (Cambridge: Cambridge University Press, 1994).

Hale, David George, *Body Politic: A Political Metaphor in Renaissance English Literature* (The Hague: Mouton, 1971).

Hallissy, Margaret, *Venomous Woman: Fear of the Female in Literature* (Westport: Greenwood, 1987).

Halperin, David M., 'Forgetting Foucault: acts, identities, and the histories of sexuality', *Representations*, 63 (1998), 93–120.

Hanawalt, Barbara A., *The Ties that Bound: Peasant Families in Medieval England* (New York: Oxford University Press, 1986).

—— *'Of Good and Ill Repute': Gender and Social Control in Medieval England* (New York: Oxford University Press, 1998).

Hardin, Richard F., 'Chronicles and mythmaking in Shakespeare's Joan of Arc', *Shakespeare Survey*, 42 (1989/90), 25–35.

Harding, Wendy, 'Body into text: *The Book of Margery Kempe*', in Linda Lomperis and Sarah Stanbury (eds), *Feminist Approaches to the Body in Medieval Literature* (Philadelphia: University of Pennsylvania Press, 1993), pp. 168–87.

Hayward, Paul, 'Suffering and innocence in Latin sermons for the Feast of the Holy Innocents, *c.*400–800', *Studies in Church History*, 31 (1994), 67–80.

Heffernan, Thomas J., *Sacred Biography: Saints and their Biographers in the Middle Ages* (New York: Oxford University Press, 1988).

Heller, Wendy Beth, *Chastity, Heroinics and Culture: Women and the Opera of Seventeenth Century Venice* (Ann Arbor: University of Michigan Press, 1997).

Helmholz, R. H., *Marriage Litigation in Medieval England* (Cambridge: Cambridge University Press, 1974).

Heng, Geraldine, 'The romance of England: *Richard Coer de Lyon*, Saracens, Jews, and the politics of race and nation', in Jeffrey Jerome Cohen (ed.), *The Postcolonial Middle Ages* (New York: St Martin's Press, 2000), pp. 135–71.

Heningham, Eleanor K., 'The literary unity, the date and the purpose of the Lady Edith's book, "The Life of King Edward who rests at Westminster"', *Albion*, 7 (1975), 24–40.

Henningfeld, Diane Andrews, 'Contextualising rape: sexual violence in Middle English literature' (unpublished doctoral thesis, Michigan State University, 1994).

Hodgson, Miranda, 'Impossible women: Ælfric's *sponsa Christi* and "la mystérique"', *Medieval Feminist Forum*, 33 (2002), 12–21.

Hollywood, Amy, *Sensible Ecstasy: Mysticism, Sexual Difference, and the Demands of History* (Chicago: University of Chicago Press, 2002).

Horvat, Frank, and Michel Pastoureau, *Figures romanes* (Paris: Seuil, 2001).

Hughes, Jonathan, *Pastors and Visionaries: Religion and Secular Life in Late Medieval Yorkshire* (Woodbridge: Boydell, 1988).

—— *Arthurian Myths and Alchemy: The Kingship of Edward IV* (Stroud: Sutton, 2002).

Hunt, Leon, 'What are big boys made of? *Spartacus, El Cid*, and the male epic', in Pat Kirkham and Janet Thumim (eds), *You Tarzan: Masculinity, Movies, and Men* (London: Lawrence & Wishart, 1993), pp. 65–83.

Hunt, Tony, 'The Song of Songs and courtly literature', in Glyn S. Burgess and Robert Taylor (eds), *Court and Poet* (Liverpool: ARCA, 1981), pp. 189–96.

—— 'Anecdota Anglo-Normannica', *Yearbook of English Studies*, 15 (1985), 1–17.

Innes-Parker, Catherine, 'Sexual violence and the female reader: symbolic "rape" in the saints' lives of the Katherine group', *Women's Studies*, 24 (1995), 205–17.

Irigaray, Luce, 'Così fan tutti', in *This Sex which is Not One*, trans. Catherine Porter (Ithaca, NY: Cornell University Press, 1985), pp. 86–105.

Ives, E. W., ' "Agaynst taking awaye of women": the inception and operation of the Abduction Act of 1487', in R. J. Knecht Ives, and J. J. Scarisbrick (eds), *Wealth and Power in Tudor England* (London: Athlone, 1978), pp. 21–44.

Jacquart, Danielle, and Claude Thomasset, *Sexuality and Medicine in the Middle Ages*, trans. Matthew Adamson (Cambridge: Polity Press, 1988).

Jarman, A. O. H., and Gwilym Rees Hughes, *A Guide to Welsh Literature*, vol. 1 (Swansea: Davies, 1976).

Jenkins, Dafydd, *Cyfraith Hywel: Rhagarweiniad i Gyfraith Gynhenid Cymru'r Oesoedd Canol* (Llandysul: Gwasg Gomer, 1970).

—— and Morfydd E. Owen, *The Welsh Law of Women* (Cardiff: University of Wales Press, 1980).

Johns, Catherine, *Sex or Symbol? Erotic Images of Greece and Rome* (London: British Museum, 1982).

Johnson, Willis, 'The myth of Jewish male menses', *Journal of Medieval History*, 24 (1998), 273–95.

Johnston, Dafydd (ed.), *Canu Maswedd yr Oesoedd Canol / Medieval Welsh Erotic Poetry* (Cardiff: Tafol, 1991).

Jones, E. D., 'The medieval leyrwite: a historical note on female fornication', *English Historical Review*, 107 (1992), 945–53.

Jones, Ida B. 'Hafod 16 (A mediaeval Welsh medical treatise)', *Études celtiques*, 7 (1955/6), 46–75, 270–339.

—— 'Hafod 16 (*suite*)' and 'Hafod 16 (*suite et fin*)', *Études celtiques*, 8 (1958/9), 66–97, 346–93.

Jones, Thomas Gwynn, *Welsh Folklore and Folk Custom* (London: Methuen, 1930).

Jones, Timothy S., and David A. Sprunger (eds), *Marvels, Miracles and Monsters: Studies in the Medieval and Early Modern Imaginations* (Kalamazoo: Medieval Institute Publications, 2002).

Jordan, Mark D., *The Invention of Sodomy in Christian Theology* (Chicago: University of Chicago Press, 1997).

Kappler, Claude, *Monstres, démons et merveilles à la fin du Moyen Âge* (Paris: Payot, 1980).

Karras, Ruth Mazo, 'Review essay: Active/passive, acts/passions: Greek and Roman sexualities', *American Historical Review*, 105 (2000), 1250–65.

Kase, N. G., A. B. Weingold et al., *The Principles and Practice of Clinical Gynaecology* (Edinburgh: Churchill Livingstone, 1990).

Kay, Sarah, 'The sublime body of the martyr: violence in early romance saints' lives', in Richard W. Kaeuper (ed.), *Violence in Medieval Society* (Woodbridge: Boydell, 2000), pp. 3–20.

Kealey, Edward J., *Medieval Medicus: A Social History of Anglo-Norman Medicine* (Baltimore: Johns Hopkins University Press, 1981).

Kelly, Eamonn P., *Sheela-na-Gigs: Origins and Functions* (Dublin: Country House, in association with The National Museum of Ireland, 1996).

Kelly, Henry A., 'English kings and the fear of sorcery', *Medieval Studies*, 39 (1977), 206–38.

—— 'Statutes of rapes and alleged ravishers of wives: a context for the charges against Thomas Malory, knight', *Viator*, 28 (1997), 361–419.

—— 'Meanings and uses of *raptus* in Chaucer's time', *Studies in the Age of Chaucer*, 20 (1998), 101–65.

Kelly, Kathleen Coyne, 'Menaced masculinity and imperiled virginity in the *Morte Darthur*', in Kelly and Marina Leslie (eds), *Menacing Virgins: Representing Virginity in the Middle Ages and Renaissance* (London: Associated University Presses, 1999), pp. 97–114.

—— 'Useful virgins in medieval hagiography', in Cindy L. Carlson and Angela Jane Weisl (eds), *Constructions of Widowhood and Virginity in the Middle Ages* (London: Macmillan, 1999), pp. 135–64.

—— *Performing Virginity and Testing Chastity in the Middle Ages* (London: Routledge, 2000).

—— and Marina Leslie, 'Introduction: the epistemology of virginity', in Kelly and Leslie (eds), *Menacing Virgins: Representing Virginity in the Middle Ages and Renaissance* (London: Associated University Presses, 1999), pp. 15–25.

—— and Marina Leslie (eds), *Menacing Virgins: Representing Virginity in the Middle Ages and Renaissance* (London: Associated University Presses, 1999).

King, Helen, *Hippocrates' Woman: Reading the Female Body in Ancient Greece* (London: Routledge, 1998).

Kingsford, Charles Lethbridge, *English Historical Literature in the Fifteenth Century* (Oxford: Clarendon Press, 1913).

Kipnis, Laura, *Bound and Gagged: Pornography and the Politics of Fantasy in America* (New York: Grove Press, 1996).

Kittel, Ruth, 'Rape in thirteenth-century England: a study of the common-law courts', in D. Kelly Weisberg (ed.), *Women and the Law: A Social Historical Perspective*, 2 vols (Cambridge, MA: Schenkman, 1982), vol. 2, pp. 101–15.

Kittredge, G. L., *Witchcraft in Old and New England* (Cambridge, MA: Harvard University Press, 1928).

Kripal, Jeffrey J., *Roads of Excess, Palaces of Wisdom: Eroticism and*

Reflexivity in the Study of Mysticism (Chicago: University of Chicago Press, 2001).

Kuefler, Matthew S., 'Castration and eunuchism in the Middle Ages', in Vern L. Bullough and James A. Brundage (eds), *Handbook of Medieval Sexuality* (New York: Garland, 1996), pp. 279–306.

Lacan, Jacques, *Le Séminaire, livre XX, Encore*, ed. Jacques-Alain Miller (Paris: Seuil, 1975).

—— *Feminine Sexuality: Jacques Lacan and the* école freudienne, ed. Juliet Mitchell and Jacqueline Rose (London: Macmillan, 1982).

Lampert, Lisa, 'The once and future Jew: the Croxton *Play of the Sacrament*, Little Robert of Bury and historical memory', *Jewish History*, 15 (2001), 235–55.

Langmuir, Gavin I., *History, Religion, and Antisemitism* (London: I. B. Tauris, 1990).

Laqueur, Thomas, *Making Sex: Body and Gender from the Greeks to Freud* (Cambridge, MA: Harvard University Press, 1990).

Lascault, Gilbert, *Le Monstre dans l'art occidental* (Paris: Klincksieck, 1973).

Last, R. J., *Last's Anatomy: Regional and Applied* (Edinburgh: Churchill Livingstone, 1990), 8th edn by R. M. H. McMinn.

Lastique, Esther, and Helen Rodnite Lemay, 'A medieval physician's guide to virginity', in Joyce E. Salisbury (ed.), *Sex in the Middle Ages: A Book of Essays* (New York: Garland, 1991), pp. 56–82.

Lawton, David, *Faith, Text and History: The Bible in English* (Charlottesville: University Press of Virginia, 1990).

Lea, Henry Charles, *A History of Sacerdotal Celibacy in the Christian Church*, 2 vols (London: Williams & Norgate, 1907).

Leclercq, Jean, *Monks and Love in Twelfth-Century France: Psycho-Historical Essays* (Oxford: Clarendon Press, 1979).

Lees, Clare A., 'Engendering religious desire: sex, knowledge, and Christian identity in Anglo-Saxon England', *Journal of Medieval and Early Modern Studies*, 27 (1997), 17–46.

—— and Gillian R. Overing, 'Before history, before difference: bodies, metaphor, and the Church in Anglo-Saxon England', *Yale Journal of Criticism*, 11 (1998), 315–34.

Lees, Sue, *Carnal Knowledge: Rape on Trial* (London: Hamish Hamilton, 1996).

Leiris, Michel, *Mots sans mémoire* (Paris: Gallimard, 1969).

Lemay, Helen Rodnite, 'William of Saliceto on human sexuality', *Viator*, 12 (1981), 165–81.

Le Roux, Françoise, and Christian-J. Guyonvarch, *Les Fêtes celtiques* (Rennes: Éditions Ouest-France Université, 1995).

Levine, Joseph M., *Humanism and History: Origins of Modern English Historiography* (Ithaca, NY: Cornell University Press, 1987).

Lévy, Jean-Philippe, 'L'officialité de Paris et les questions familiales à la fin du XIVe siècle', in *Études d'histoire du droit canonique dédiées à Gabriel le Bras*, 2 vols (Paris: Sirey, 1965), vol. 2, pp. 1265–94.

Lewis, Katherine J., *The Cult of St Katherine of Alexandria in Late Medieval England* (Woodbridge: Boydell, 2000).

—— ' "Lete me suffre": reading the torture of St Margaret of Antioch in late medieval England', in Jocelyn Wogan-Browne et al. (eds), *Medieval Women: Texts and Contexts in Late Medieval Britain: Essays for Felicity Riddy* (Turnhout: Brepols, 2000), pp. 69–82.

—— 'Becoming a virgin king: Richard II and Edward the Confessor', in Samantha J. E. Riches and Sarah Salih (eds), *Gender and Holiness: Men, Women and Saints in Late Medieval Europe* (London: Routledge, 2002), pp. 86–100.

Leyser, C., 'Masculinity in flux: nocturnal emission and the limits of celibacy in the early Middle Ages', in D. M. Hadley (ed.), *Masculinity in Medieval Europe* (London: Longman, 1999), pp. 103–20.

Lipscomb, Lan, 'A distinct legend of the ring in the *Life of Edward the Confessor*', *Medieval Perspectives*, 6 (1992), 45–57.

Lochrie, Karma, *Margery Kempe and Translations of the Flesh* (Philadelphia: University of Pennsylvania Press, 1991).

—— 'Mystical acts, queer tendencies', in Lochrie, Peggy McCracken and James A. Schultz (eds), *Constructing Medieval Sexuality* (Minneapolis: University of Minnesota Press, 1997), pp. 180–200.

—— *Covert Operations: The Medieval Uses of Secrecy* (Philadelphia: University of Pennsylvania Press, 1999).

Loughlin, Marie H., *Hymeneutics: Interpreting Virginity on the Early Modern Stage* (Lewisburg: Bucknell University Press, 1997).

McAll, Christopher, 'The normal paradigms of a woman's life in the Irish and Welsh law texts', in Dafydd Jenkins and Morfydd E. Owen (eds), *The Welsh Law of Women* (Cardiff: University of Wales Press, 1980), pp. 7–22.

McAvoy, Liz Herbert, and Teresa Walters (eds), *Consuming Narratives: Gender and Monstrous Appetites in the Middle Ages and Renaissance* (Cardiff: University of Wales Press, 2002).

Mac Cana, Proinsias, *Celtic Mythology* (London: Chancellor, 1996).

MacCulloch, John Arnott, *Celtic Mythology* (London: Constable & Co., 1918).

MacGibbon, David, *Elizabeth Woodville, 1437–1492: Her Life and Times* (London: Arthur Barker, 1938).

McInerney, Maud Burnett, ' "In the meydens womb": Julian of Norwich and the poetics of enclosure', in John Carmi Parsons and Bonnie Wheeler (eds), *Medieval Mothering* (New York: Garland, 1996), pp. 157–83.

—— 'Like a virgin: the problem of male virginity in the *Symphonia*', in McInerney (ed.), *Hildegard of Bingen: A Book of Essays* (New York: Garland, 1998), pp. 133–54.

—— 'Rhetoric, power and integrity in the passion of the virgin martyr', in Kathleen Coyne Kelly and Marina Leslie (eds), *Menacing Virgins: Representing Virginity in the Middle Ages and Renaissance* (London: Associated University Presses, 1999), pp. 50–70.

McMahon, Joanne, and Jack Roberts, *The Sheela-na-Gigs of Ireland and Britain: The Divine Hag of the Christian Celts, an Illustrated Guide* (Cork: Mercier Press, 2000).

McNamara, Jo Ann, 'Chaste marriage and clerical celibacy', in Vern L. Bullough and James A. Brundage (eds), *Sexual Practices and the Medieval Church* (Buffalo, NY: Prometheus Books, 1982), pp. 22–33.

—— *A New Song: Celibate Women in the First Three Christian Centuries* (New York: Haworth Press, 1983).

—— 'The *Herrenfrage*: the restructuring of the gender system, 1050–1150', in Clare A. Lees (ed.), *Medieval Masculinities: Regarding Men in the Middle Ages* (Minneapolis: University of Minnesota Press, 1994), pp. 3–29.

—— *Sisters in Arms: Catholic Nuns through Two Millennia* (Cambridge, MA: Harvard University Press, 1996).

—— 'An unresolved syllogism: the search for a Christian gender system', in Jacqueline Murray (ed.), *Conflicted Identities and Multiple Masculinities: Men in the Medieval West* (New York: Garland, 1999), pp. 1–24.

Mason, Emma, *Westminster Abbey and its People, c.1050–c.1216* (Woodbridge: Boydell, 1996).

Mate, Mavis E., *Daughters, Wives and Widows after the Black Death: Women in Sussex, 1350–1535* (Woodbridge: Boydell, 1998).

Matter, E. Ann, *The Voice of my Beloved: The Song of Songs in Western Medieval Christianity* (Philadelphia: University of Pennsylvania Press, 1990).

Mazzoni, Cristina, *Saint Hysteria: Neurosis, Mysticism and Gender in European Culture* (Ithaca, NY: Cornell University Press, 1996).

Mellars, Paul, 'The Upper Palaeolithic revolution', in Barry Cunliffe (ed.), *The Oxford Illustrated Prehistory of Europe* (Oxford: Oxford University Press, 1994), pp. 42–79.

Mellinkoff, Ruth, *Outcasts: Signs of Otherness in Northern European Art of the Late Middle Ages*, 2 vols (Berkeley: University of California Press, 1993).

Meltzer, Françoise, *For Fear of the Fire: Joan of Arc and the Limits of Subjectivity* (Chicago: University of Chicago Press, 2001).

Menache, Sophia, 'The king, the church and the Jews: some considerations on the expulsions from England and France', *Journal of Medieval History*, 13 (1987), 223–36.

—— 'Matthew Paris's attitudes towards Anglo-Jewry', *Journal of Medieval History*, 23 (1997), 139–62.

Mews, Constant (ed.), *Listen Daughter: The* Speculum Virginum *and the*

Formation of Religious Women in the Middle Ages (New York: Palgrave, 2001).

Miles, Margaret R., *Carnal Knowing: Female Nakedness and Religious Meaning in the Christian West* (Boston: Beacon Press, 1989).

Miller, Julie B., 'Eroticized violence in medieval women's mystical literature: a call for a feminist critique', *Journal of Feminist Studies in Religion*, 15 (1999), 25–49.

Miller, Nancy Weitz, 'Metaphor and the mystification of chastity in Vives's *Instruction of a Christen Woman*', in Kathleen Coyne Kelly and Marina Leslie (eds), *Menacing Virgins: Representing Virginity in the Middle Ages and Renaissance* (London: Associated University Presses, 1999), pp. 132–45.

Mills, Robert, 'Visions of excess: pain, pleasure and the penal imaginary in late-medieval art and culture' (unpublished Ph.D. thesis, University of Cambridge, 2000).

—— ' "Whatever you do is a delight to me!": masculinity, masochism and queer play in representations of male martyrdom', *Exemplaria*, 13 (2001), 1–37.

—— 'A man is being beaten', in Rita Copeland, David Lawton and Wendy Scase (eds), *New Medieval Literatures*, vol. 5 (Oxford: Oxford University Press, 2002), pp. 115–54.

—— 'Ecce homo', in Samantha J. E. Riches and Sarah Salih (eds), *Gender and Holiness: Men, Women and Saints in Late Medieval Europe* (London: Routledge, 2002), pp. 152–73.

Minnis, Alastair J., and A. B. Scott (eds), with the assistance of David Wallace, *Medieval Literary Theory and Criticism, c.1100–c.1375: The Commentary Tradition* (Oxford: Clarendon Press, 1988).

Minnis, A. J., '*De impedimento sexus*: women's bodies and medieval impediments to female ordination', in Peter Biller and Minnis (eds), *Medieval Theology and the Natural Body* (Woodbridge: York Medieval Press, 1997), pp. 109–39.

Mitchell, Sally, *The Fallen Angel; Chastity, Class and Women's Reading 1835–1880* (Bowling Green: Bowling Green University Popular Press, 1981).

Moorcraft, Paul L., *Anchoress of Shere* (Shere: Millstream Press, 2000).

Moore, Grace E., *The Middle English Verse Life of Edward the Confessor* (Philadelphia: University of Pennsylvania, 1942).

Morgan, Nigel, 'Longinus and the wounded heart', *Wiener Jahrbuch für Kunstgeschichte*, 46 (1993/4), 507–18.

Morgan, Robin, 'Theory and practice: pornography and rape', in Laura Lederer (ed), *Take Back the Night: Women on Pornography* (New York: William Morrow, 1980), pp. 125–47.

Mozley, J. F., *John Foxe and his Book* (London: SPCK, 1940).

Murray, Jacqueline, 'Twice marginal and twice invisible: lesbians in the

Middle Ages', in Vern L. Bullough and James A. Brundage (eds), *Handbook of Medieval Sexuality* (New York: Garland, 1996), pp. 191–222.

—— (ed.), *Conflicted Identities and Multiple Masculinities: Men in the Medieval West* (New York: Garland, 1999).

—— 'Supernatural castration: a response to masculine sexual anxiety in the Middle Ages', unpublished conference paper delivered at The Queer Middle Ages Conference, CUNY Graduate Center, New York, NY, October 1997.

—— 'Mystical castration: some reflections on Peter Abelard, Hugh of Lincoln and sexual control', in Murray (ed.), *Conflicted Identities and Multiple Masculinities: Men in the Medieval West* (New York: Garland, 1999), pp. 73–91.

—— '"The law of sin that is in my members": the problem of male embodiment', in Samantha J. E. Riches and Sarah Salih (eds), *Gender and Holiness: Men, Women and Saints in Late Medieval Europe* (London: Routledge, 2002), pp. 9–22.

Myers, A. R., *Crown, Household and Parliament in Fifteenth-Century England*, ed. Cecil H. Clough (London: Hambledon, 1985).

Neale, Steve, 'Masculinity as spectacle: reflections on men and mainstream cinema', *Screen*, 24 (1983), 2–16.

Neubauer, Hans-Joachim, *The Rumour: A Cultural History*, trans. Christian Braun (London: Free Association Books, 1999).

Neumann, Erich, *The Great Mother: An Analysis of the Archetype*, trans. Ralph Manheim (Princeton: Princeton University Press, 1963).

Newman, Barbara, 'Flaws in the golden bowl: gender and spiritual formation in the twelfth century', *Traditio*, 45 (1989/90), 111–46.

—— *From Virile Woman to WomanChrist: Studies in Medieval Religion and Literature* (Philadelphia: University of Pennsylvania Press, 1995).

Nora, Pierre (ed.), *Realms of Memory: Rethinking the French Past*, vol. 1, *Conflicts and Divisions*, trans. Arthur Goldhammer (New York: Columbia University Press, 1996).

North, Tim, 'Legerwite in the thirteenth and fourteenth centuries', *Past and Present*, 111 (1986), 3–16.

Nye, Robert A., 'Introduction', in Nye (ed.), *Sexuality* (Oxford: Oxford University Press, 1999), pp. 3–18.

O'Donovan, John, *Ordnance Survey Letters, Co. Tipperary* (Dublin: typed copy, 1840).

Otis, Leah Lydia, *Prostitution in Medieval Society: The History of an Urban Institution in Languedoc* (Chicago: University of Chicago Press, 1985).

Otter, Monika, 'Closed doors: an epithalamium for Queen Edith, widow and virgin', in Cindy L. Carlson and Angela Jane Weisl (eds), *Constructions of Widowhood and Virginity in the Middle Ages* (Basingstoke: Macmillan, 1999), pp. 63–92.

Owen, Morfydd E., 'Meddygon Myddfai: a preliminary survey of some medieval medical writing in Welsh', *Studia Celtica*, 10 (1975/6), 210–33.

—— 'Shame and reparation: women's place in the kin', in Dafydd Jenkins and Morfydd E. Owen, *The Welsh Law of Women* (Cardiff: University of Wales Press, 1980), pp. 40–68.

Parker, Patricia A., *Literary Fat Ladies: Rhetoric, Gender, Property* (London: Methuen, 1987).

—— 'Virile style', in Louise Fradenburg and Carla Freccero (eds), with the assistance of Kathy Lavezzo, *Premodern Sexualities* (New York: Routledge, 1996), pp. 201–22.

Partner, Nancy F., 'Reading *The Book of Margery Kempe*', *Exemplaria*, 3 (1991), 29–66.

—— 'Did mystics have sex?', in Jacqueline Murray and Konrad Eisenbichler (eds), *Desire and Discipline: Sex and Sexuality in the Premodern West* (Toronto: University of Toronto Press, 1996), pp. 296–311.

Patterson, Annabel, *Reading Holinshed's Chronicles* (Chicago: University of Chicago Press, 1994).

Patterson, Lee, 'Chaucer's Pardoner on the couch: Psyche and Clio in medieval literary studies', *Speculum*, 76 (2001), 638–80.

Patterson, Nerys W., 'Honour and shame in medieval Welsh society', *Studia Celtica*, 16/17 (1981/2), 73–103.

Payer, Pierre J., *The Bridling of Desire: Views of Sex in the Later Middle Ages* (Toronto: University of Toronto Press, 1993).

Pearson, Ann, 'Reclaiming the *sheela-na-gigs*: goddess imagery in medieval sculptures of Ireland', *Canadian Woman Studies/Les Cahiers de la femme*, 17 (1997), 20–4.

Phillips, Kim M., 'Written on the body: reading rape from the twelfth to fifteenth centuries', in Noël James Menuge (ed.), *Medieval Women and the Law* (Woodbridge: Boydell, 2000), pp. 125–44.

—— *Medieval Maidens: Young Women and Gender in England, 1270–1540* (Manchester: Manchester University Press, 2003).

—— and Barry Reay, 'Introduction: sexualities in history', in Phillips and Reay (eds), *Sexualities in History: A Reader* (New York: Routledge, 2002), pp. 1–23.

Poos, L. R. and R. M. Smith, ' "Legal windows onto historical populations"? Recent research on demography and the manor court in medieval England', *Law and History Review*, 2 (1984), 128–52.

Post, J. B., 'Ravishment of women and the Statutes of Westminster', in J. H. Baker (ed.), *Legal Records and the Historian* (London: Royal Historical Society, 1978), pp. 150–64.

—— 'Sir Thomas West and the Statute of Rapes, 1382', *Bulletin of the Institute for Historical Research*, 53 (1980), 24–30.

Pouchelle, Marie-Christine, *The Body and Surgery in the Middle Ages*, trans. Rosemary Morris (Oxford: Polity Press, 1990).

Power, Eileen, *Medieval Women*, ed. M. M. Postan (Cambridge: Cambridge University Press, 1975).

Rahman, Anika, and Nahid Toubia, *Female Genital Mutilation: A Guide to Laws and Policies Worldwide* (New York: Zed Books, 2000).

Raknem, Ingvald, *Joan of Arc in History, Legend and Literature* (Oslo: Universitetsforlaget, 1971).

Rambuss, Richard, *Closet Devotions* (Durham, NC: Duke University Press, 1998).

Rawcliffe, Carole, *Medicine and Society in Later Medieval England* (Stroud: Sutton, 1997).

—— 'Women, childbirth and religion in later medieval England', in D. Wood (ed.), *Women and Religion in Medieval England* (Oxford: Oxford University Press, forthcoming).

Raymo, Robert, 'Works of religious and philosophical instruction', in Albert E. Hartung (gen. ed.), *Manual of the Writings in Middle English* (Hamden: Connecticut Academy of Arts and Sciences, 1983–), vol. 7, pp. 2255–378.

Razi, Zvi, 'The Toronto School's reconstitution of medieval peasant society: a critical view', *Past and Present*, 85 (1979), 141–57.

—— *Life, Marriage and Death in a Medieval Parish: Economy, Society and Demography in Halesowen 1270–1400* (Cambridge: Cambridge University Press, 1980).

—— 'Family, land and the village community in later medieval England', *Past and Present*, 93 (1981), 3–36.

—— 'The struggles between the abbots of Halesowen and their tenants in the thirteenth and fourteenth centuries', in T. H. Aston et al. (eds), *Social Relations and Ideas: Essays in Honour of R. H. Hilton* (Cambridge: Cambridge University Press, 1983), pp. 151–67.

Rees, Emma L. E., 'Sheela's voracity and Victorian veracity', in Liz Herbert McAvoy and Teresa Walters (eds), *Consuming Narratives: Gender and Monstrous Appetite in the Middle Ages and the Renaissance* (Cardiff: University of Wales Press, 2002), pp. 116–27.

Riches, Samantha J. E., *St George: Hero, Martyr and Myth* (Stroud: Sutton, 2000)

—— 'St George as virgin martyr', in Riches and Sarah Salih (eds), *Gender and Holiness: Men, Women and Saints in Late Medieval Europe* (London: Routledge, 2002), pp. 65–85.

Ridyard, Susan J., '*Condigna veneratio*: post-conquest attitudes to the saints of the Anglo-Saxons', *Anglo-Norman Studies*, 9 (1987), 179–206.

—— *The Royal Saints of Anglo-Saxon England: A Study of West Saxon and East Anglian Cults* (Cambridge: Cambridge University Press, 1988).

Robertson, Duncan, *The Medieval Saints' Lives: Spiritual Renewal and Old*

French Literature, Edward C. Armstrong Monographs on Medieval Literature, 8 (Levington: French Forum, 1995).

Robinson, J. Armitage, 'Westminster in the twelfth century: Osbert of Clare', *Church Quarterly Review*, 68 (1909), 336–56.

Rogers, John, 'The enclosure of virginity: the poetics of sexual abstinence in the English revolution', in Richard Burt and John Michael Archer (eds), *Enclosure Acts: Sexuality, Property and Culture in Early Modern England* (Ithaca, NY: Cornell University Press, 1994), pp. 229–50.

Ross, Anne, *Pagan Celtic Britain: Studies in Iconography and Tradition* (London: Routledge & Kegan Paul; New York: Columbia University Press, 1967).

—— 'The divine hag of the pagan Celts', in Venetia Newall (ed.), *The Witch Figure* (London: Routledge & Kegan Paul, 1973), pp. 139–64.

Rossiaud, Jacques, *Medieval Prostitution*, trans. Lydia G. Cochrane (London: Blackwell, 1988).

Rubin, Miri, 'Choosing death? Experiences of martyrdom in late medieval Europe', in Diane Wood (ed.), *Martyrs and Martyrologies*, Studies in Church History, 30 (Oxford: Blackwell, 1993), pp. 153–83.

—— *Gentile Tales: The Narrative Assault on Late Medieval Jews* (New Haven: Yale University Press, 1999).

Russell, Jeffrey Burton, *Witchcraft in the Middle Ages* (Ithaca, NY: Cornell University Press, 1972).

Said, Edward W., *Orientalism: Western Conceptions of the Orient* (London: Penguin, 1978).

Saint-Paul, Thérèse, 'The magical mantle, the drinking horn and the chastity test: a study of a "tale" in Arthurian Celtic literature' (unpublished doctoral thesis, University of Edinburgh, 1987).

Salih, Sarah, 'Performing virginity: sex and violence in the *Katherine Group*', in Cindy L. Carlson and Angela Jane Weisl (eds), *Constructions of Widowhood and Virginity in the Middle Ages* (New York: St Martin's Press, 1999), pp. 95–112.

—— *Versions of Virginity in Late Medieval England* (Cambridge: Brewer, 2001).

—— 'Monstrous virginity: St Aelred writes the nuns of Watton', in Kate Boardman, Catherine Emerson and Adrian Tudor (eds), *Framing the Text: Reading Tradition and Image in Medieval Europe*, *Mediaevalia*, 20 (2001), 49–72.

—— 'Queering *sponsalia Christi*: virginity, gender and desire in the early Middle English anchoritic texts', in Rita Copeland, David Lawton and Wendy Scase (eds), *New Medieval Literatures*, vol. 5 (Oxford: Oxford University Press, 2002), pp. 155–75.

Salisbury, Joyce E., *Church Fathers, Independent Virgins* (London: Verso, 1991).

Sanderson, Lillian Passmore, *Against the Mutilation of Women: The Struggle to End Unnecessary Suffering* (London: Ithaca Press, 1981).

Saunders, Corinne, *Rape and Ravishment in the Literature of Medieval England* (Cambridge: Brewer, 2001).

Scammell, Jean, 'Freedom and marriage in medieval England', *Economic History Review*, 2nd ser., 27 (1974), 523–37.

—— 'Wife-rents and merchet', *Economic History Review*, 2nd ser., 29 (1976), 487–90.

Scarry, Elaine, *The Body in Pain: The Making and Unmaking of the World* (New York: Oxford University Press, 1985).

Schibanoff, Susan, 'True lies: transvestism and idolatry in the trial of Joan of Arc', in Bonnie Wheeler and Charles T. Wood (eds), *Fresh Verdicts on Joan of Arc* (New York: Garland, 1996), pp. 31–60.

—— 'Worlds apart: orientalism, antifeminism and heresy in Chaucer's *Man of Law's Tale*', *Exemplaria*, 8 (1996), 59–96.

Scholz, Bernhard W., 'The canonization of Edward the Confessor', *Speculum*, 36 (1961), 38–60.

Schulenberg, Jane Tibbetts, 'Saints and sex, *ca.*500–1100: striding down the nettled path of life', in Joyce E. Salisbury (ed.), *Sex in the Middle Ages: A Book of Essays* (New York: Garland, 1991), pp. 203–31.

Schwyzer, Philip, 'Purity and danger on the west bank of the Severn: the cultural geography of *A Masque Presented at Ludlow Castle, 1634*', *Representations*, 60 (1997), 22–48.

Scofield, Cora L., *The Life and Reign of Edward the Fourth, King of England and of France and Lord of Ireland*, 2 vols (London: Cass, 1967).

Scott, Jim, 'Everyday forms of peasant resistance', *Journal of Peasant Studies*, 13 (1986), 5–35.

Scott, Joan W., 'Gender: a useful category of historical analysis', *American Historical Review*, 91 (1986), 1053–75.

Searle, Eleanor, 'Freedom and marriage in medieval England: an alternative hypothesis', *Economic History Review*, 2nd ser., 29 (1976), 482–6.

Sheehan, Elizabeth A., 'Victorian clitoridectomy: Isaac Baker Brown and his harmless operative procedure', in Roger N. Lancaster and Micaela di Leonardo (eds), *The Gender/Sexuality Reader* (New York: Routledge, 1997).

Shell-Duncan, Bettina, and Ylva Hernlund, 'Female "circumcision" in Africa: dimensions of the practice and debates', in Shell-Duncan and Hernlund (eds), *Female 'Circumcision' in Africa: Culture, Controversy, and Change* (Boulder, CO: Rienner, 2000), pp. 1–38.

Sissa, Giulia, *Greek Virginity*, trans. Arthur Goldhammer (Cambridge, MA: Harvard University Press, 1990).

Smith, Anthony D., *Myths and Memories of the Nation* (Oxford: Oxford University Press, 1999).

Smith, David M., *A Guide to the Archives of the Company of Merchant Adventurers of York*, Borthwick Texts and Calendars, 16 (York: University of York, 1990).

Spearing, A. C., '*The Book of Margery Kempe*; or, the diary of a nobody', *Southern Review*, 38 (2002), 625–35.

Spiegel, Gabrielle M., *The Past as Text: The Theory and Practice of Medieval Historiography* (Baltimore: Johns Hopkins University Press, 1997).

Spivak, Gayatri Chakravorty, 'Can the subaltern speak? Speculations on widow-sacrifice', *Wedge* 7/8 (1985), 120–30.

—— 'Can the subaltern speak?' in Cary Nelson and Lawrence Grossberg (eds), *Marxism and the Interpretation of Culture* (Basingstoke: Macmillan, 1988), pp. 271–313.

—— *The Spivak Reader: Selected Works of Gayatri Chakravorty Spivak*, ed. Donna Landry and Gerald Maclean (London: Routledge, 1996).

Stafford, Pauline, *Queen Emma and Queen Edith: Queenship and Women's Power in Eleventh-Century England* (Oxford: Blackwell, 1997).

Stallybrass, Peter, 'Patriarchal territories: the body enclosed', in Margaret W. Ferguson, Maureen Quilligan and Nancy J. Vickers (eds), *Rewriting the Renaissance: The Discourses of Sexual Difference in Early Modern Europe* (Chicago: University of Chicago Press, 1986), pp. 123–42.

Stein, Robert M., 'Making history English: cultural identity and historical explanation in William of Malmesbury and Lamon's *Brut*', in Sylvia Tomasch and Sealy Gilles (eds), *Text and Territory: Geographical Imagination in the European Middle Ages* (Philadelphia: University of Pennsylvania Press, 1998), pp. 97–115.

Steinberg, Leo, *The Sexuality of Christ in Renaissance Art and Modern Oblivion*, 2nd edn (Chicago: University of Chicago Press, 1995).

Stock, Lorraine K., 'The hag of Castle Hautdesert: the Celtic sheela-na-gig and the *Auncian* in *Sir Gawain and the Green Knight*', in Bonnie Wheeler and Fiona Tolhurst (eds), *On Arthurian Women: Essays in Memory of Maureen Fries* (Dallas: Scriptorium Press, 2001), pp. 121–48.

Strohm, Paul, *Theory and the Premodern Text* (Minneapolis: University of Minnesota Press, 2000).

Sturges, Robert S., 'The Pardoner, veiled and unveiled', in Jeffrey Jerome Cohen and Bonnie Wheeler (eds), *Becoming Male in the Middle Ages* (New York: Garland, 1997), pp. 261–77.

Sunder Rajan, Rajeswari, *Real and Imagined Women: Gender, Culture and Postcolonialism* (London: Routledge, 1993).

Sutton, Anne F., and Livia Visser-Fuchs, ' "A most benevolent queen": Queen Elizabeth Woodville's reputation, her piety and her books', *The Ricardian*, 129 (1995), 214–45.

Taylor, Andrew, 'Reading the dirty bits', in Jacqueline Murray and Konrad Eisenbichler (eds), *Desire and Discipline: Sex and Sexuality in the Premodern West* (Toronto: University of Toronto Press, 1996), pp. 280–95.

Thomas, Graham C. G., 'Chwedlau Tegau Eurfron a Thristfardd bardd Urien Rheged', *Bulletin of the Board of Celtic Studies*, 24 (1970), 1–9.

Thompson, Anne B., 'The legend of St Agnes: improvisation and the practice of hagiography', *Exemplaria*, 13 (2001), 355–97.

Thomson, Rodney M., 'Two versions of a saint's life from St Edmund's Abbey: changing currents in twelfth century monastic style', *Revue Bénédictine*, 84 (1974), 383–408.

Thorndike, Lynn, *A History of Magic and Experimental Science*, 8 vols (New York: Columbia University Press, 1923–58).

Todd, Jan (ed.), *Women Writers Talking* (New York: Holmes & Meier, 1983).

Tomasch, Sylvia, 'Postcolonial Chaucer and the virtual Jew', in Jeffrey Jerome Cohen (ed.), *The Postcolonial Middle Ages* (New York: St Martin's Press, 2000), pp. 243–60.

Toubia, N., and S. Izett, *Female Genital Mutilation: An Overview* (Geneva: WHO, 1998).

Traister, Barbara H., '"Matrix and the pain thereof": a sixteenth-century gynaecological essay', *Medical History*, 35 (1991), 436–51.

Turner, Denys, *Eros and Allegory: Medieval Exegesis of the Song of Songs* (Kalamazoo: Cistercian Publications, 1995).

Turville-Petre, Thorlac, *England the Nation: Language, Literature, and National Identity, 1290–1340* (Oxford: Clarendon Press, 1996).

T. W., 'Influence of medieval upon Welsh literature', *Archaeologia Cambrensis*, ser. 3, 9 (1863), 7–40.

Valente, Roberta Louise, 'Merched y Mabinogi: women and the thematic structure of the Four Branches' (unpublished doctoral thesis, Cornell University, 1986).

Vickers, Brian, 'On the practicalities of Renaissance rhetoric', in Vickers (ed.), *Rhetoric Revalued: Papers from the International Society for the History of Rhetoric*, Medieval and Renaissance Texts and Studies, 19 (Binghamton, NY: Centre for Medieval and Early Renaissance Studies, 1982), pp. 133–41.

Vitz, Evelyn Birge, 'Rereading rape in medieval literature: literary, historical and theoretical reflections', *Romanic Review*, 88 (1997), 1–26.

Voaden, Rosalynn, 'Beholding men's members: the sexualizing of transgression in *The Book of Margery Kempe*', in Peter Biller and A. J. Minnis (eds), *Medieval Theology and the Natural Body* (Woodbridge: York Medieval Press, 1997), pp. 175–90.

Wade-Evans, Arthur W., *Medieval Welsh Law* (Oxford: Clarendon Press 1909).

Warnatsch, O., 'Der Mantel, Bruchstück eines Lanzeletrones des H. von dem Türlîn (nebst einer Abhandlung über die Sage vom Trinkhorn und Mantel und die Quelle der Krone)', in *Germanische Abhandlungen*, ed. K. Weinhold, vol. 2 (Breslau: Koebner, 1883).

Warner, Marina, *Joan of Arc: The Image of Female Heroism* (London: Vintage, 1991).

Watson, Nicholas, 'Censorship and cultural change in late-medieval England: vernacular theology, the Oxford translation debate, and Arundel's Constitutions of 1409', *Speculum*, 70 (1995), 822–64.

Waugh, W. T., 'Joan of Arc in English sources of the fifteenth century', in J. G. Edwards, V. H. Galbraith and E. F. Jacob (eds), *Historical Essays in Honour of James Tait* (Manchester: Subscribers, 1933), pp. 387–98.

Weir, Anthony, and James Jerman, *Images of Lust: Sexual Carvings on Medieval Churches* (London: Routledge, 1999).

Weissman, Hope Phyllis, 'Margery Kempe in Jerusalem: *hysterica compassio* in the late Middle Ages', in Mary J. Carruthers and Elizabeth D. Kirk (eds), *Acts of Interpretation: The Text in its Contexts* (Norman, OK: Pilgrim Books, 1982), pp. 201–18.

Wenzel, Siegfried, *Verses in Sermons: 'Fasciculus Morum' and its Middle English Poems* (Cambridge, MA: Mediaeval Academy of America, 1978).

Wilkins, Nigel, *Nicolas Flamel: Des livres et de l'or* (Paris: Imago, 1993).

Williams, David, *Deformed Discourse: The Function of the Monster in Medieval Thought and Literature* (Exeter: University of Exeter Press, 1996).

Williams, Mary, 'Buched Meir Wyry', *Revue Celtique*, 33 (1912), 207–38.

Winstead, Karen A., 'Capgrave's St Katherine and the perils of gynecocracy', *Viator*, 25 (1994), 361–76.

—— *Virgin Martyrs: Legends of Sainthood in Late Medieval England* (Ithaca, NY: Cornell University Press, 1997).

Wogan-Browne, Jocelyn, 'Saints' lives and the female reader', *Forum for Modern Language Studies*, 27 (1991), 314–32.

—— 'The apple's message: some post-conquest accounts of hagiographic transmission', in Alistair Minnis (ed.), *Late Medieval Religious Texts and their Transmissions* (Cambridge: Brewer, 1993), pp. 39–53.

—— '"Clerc u lai, muine u dame": women and Anglo-Norman hagiography in the twelfth and thirteenth centuries', in Carol M. Meale (ed.), *Women and Literature in Britain 1150–1500* (Cambridge: Cambridge University Press, 1993), pp. 61–85.

—— '"Bet . . . to rede . . . on holy seyntes lyves": romance and hagiography again', in Carol M. Meale (ed.), *Readings in Medieval English Romance* (Cambridge: Brewer, 1994), pp. 83–97.

—— 'Chaste bodies: frames and experiences', in Sarah Kay and Miri Rubin (eds), *Framing Medieval Bodies* (Manchester: Manchester University Press, 1994), pp. 24–42.

—— 'The virgin's tale', in Ruth Evans and Lesley Johnson (eds), *Feminist Readings in Middle English Literature: The Wife of Bath and All her Sect* (London: Routledge, 1994), pp. 165–94.

—— 'Outdoing the daughters of Syon? Edith of Wilton and the representation of female community in fifteenth-century England', in Wogan-Browne et al. (eds), *Medieval Women: Texts and Contexts in Late*

Medieval Britain: Essays for Felicity Riddy (Turnhout: Brepols, 2000), pp. 393–409.

—— *Saints' Lives and Women's Literary Culture, c.1150–1300: Virginity and its Authorizations* (Oxford: Oxford University Press, 2001).

—— 'Virginity always comes twice', in Louise D'Arcens and Juanita Ruys (eds), *'Maistresse of My Wit': The Modern Study of Medieval Women* (Turnhout: Brepols, forthcoming).

Wolfthal, Diane, *Images of Rape: The 'Heroic' Tradition and its Alternatives* (Cambridge: Cambridge University Press, 1999).

Wulff, F. A., 'Le conte du mantel, texte français des dernières années du XIIe siècle', *Romania*, 14 (1885), 343–80.

Wunderli, Richard M., *London Church Courts and Society on the Eve of the Reformation* (Cambridge, MA: Mediaeval Academy of America, 1981).

Yohe, Katherine M., 'Sexual attraction and the motivations for love and friendship in Aelred of Rievaulx', *American Benedictine Review*, 46 (1995), 283–307.

Zuckerman, Lord, with Deryck Darlington and F. Peter Lisowski, *A New System of Anatomy: A Dissector's Guide and Atlas* (Oxford: Oxford University Press, 1961: 2nd edn, 1981).

Websites

Theatana, Kathryn Price, 'Síla na Géige: Sheela na Gig and sacred space', http://www.bandia.net/sheela/LanguageNote

http://www.geocities.com/Wellesley/1752/sheela.html [Larissa Brown's Website]

http://www.jharding.demon.co.uk/index.htm [Megalithica]

http://www.lib.cam.ac.uk/cgi-bin/Ee.3.59/browse?0

http://www.members.tripod.com/~taramc/sheelas.html [Tara McLoughlin's Sheela-na-gig Website]

http://www.sheelanagig.org/ [The Sheela Na Gig project]

http:///www.upnaway.com/~pixiecat/cat/Sheela.html [The Sheela page]

Films

Anchoress, dir. Chris Newby (1993)
Scream, dir. Wes Craven (1996)

INDEX

Numbers in bold type indicate illustrations

Abbott, Elizabeth, 10
abduction, 61, 81–6
Abelard, Peter, 108
abortion, 62
Abraham, The Book of, 144
Abulafia, Anna, 239
Adelidis, abbess of Barking, 137, 237
Adventure of the Sons of Echu Muigmedóin, 41
Ælfric, 210
Aelred of Rievaulx, 8, 19–20, 24, 120–1, 122, 127–32, 237
Aers, David, 18
Agatha, St, 175, 190
Agnes, St, 168, 175, 189–95, 196–204, **198**, **199**, **200**, 209, 210
Ailes, M. J., 30
Alain de Lille, 117, 221
Albert the Great, 17, 71
alchemy, 9, 140–61, 238
Aldhelm, 232
Alexander III, Pope, 121, 131
Alexis, St, 105
Ambrose, St, 195
Ammonius, St, 104
amobr, 59, 73; *see also* leyrwite
Ana/Anu, 40
Anastasia, St, 190
anchoritism, 20, 150–1
Ancrene Wisse, 20, 150, 172, 210
Andersen, Jørgen, 35, 47
Andrew, St, 116
Anne, St, 137
Anthony, St, 106
anti-semitism, 9, 168–73, 176–81, 203, 212, 239–41
Aranrhod, 40, 60–3, 66

Arthur, King, 65–6, 159
Arthurian legend, 9, 26, 42, 65–8, 147, 153–4, 159–60
asceticism, 102–5, 107, 109–11
Ashby, George, 153
Ashton, Gail, 3, 188, 193–4, 211
Auchinleck manuscript, 203
Augustine of Hippo, 20, 110, 178
Avicenna, 149

Bacon, Roger, 141, 143, 144, 146
Bakhtin, Mikhail, 46, 48
Baldwin, John W., 27–8
Bale, John, 218, 219, 228
Bale, Robert, 157
banshee, 42
baptism, 178, 180
Barbara, St, 168, 204, **205**
Barlow, Frank, 119, 120, 122, 123, 125, 132
Bartlett, Robert, 137
Beattie, Cordelia, 93
Beaufort, Margaret, 157
Bede, 103, 237
Benedict, St, 104, 105
Bennett, Judith M., 90
Bernard of Clairvaux, 19, 24, 25, 105, 109–11, 116
Bernau, Anke, 20, 237
Bernini, Lorenzo, 49
bestiary, 6, 45–6
Bible,
    2 Corinthians, 128
    Ecclesiasticus, 128
    John, 232
    1 Kings, 136
    Matthew, 108
    Numbers, 74

Song of Songs, 14, 23, 194, 240
1 Timothy, 219
2 Timothy, 219
see also Pamplona Bible
Biddick, Kathleen, 176–7, 185, 206
Biket, Robert, 65–6
Blacman, John, 153, 154
Blake, Thomas, 160
Bloch, R. Howard, 68, 109, 208
Bokenham, Osbern, 175, 190–204, 210
'Boy and the Mantle, The', 65
Bracton, 84–5
Branwen, 42
Brigid, St, 40–1, 53
Brihtwald, bishop of Wiltshire, 121–4, 128
Britton, 84
Brut, 155, 214, 227
Buched Meir, 57
Buchet, John, 223
Bullough, Bonnie, 179
Bullough, Vern, 179
Butler, Judith, 181, 194
Bynum, Caroline Walker, 18–19, 30, 206, 239

cabbalah, 31
Caciola, Nancy, 29
Caesarius of Heisterbach, 103, 105–6, 107–8, 109
Cailleach Bhéirre, 42
Camille, Michael, 14, 46–8
canonization, 120–1, 125, 131, 174
Capgrave, John, 25, 153
Carlson, Cindy, 4, 5
Carpenter, Christine, 1
Carpenter, Richard, 143
Cassian, 108
castration, 25, 35, 38–9, 84, 107–8, 110–13
Catherine of Siena, 150
Caviness, Madeline H., 28
Caxton, William, 214, 216, 217
Cazelles, Brigitte, 187
Cecilia, St, 175, 178
Charles VI of France, 197

chastity belts, 1
Chaucer, Geoffrey, 7, 53, 172, 175, 178
Chester cycle play, 58, 241
childbirth, 41–2, 60–1, 147, 150
childwite, 90
Christ, 3, 6, 7, 14, 25, 45, 122, 129, 150–1, 172–4, 175, 179, 189–90, 194–5, 197, 202–3, 235, 240–1
Christina of Markyate, 25–7
Christine de Pisan, 193
Christine, St, 117, 174, 177–9, 210
Christopher, St, 105
Chwedl Tegau Eurfron, 66–7
Cicero, 231
Cixous, Hélène, 214
Cobham, Eleanor, duchess of Gloucester, 156, 157, 159
Collen, St, 58
colonialism, 202, 206
Compostela, 37
confession, 24, 149
conversion, 40–1, 43–4, 174, 179
Corpus Christi, 175–6
Cothi, Lewys Glyn, 67
cross-dressing, 215, 216, 220–2, 237
Croxton Play of the Sacrament, 169, 182–3
Croyland Chronicle, 156
Cúchulainn, 42

Dafydd ab Edmwnd, 67
Dafydd ap Gwilym, 66
Daria, St, 190
Dastin, John, 143
Davidson, H. R. Ellis, 43
Davies, Robert Rees, 59, 65
Davis, Kathleen, 170
de Certeau, Michel, 227
De haeretico comburendo, 203
Dee, Joan, 145
Dee, John, 145
defloration, 34–5, 63–4, 72–3, 82–7, 89, 92, 129, 242, 244
del Monte, Piero, 153
Delany, Sheila, 232
Derrida, Jacques, 170–1, 214, 221

Destruction of Da Derga's Hostel, 42
Diana, goddess, 40
Diana, princess of Wales, 252
Dionysius, Pseudo-, 44
Dollimore, Jonathan, 180
Donne, John, 236
droit de seigneur, 1
Dumoulié, Camille, 38

Edith, Queen, 120–5, 127–31, 138
Edith of Wilton, 173
Edward IV, 9, 142, 143, 146–7, 154–5, 156, 157–61
Edward of Lancaster, 153
Edward the Confessor, 8, 119–32, 138, 237
Edwardus Dei Gracia, 154
Einbinder, Susan, 241
Elias, 240
Elizabeth I, 215
Elizabeth of York, 155
Elliott, Alison, 192
Elliott, Dyan, 3, 4, 112
enclosure, 24, 151
English Chronicle, 156
Epp, Garrett P. J., 29
Estoire de Seint Aedward, 131
Ethelbert, St, 127
Etheldreda, St, 237
eucharist, 9, 102, 167–70, 172–3, 175–81, 185, 239
Eusebius, St, 107
Evans, Ruth, 215
Eve, 67
exhibitionism, 7, 37–9, 43, 47, 52
Exposition of the Hieroglyphicall Figures, 144
Eye (Suffolk), 201

Fabyan, Robert, 228
Fergus, 41
Ferguson, Margaret W., 2
fertility, 6, 36–7, 40–2, 47, 49, 53, 63, 64, 73, 123, 131, 143–6, 148, 238, 242
fidelity, 65–9, 121
Firth, Katherine R., 231

Flamel, Nicholas, 144
Flamel, Peronelle, 144
Fleming, Richard, 223
Fleta, 84
foot-holding, 40, 58–60, 62
Fortescue, John, 88
Fortescue, Sir John, 153, 159
Foucault, Michel, 108, 116–17
Fourth Lateran Council, 171
Foxe, John, 180, 218, 231
Fradenburg, Louise, 171, 183
Francke, Meister, 204, **205**
Franks Casket, 43
Freud, Sigmund, 16, 19–20, 31, 34–5, 37–9, 42

Galahad, 9, 154
Galen of Pergamum, 69, 71, 145–6, 149, 152
Garber, Marjorie, 172
Gaunt, Simon, 22, 28, 191
genital mutilation, 247–8, 253
Geoffrey of Monmouth, 66, 227, 229
George, duke of Clarence, 159–61
George, St, 159
Gerald of Aurillac, 109, 126
Gerald of Wales, 24, 74, 102–14, 115, 117–18, 137
Gerson, Jean, 15–16, 21
Gilbert of Sempringham, 22–7
Gilbertus Anglicus, 71
Gilfaethwy, 58–62
Gilles de Rais, 152
Glanvill, 84
goddesses, 36–44, 48–9, 53, 189
Godric (of Finchale?), 104
Godwin, earl of Wessex, 120, 122
Goewin, 58–62
Goldberg, P. J. P., 90
Gombrich, E. H., 38
Grafton, Richard, 228
Gransden, Antonia, 218, 225, 231
Gratian, 85
Gravdal, Kathryn, 190–1, 236, 237
Gray's Anatomy, 243–7, **246**, 252–3
Green, Miranda, 39–41, 44, 53
Greer, Germaine, 14

Gregory the Great, Pope, 43, 108
Grosseteste, Robert, 240–1
Guinevere (Gwenhwyfar), 66–8, 159
Guto'r Glyn, 67
Guyonvarch, Christian-J., 53
Gwallter Mechain, 66, 67
Gwydion, 58–62

Hackett, Helen, 215, 228
Hadewijch, 150
Hadfield, Andrew, 231
hagiography, 3–4, 22–7, 46, 48, 60, 104–11, 119–32, 168–81, 187–207, **198**, **199**, **200**, **205**, 210, 218, 237, 249
Hakluyt, Richard, 218
Halesowen, 89–93, 94
Hali Meiðhad, 6, 23, 248–9
Hall, Edward, 214, 216–20, 222–4
Hanawalt, Barbara, 90
Hardin, Richard, 216, 233
Harding, Wendy, 28
Harrison, William, 231
Hattecliffe, William, 153
Heffernan, Thomas J., 249
Heinrich von dem Türlîn, 65
Helen of Troy, 237
Henry V, 152
Henry VI, 9, 142, 152–6, 161, 223
heresy, 171, 203–4, 241
hermaphroditism, 6, 161
Herodotus, 69
heterosexuality, 3, 140, 146–50
Hildebert, bishop of Le Mans, 111–12
Hildegard of Bingen, 5, 152
Hoccleve, Thomas, 215
Holinshed, Raphael, 214, 216–21, 223–4, 227, 233
Hollywood, Amy, 31
homosexuality, 29–30, 149–50, 247
homunculus, 144–5, 150
Humphrey, duke of Gloucester, 147, 156–7
Hunt, Leon, 104
Huth Merlin, 66

hymen, 5–6, 64, 103, 149, 170, 242–4, 247, 252
hysteria, 21, 148, 247

Imbolc, 41, 53
imitatio Christi, 9, 18, 191
impotence, 9, 87, 155
incorruption, 120, 123–5, 130–1
infidelity, 65–70
Innocent II, Pope, 121
Irigaray, Luce, 49, 193–4
Isidore of Seville, 110, 231

Jacobus de Voragine, 103–9, 116, 117, 175, 189–90
Jacquetta of Luxembourg, 157–60
James, St, 108
Jean, duc de Berry, 197
Jenkins, Dafydd, 65
Jeremiah, 240
Jerman, James, 52, 55
Jerome, St, 3, 110, 112, 211
Jews, 9, 167–74, 176–81, 212, 237, 239–40
Joan of Arc, 6, 9, 152, 206, 214–27, 232, 233, 237
John the Evangelist, St, 130, 138
Johns, Catherine, 37
Jones, E. D., 90
Josaphat, St, 106
Joseph, St, 57–8
jouissance, 35, 49, 177
Journal d'un bourgeois de Paris, 214, 216
Judaism, 240–1
Julian of Norwich, 151–2
Juliana, St, 168, 180, 190
Juno, 40
Justina, St, 109, 190

Kappler, Claude, 38–9
Karras, Ruth Mazo, 26
Katherine Group, 15, 48, 172, 203
Katherine, St, 3, 153, 168, 174, 180, 203, 237
Kelly, Eamonn P., 43
Kelly, Edmund, 145

Kelly, Kathleen Coyne, 4–5, 8, 56, 64, 66, 68–9, 72, 103–5, 109, 111, 113, 117, 126, 175, 209–10, 211, 225
Kempe, Margery, 16–18, 81, 170–1, 173–4, 177, 203
Kilpeck, 36
Kripal, Jeffrey J., 28, 30, 31
Kymer, Gilbert, 147, 156

Lacan, Jacques, 21, 45, 49
Lai du Cort Mantel, 65–6
Lancelot, 147
Laqueur, Thomas, 244
Lascault, Gilbert, 39
Last's Anatomy, 244–5
Lawton, David A.,14
Le Roux, Françoise, 53
Leclercq, Jean, 19, 25
Leiris, Michel, 39
Leslie, Marina, 4, 225
Levine, Joseph M., 230
Lewis, G. R., 36
Lewis, Katherine J., 3, 5
leyrwite, 8, 89–93, 97; *see also* amobr
Livre de Caradoc, Le, 66
Llyfr Coch Hergest, 70–1
Llyfr Cyfnerth, 62
Llyfr Iorwerth, 60
Lochrie, Karma, 30
Louis VII, 105
Lucy, St, 190, 210
Lull, Raymund, 143
Lydgate, John, 169, 174–5

Mabinogi, 40, 53, 58–63, 69
Mac Cana, Proinsias, 40, 53
MacCulloch, John Arnott, 61
Macha, goddess, 41
MacKillop, James, 51, 53
Macrobius, 231
Malleus maleficarum, 38
Malory, Thomas, 26, 147, 160
Mandeville's Travels, 6, 27, 247
Mannyng, Robert, 87–8
Margaret of Anjou, 152–3, 156–7

Margaret of Oignt, 151
Margaret, St, 168–9, 172, 174–5, 180, 190, 203, 212
marginalia, 46
Maria Prophetissa, 141
marriage, 3, 35, 56, 59, 61, 63–4, 68, 73, 86–9, 94, 121–5, 127–31, 143, 153, 154–5, 157–61, 171–2, 183–4, 232, 239
martyrdom, 9, 121, 131, 168–70, 177–9, 187–207, **198**, 236
Mary, Virgin, 5, 7, 40, 57–8, 67, 107, 123, 137, 150, 215, 228, 229, 237, 238, 240–1
masturbation, 15, 112, 149–50, 247
Math, 40, 58–62
Matrona, goddess, 51
McAll, Christopher, 62
McInerney, Maud Burnett, 5, 103, 113, 114
McMahon, Joanne, 39, 43
Medusa, 38, 42, 247
Melangell, St, 60
Mellars, Paul, 37
Meltzer, Françoise, 210, 221, 213, 232
Melusine, 6, 157–60, **158**
menstruation, 35, 71–2, 144–6, 151–2, 159, 173, 179–80, 244
mermaids, 37, 52
Mews, Constant, 241
Miles, Margaret, 48
Miller, Julie B., 15
Mills, Robert, 4, 11, 19, 30, 236
Minerva-Pallas, 40
Minnis, Alastair, 231
Miriam, 141
Mirror of Justices, The, 84–5
monks, 15, 104–12, 114
monstrosity, 6, 33–5, 39, 42, 44–9, 238, 247
Moorcraft, Paul L., 1
Morgan le Fay, 42, 66, 160
Morrigan, the, goddess, 41
Murray, Jacqueline, 25, 28, 108, 112
Muslims, 174, 203, 212
mysticism, 7, 14–23, 25–6, 47, 108, 112, 141, 150–2, 176, 238

mythology, 8, 35–7, 40–2, 176

nakedness, 42, 48, 191, 193, 214, 221, 225
Neale, Steve, 104
Neville, Richard, earl of Warwick, 157–9
Niall, 41
Nicholas of Florence, 71, 72
Nora, Pierre, 215, 226
North Elmham, Norfolk, 202
North, Tim, 89
Norton, Thomas, 144
N-Town cycle play, 58, 241
nuns, 16, 24, 41, 73, 84, 105, 107, 109, 149, 191

Odo of Cluny, 109
O'Donovan, John, 50
orgasm, 17–18, 49, 111–12, 145, 150
Orientalism, 206
Origen, 108, 113
Osbert of Clare, 8, 120–32, 136, 137, 237
Otter, Monika, 123
Owen, Morfydd E., 69

paganism, 36–44, 168–9, 172, 174, 189, 237
Pamplona Bible, 197, **199**, **200**
Paris, William, 177–9
Parker, Patricia, 220, 222
Partner, Nancy F., 16–18, 239
Patterson, Nerys W., 64
Payer, Pierre J., 111, 122
Pearl, 7
Pearson, Ann, 51
penance, 59–60, 156
Peter, St, 121
pilgrimage, 33, 37, 108, 125, 128, 130, 196
Placita Corone, 84
Poos, L. R., 90, 92
pornography, 3–4, 36, 48, 187, 204
Pouchelle, Marie-Christine, 244
Power, Eileen, 248
pregnancy, 34, 41, 58, 61–2, 63, 69–70, 73, 91, 103, 143–6, 214, 216
Preiddeu Annwn, 40
prostitution, 59, 84, 87, 105, 143, 179–80, 186, 189–90
Protestantism, 215, 239
Pseudo-Dionysius, *see* Dionysius, Pseudo-
Pythia, 33

Raknem, Ingvald, 233
Ralegh, Walter, 229
Ralph of Hengham, 85
Rambuss, Richard, 19
rape, 3, 56, 58, 59, 61, 81–8, 96, 97, 109, 187, 189–92, 201, 236
Razi, Zvi, 90, 92
Red Book of Hergest, *see Llyfr Coch Hergest*
Rees, Emma, L. E., 36, 50, 51
Reformation, 215, 218
representation, 2, 5–8, 38–9, 44–6, 49, 128, 216–17, 219–27, 238
rhetoric, 206, 217–26, 232
Richard II, 5, 131
Richard of Cirencester, 122, 124, 129, 135
Richard, duke of York, 153
Riches, Samantha J. E., 31
Ricoeur, Paul, 220
Ridyard, Susan J., 127
Ripley, George, 141–3, 145–6, 152–5, 157, **158**, 161
Rober le Chapelain, 171–2, 183–4
Roberts, Jack, 39, 43
Roby, Douglass, 19–20
Roger of Howden, 146
Romance of the Rose, 17
Ross, Anne, 36–7, 39–41, 51
Rossetti, Christina, 14
Royal Gold Cup, British Museum, 197, **198**
Rubin, Miri, 168, 179, 182, 212

sacraments, 171–2, 175–6
    see also baptism, confession, eucharist, marriage, penance
Said, Edward, 206

Saint-Paul, Thérèse, 68
Salih, Sarah, 48, 80–1, 126, 131, 211, 233, 236, 249
Salome, 58
sati, 9, 188, 195–7, 201–2, 236
Scammell, Jean, 90
Scarry, Elaine, 192
Scott, Jim, 90
Scream, 1
Schibanoff, Susan, 212
Searle, Eleanor, 90
Secreta secretorum, 146
Secrets of Women, The, 70, 146
Seinte Margarete, 168, 172, 174
Sekenesse of Wymmen, The, 147–50
sexual identity, 2, 19, 80–1, 146–50, 169–70
sexuality, 7, 8, 14–27, 33–43, 45, 47–9, 57, 80–1, 102–14, 140–61, 169, 179–80, 190, 238, 242
Shakespeare, William, 180–1
sheela-na-gig, 6, 7, 33–8, **34**, 42–4, 47–9, 238, 250
Sir Gawain and the Green Knight, 42
Sissa, Giulia, 6, 33
Smith, R. M., 90, 92
Soranus, 72
South English Legendary, 190–1, 209
Southwell, Thomas, 156
sovereignty, goddess of, 6, 37, 40–2, 51
Spearing, A. C., 29
Spears, Britney, 1
Spiegel, Gabrielle M., 231
Spivak, Gayatri Chakravorty, 188, 202, 206
Stacy, Dr, 160
Steinberg, Leo, 19
Stephen, King, 120
Stock, Lorraine K., 42, 50, 51
Stow, John, 228
Sunder Rajan, Rajeswari, 196–201

Taliesin, 42, 54
Tegau Eurfron, 65–8
Tertullian, 6, 47, 81, 187
Theatana, Kathryn Price, 51

Theodora, St, 190
Theresa, St, 49
Thomas, archbishop of York, 146
Thompson, Anne B., 209
Thompson, Stith, 61
Tillet, John, 219
Tomasch, Sylvia, 172–3
Tostig, earl of Northumbria, 121
Treatise of Woman's Sicknesse, 148
Trotula, 147–9, 163, 242, 247
Tudur Penllyn, 67

Ulrich von Zatzikhoven, 65
Ursula, St, 190

Valente, Roberta, 59
Venus figurines, 37
Vergil, Polydore, 214, 217–19, 231
Vernon manuscript, 175
Vesta, 189
vestals, 41
Vickers, Brian, 217
violence, 3, 6, 9, 48, 84, 91, 126, 168–74, 177–80, 187–95, 197–203, **198**, **200**, 210, 247
Virgin of Antioch, 190
virginity
    clerical, 3, 4, 8, 22–25, 102–14, 115, 117, 146
    as commodity, 5, 8, 73, 86–9
    consecrated, 3, 15, 24, 80–1, 235–6
    feminine, 2–4, 6–9, 25–6, 33–5, 37–8, 40–2, 44, 48–9, 56–73, 80–95, 103–4, 109, 112–13, 122–6, 128–9, 149–52, 168–80, 187–207, 214–27, 234–8, 240–1
    in hagiography, 3–9, 22–7, 40, 48, 60, 104–11, 119–32, 168–81, 187–207, 215, 236–9
    kingly, 5, 8–9, 119–32, 153–4, 237
    legal, 4, 6, 8, 63–5, 81–95, 235
    loss of, *see* defloration
    marital, 3–4, 87, 121–5, 127–31, 153, 237
    masculine, 4–5, 7–9, 22–5, 96, 102–14, 119–32, 146, 153–4, 236–7

medical, 9, 69–73, 105, 146–50, 242–8

modern, 1, 6, 10, 242–8

monstrous, 6, 33–5, 37–9, 41–3, 161, 238

and nation, 5, 9, 59, 148, 173, 215–27, 229, 231, 237–8

pre-marital, 6, 8, 56–9, 63–5, 70–3, 80–95, 149–50

studies of, 1–7, 10, 80–1, 187–9, 234–42, 250–1

testing of, 2, 5–6, 8, 56–73, 74, 78, 87, 104, 214, 217, 221, 223–5, 239–42

theories of, 2–7, 15–16, 33–5, 44–9, 71–2, 80–1, 103–4, 108–14, 147, 170–1, 187–9, 215–16, 233, 234–42

variants of, 2–9

Vita Ædwardi regis qui apud Westmonasterium requiescit, 120–4, 131

Vitz, Evelyn Birge, 3–4

Wake, Thomas, 159

Walter of Wimborne, 85

Weir, Anthony, 52, 55

Weisl, Angela Jane, 4

Weissman, Hope Phyllis, 28

Welsh laws of court, 60

Westminster Abbey, 8, 120–1, 124–7, 131–2

Widdecombe, Ann, 1

William of Malmesbury, 138, 238

William of Newburgh, 146, 240–1

William of Saliceto, 71

Williams, David, 44–6

Wilson, Thomas, 220

Winstead, Karen, 3, 5, 188, 211

witchcraft, 38–9, 140, 155–61, 190

Wogan-Browne, Jocelyn, 4, 5, 10–11, 171, 173, 184, 187, 212, 213

Wohunge of ure Lauerd, Þe, 18

Wolfthal, Diane, 201

Woodville, Elizabeth, 155, 157–60

Wulfstan, St, 126–7

Yohe, Katherine M., 30

York Barber Surgeons, Book of the, 154

York cycle play, 173

Zosimos of Panoplis, 141